HOW TO MAKE
NURSING DIAGNOSIS
WORK Administrative and Clinical Strategies

HOW TO MAKE NURSING DIAGNOSIS

WORK Administrative and Clinical Strategies

Emmy Miller, R.N., M.N.
Doctoral Student
Virginia Commonwealth University
Medical College of Virginia
Richmond, Virginia
Formerly Clinical Nurse Specialist
Neuroscience Nursing
Medical College of Virginia Hospitals
Richmond, Virginia

APPLETON & LANGE
Norwalk, Connecticut/San Mateo, California

0-8385-1608-4

89 90 91 92 93 / 10 9 8 7 6 5 4 3 2 1

Prentice Hall International (UK) Limited, London
Prentice Hall of Australia Pty. Limited, *Sydney*
Prentice Hall Canada, Inc., *Toronto*
Prentice Hall Hispanoamericana, S.A., *Mexico*
Prentice Hall of India Private Limited, *New Delhi*
Prentice Hall of Japan, Inc., *Tokyo*
Simon & Schuster Asia Pte. Ltd., *Singapore*
Editora Prentice Hall do Brasil Ltda., *Rio de Janeiro*
Prentice Hall, *Englewood Cliffs, New Jersey*

Library of Congress Cataloging-in-Publication Data
How to make nursing diagnosis work.
    Includes index.
    1. Diagnosis. 2. Nursing. I. Miller, Emmy.
[DNLM: 1. Nursing Diagnosis. WY 100 D537]
RT48.D47   1989   616.07′5   88-34980
ISBN 0-8385-1608-4

Acquisitions Editor: Janet Foltin
Production Editor: Lauren Manjoney
Designer: Steven M. Byrum

PRINTED IN THE UNITED STATES OF AMERICA

This book is dedicated to nurses and patients in the hopes
that it may make a small contribution toward improving the
circumstances and experiences of both.

Contributors

Katherine Norfleet Berry, R.N., M.S.
Clinical Nurse Specialist
Psychiatric Nursing
Medical College of Virginia Hospitals
Richmond, Virginia

Brenda B. Colley, R.N., M.S.N.
Director of Surgical Nursing
Medical College of Virginia Hospitals
Richmond, Virginia

Sherry Williams Fox, R.N., B.S.N.
Critical Care Educator
Department of Nursing Education
Medical College of Virginia
Richmond, Virginia

John A. Horton, M.S.
Manager, Mid-Atlantic Health Care Consulting Practice
Arthur Young
Atlanta, Georgia

Catherine S. Kedy, R.N., M.S.
Psychiatric Liaison Clinical Nurse Specialist
Medical College of Virginia Hospitals
Richmond, Virginia

Carolyn C. Lavecchia, R.N., M.S., F.N.P., J.D.
Emroch & Williamson, Attorneys at Law
Richmond, Virginia
Formerly Assistant Professor of Nursing
Virginia Commonwealth University
Medical College of Virginia

Dana Moriconi, R.N., M.B.A.
Nursing Quality Assurance
Medical College of Virginia Hospitals
Richmond, Virginia

Judith Rocchiccioli, R.N., M.S.N.
Educational Consultant
Department of Nursing Education
Medical College of Virginia Hospitals
Richmond, Virginia

Pamela H. Shurett, R.N., M.N.
Instructor
Department of Nursing
Garland County Community College
Hot Springs, Arkansas

Reviewers

Deborah R. Bailey, R.N., M.S.
Associate Director of Nursing
Northeast Georgia Medical Center
Gainesville, Georgia

Kathy V. Gettrust, R.N., B.S.N.
Instructor
Allied Health Program
Waukesha County Technical College
Pewaukee, Wisconsin

Brenda Ann Patterson, R.N., M.S.N.
Clinical Nurse Specialist
Vanderbilt University Hospital
Nashville, Tennessee

Sue Popkess-Vawter, R.N., Ph.D.
Associate Professor
School of Nursing
College of Health Sciences
The University of Kansas
Kansas City, Kansas

Contents

Preface

How to Make Nursing Diagnosis Work: Administrative and Clinical Strategies is a book born out of the experiences, excitement, and challenges of trying to do just that—make nursing diagnosis *work* in clinical nursing practice. It sometimes seems that the concept of nursing diagnosis has taken the world of nursing by storm, yet the pragmatic, operational knowledge and information that nurses need to use nursing diagnoses effectively and easily in clinical nursing practice is hard to find. This book is designed to provide that knowledge and information for nurses in clinical practice, nursing administration, and education who want to make nursing diagnosis a viable clinical tool for nursing practice.

As the concept of nursing diagnosis has become clearer, and more nursing diagnoses are identified, the questions that nurses have about nursing diagnosis are changing. The issue is no longer one of "Do nurses diagnose?" or "What *is* nursing diagnosis?" Today, the question is, "What do I *do* with nursing diagnosis and *how* do I do it?"

The purpose of this book is to answer some of these questions. The major premise of this book is that thinking leads to doing; how nurses think about patient conditions and available strategies to address these will ultimately determine the type, variety, and eventual success of nursing care. Nursing diagnosis can be utilized as a significant and effective tool to organize nursing thinking and the clinical practice that results from these thinking processes.

In Part I: Introduction of Nursing Diagnosis and Diagnosis-based Nursing Practice, the concept of nursing diagnosis will be examined and the foundation that it offers for diagnosis-based nursing practice will be presented. In diagnosis-based nursing practice, the activities of the professional nurse are guided by the patient conditions described with nursing diagnoses, instead of focusing only on the need to accomplish the tasks, duties, and responsibilities of delegated medical activities or organizational routines. Diagnosis-based nursing practice, rather than task-based nursing practice, offers a number of benefits for patients, for the nurses who care for them, and the health care organizations where nursing care is delivered.

The implementation of nursing diagnosis is a critical first step toward diagnosis-based nursing practice and the benefits that accompany it. If implementation is to be successful, however, nursing diagnosis must be incorporated into the clinical practice systems and culture of the organization, not simply added on to the nurse's already busy list of activities. In Part II: Planning and Preparing for the Implementation of Nursing Diagnosis and Diagnosis-based Nursing Practice, strategies for incorporating nursing diagnosis into the clinical nursing practice models, documentation framework, quality assurance program, and the information systems of the nursing organization will be presented. Educational and legal issues are also examined for their roles and importance in the use of nursing diagnoses.

The implementation strategies discussed in Part II include educational strategies, clinical strategies, systems strategies, and administrative strategies. An essential aspect of the use of nursing diagnosis in clinical practice is that making nursing diagnoses is a cognitive skill; as such, knowledge about nursing diagnoses and the clinical conditions of patients must be applied in the clinical setting, at the bedside. If *only* educational strategies are used, the implementation effort is very likely to be unsuccessful in changing behavior because the skill development aspect of nursing diagnosis was not addressed. Similarly, using an implementation approach that does not support the nurses' use of nursing diagnosis through appropriate documentation frameworks, staffing and assignment patterns, quality assurance monitoring, and job description criteria is also unlikely to succeed; assuming that the nurses have the requisite diagnostic skill, there is no place in the clinical practice systems or culture that supports or encourages them in using nursing diagnosis.

In order to move successfully from task-based nursing practice to diagnosis-based nursing practice, a variety of strategies will be required. Furthermore, the combined efforts of nurses in clinical practice and nursing administrators are necessary. If nursing diagnosis is viewed *only* as a clinical issue, it will be difficult to accomplish the necessary changes in clinical practice systems to support nurses in using nursing diagnosis. On the other hand, if nursing diagnosis is perceived as an "administrative mandate," rather than as a tool for clinical thinking in nursing, then success is equally unlikely.

A critical aspect of the success of any implementation program for nursing diagnosis is the collaborative efforts of clinicians and administrators and a set of shared values that are clearly defined. Viewing the implementation of nursing diagnosis and the move to diagnosis-based nursing practice as an organizational change, which must be supported by individual behaviors and organizational systems and values, is a useful approach to a change project of this magnitude. This approach also suggests that implementing nursing diagnosis is not a "quick fix" for nursing practice or documentation issues, but rather a philosophical and operational commitment to professional nursing practice. Such goals can only be accomplished through a variety of strategies and the investment of clinical and administrative nurses in the organization. In Part III: Implementing Diagnosis-based Nursing Practice: Specialty Issues and Clinical Applications, some specific strategies for the implementation of nursing diagnosis in two specialty nursing areas and an example of clinical application of one nursing diagnosis are presented. The issues of applying nursing diagnoses to psychiatric patients and to critically ill patients present a number of challenges to nurses in those areas, and some exciting and interesting clinical thinking is taking place as nurses struggle with these issues. As nursing practice becomes more and more specialized, questions about the use of nursing diagnoses and the scope of nursing practice in specialty areas will continue to be raised. The answers must come from a thoughtful and analytical examination of the realities of clinical nursing practice and the patient population of concern. The chapters presented in Part III provide a representative, although not exhaustive, discussion of the issues and some strategies to address these regarding the implementation of nursing diagnoses in psychiatric nursing practice and critical care nursing practice. These areas were selected because of the author's experience with the implementation of nursing diagnoses in the clinical areas.

The implementation of nursing diagnoses, as the foundation of diagnosis-based nursing practice, offers an exciting challenge to nurses in all areas of practice. The emergence of nursing diagnoses as a consistent framework for naming the patient conditions of concern to nurses has raised questions about the terminology used by nurses, the role of nursing care planning, and ultimately the scope of nursing practice. Although the nursing diagnostic terminology is evolving and gaps exist, the only way to advance to "state of the art" nursing diagnoses is for nurses to use them in clinical nursing practice; however, this must be done thoughtfully, deliberately, and as a part of a systematic, organized approach to nursing practice in the health care delivery setting. Nursing diagnoses must be implemented and used in clinical nursing practice on a wide scale in order to discover much of the knowledge that is still needed about nursing diagnosis. Now is the time to begin this effort.

Emmy Miller, R.N., M.N.
Richmond, Virginia

Acknowledgments

My experiences and those of the chapter contributors played an important role in the development and writing of this book. Many of the ideas and strategies presented here were identified and defined as we struggled with questions about using nursing diagnoses ourselves, helping other nurses develop diagnostic skills, and supporting the use of nursing diagnoses in documentation systems and nurse–patient assignments. The Department of Nursing Services of the Medical College of Virginia Hospitals provided a rich and rewarding arena, as well as a great many excited and energetic nurses, for examining the issues and opportunities of diagnosis-based nursing practice and exploring strategies and approaches for the implementation of nursing diagnosis. Without the opportunity to put many of these ideas into practice, and the encouragement and support of many individuals, this book could not have been written.

PART I

Introduction to Nursing Diagnosis and Diagnosis-based Nursing Practice

CHAPTER 1

Introduction to Diagnosis-based Nursing Practice

Emmy Miller

Nursing diagnosis is here to stay. It is a means for nurses to identify and describe the problems that are addressed in nursing practice. Efforts to accomplish this are not new; the careful observations of Florence Nightingale, the time-motion studies of industrial engineers, and the computerized nursing intensity measures based on selected patient indicators are strategies that have attempted to define the practice of nursing and the contributions of nursing to the recovery of the patient. Nursing diagnosis is another step in this progress.

Nursing diagnosis offers a challenge for the clinical practice of nursing. The advent of standardized problem names for use in nursing practice presents an opportunity to transform clinical nursing practice. With a focus on patient problems that require nursing treatment, nursing practice becomes diagnosis-based rather than grounded in the tasks, chores, and routines that often occupy the nurse's time and energy. Diagnosis-based nursing practice is nursing at its most professional, accountable, and visible.[1] This type of nursing practice could produce tremendous benefits for patients, for nurses at all levels of skill and experience, and for the health care institutions where nurses practice.

The implementation of nursing diagnosis is the foundation of diagnosis-based nursing practice. The implementation process is not just an introduction to the concept and language of nursing diagnosis. It is an opportunity to examine nursing practice and to utilize nursing diagnosis as a vehicle to make changes in actual clinical nursing practice. These changes may range from relatively simple tasks, such as new wording of nursing care plan forms, to major change projects, such as changing the models of nursing practice in the environment.

This book presents the basis for and the steps to accomplish the implementation of nursing diagnosis in a health care institution or agency. Implementation of nursing diagnosis is much more than simply using some new terminology. A successful implementation program must define and structure clinical nursing practice so that diagnosis-based nursing practice is a reality. The organization of this information around the use of nursing diagnosis in clinical practice is the focus of this book. A starting point is the definition of nursing diagnosis.

NURSING DIAGNOSIS

In 1980, the American Nurses' Association (ANA) defined nursing as "the diagnosis and treatment of human responses to actual or potential health problems."[2] Here, nursing diagnosis refers to the patient's responses to health problems, but these are not described. The delineation of these human responses is a tremendous undertaking and one of critical significance for nursing.

In order to apply the ANA definition of nursing practice, these human responses must be identified, described, and linked with effective nursing interventions. The National Conference Groups on Nursing Diagnosis, now the North American Nursing Diagnosis Association (NANDA), began the work of determining exactly what these human responses are in the early 1970s. This has resulted in a group of 98 nursing diagnoses, arranged in a taxonomy based on human response patterns and classified by levels of abstraction.[3]

The process of identifying and classifying nursing diagnoses is just beginning, and many questions and controversies about nursing diagnosis exist. The current group of nursing diagnoses is incomplete, and many of the diagnostic labels are highly abstract. The research to define and validate these diagnoses is in its early stages. The professional debate about the content and the process of nursing diagnosis is still unresolved; however, the time has come to begin working with nursing diagnosis even as these debates continue. In fact, it will only be through use of the nursing diagnosis in clinical practice that the answers will be found.

The definition of nursing diagnosis has been, and continues to be, actively debated. One of the most widely recognized definitions is:

> Nursing diagnoses, or clinical diagnoses made by professional nurses, describe actual or potential health problems, which nurses by virtue of their education and experience are capable and licensed to treat.[4]

This definition clearly identifies that nursing diagnoses, while concerned with matters relating to health, are different from medical diagnoses, which require treatment by a physician. This distinction is a critical one and will be discussed in detail in Chapter 2.

Nursing diagnosis provides a way for nurses to name the patient problems that they deal with every day. It also distinguishes those problems that are the unique domain of nursing from the medical diagnosis. Grounded in practice reality, nursing diagnosis serves as a tool that can capture the clinical thinking of nurses who are providing care for patients and focus that thinking on solving the clearly named problems.

The addition of nursing diagnosis as a formal step into the profession's recognized thinking model, the nursing process, has provided an exciting new focus for clinical thinking in nursing. The nursing process was originally described as a four-step model: (1) assessment, (2) planning, (3) implementation of the plan, and (4) evaluation of the plan's effectiveness.[5] Inserting this diagnostic step between assessment and planning provides a critical linkage that had been absent between these components; only if the patient's problem is clearly identified will planning to solve it be effective. Nursing diagnosis, in the context of nursing process, enables the nurse to select the best nursing interventions to improve the patient's problem.

Implementation of Nursing Diagnosis

How does the implementation of nursing diagnosis differ from simply using nursing diagnosis in clinical practice? This book describes implementation as an institution or agency commitment to use nursing diagnosis and to make the necessary changes in both clinical and administrative systems that are needed to support diagnosis-based nursing practice. This contrasts significantly with the decision by an individual nurse to use nursing diagnosis, not only in the scope of the decision, but also in the possibilities of success. Every practicing nurse can recall the frustration and helplessness that results from trying to do something new or different in the absence of peer or administrative support. A well-planned and executed implementation program for the use of nursing diagnosis could avoid much of this distress and capture those energies for productive purposes.

The implementation process can begin with the use of existing nursing diagnoses to describe patients' problems encountered in nursing practice. These nursing diagnoses offer a starting point for beginning the development of diagnosis-based nursing practice. In view of the formative stage of the nursing diagnosis Taxonomy I, this is the logical starting place for large groups of nurses to begin working with nursing diagnoses.

It must be recognized that both the NANDA list and other available diagnostic labels do not represent an exhaustive listing of human responses to actual or potential health problems, and the work of identifying new diagnostic labels and refining existing nursing diagnosis is of critical importance to the profession and the practice of nursing. This work, however, must be done by clinical experts and supported by nursing research. This book will focus on the use of the existing nursing diagnostic labels in clinical practice rather than the discovery of new diagnostic labels.

Implementation: The Change to Diagnosis-based Nursing Practice

In order to obtain the maximum benefits from the use of nursing diagnosis, the implementation process should proceed as a planned change process. The type of change necessary for implementation of nursing diagnosis and the development of a diagnosis-based nursing practice is organizational change. Organizational change must encompass other levels of change if it is to be effective in accomplishing long-standing behavioral change. These other levels include changes in knowledge, changes in attitudes, and changes in individual behavior; these must occur before the goal of organizational change is reached.[6]

Change is an important and ever present part of organizational life. It may be defined as:

> to alter by substituting something else for, or by giving up for something else; to put or take another or others in place of; to make different or convert; to exchange, alter, vary, modify.[7]

In the above definition, change involves doing something different or giving up something familiar. This invariably evokes strong feelings. To counter this, the concept of planned, deliberate change has evolved. Planned change is a deliberate and collaborative effort to improve the operations of a human system, whether it be a self-system or cultural system, through the use of scientific knowledge.[8]

There are many classifications for types of change and a variety of suggested sequences for accomplishing change in the literature. For a change project of the magnitude of the implementation of nursing diagnosis, it is useful to take an eclectic approach and utilize strategies from a number of authors. One type of change has already been identified for the implementation of nursing diagnosis, organizational change. This indicates the scope of the change process and gives some idea of the magnitude of the project.

This approach to organizational change also gives some direction in relation to the sequencing of the change process as well. Before the benefits of diagnosis-based nursing practice can be gained, changes in information at all levels of nursing staff, changes in attitudes about nursing care planning and nursing diagnosis, and changes in individual nursing behavior must be accomplished. An implementation plan should include strategies to deal with all of these levels of change as well as strategies to make the overall practice environment supportive of diagnosis-based nursing practice. (See Chapter 5 for a further discussion of these concepts.)

It is also helpful to look at the implementation of nursing diagnosis and the development of a diagnosis-based nursing practice by taking a structural approach. In this approach, organizational behavioral change is effected through changes in organizational structure and relationships.[9] The most important organizational structure that must be supportive of diagnosis-based nursing practice is the model of nursing practice at the unit level.

Nursing diagnosis must be clearly identified as a responsibility of the registered nurse, and the model of practice and associated unit systems must permit and enable the RN to fulfill this. This is not the usual approach to issues of organizational structure, but it is a critical one for the implementation of nursing diagnosis. Chapter 6 discusses this approach, presenting specific assessment criteria for identifying an appropriate model, guidelines for changing models, and the unit-based structure and systems in various models that support a diagnosis-based nursing practice.

Part II discusses in detail the specific strategies and the sequencing of these for the implementation of nursing diagnosis. As in the preceding discussion, an eclectic approach is taken, and a range of options are presented whenever possible. The implementation of nursing diagnosis and the development of a diagnosis-based nursing practice environment is not a small or insignificant undertaking. Change has been described as cultural transformation, and this is not a process to be entered into lightly; however, the benefits of diagnosis-based practice are significant. An examination of the clinical nursing practice culture is a place to begin this discussion.

THE CLINICAL NURSING PRACTICE CULTURE

Consider the differences between diagnosis-based nursing practice after the implementation of nursing diagnosis and nursing practice without nursing diagnosis. The differences may be illustrated by presenting two definitions of nursing practice. The first is:

> Nursing is the diagnosis and treatment of human responses to actual or potential health problems.[10]

This definition is grounded in the concepts of professionalism and accountability. This is diametric contrast to the next definition, which states:

> The nurse's place in the division of labor is essentially that of doing in a responsible way whatever necessary things are in danger of not being done at all.[11]

While the preceding definition may offend many nurses' sensibilities, there is an unfortunate grain of truth to it.

The busy day of the staff nurse is filled with tasks, duties, and responsibilities. Many of these have to do with carrying out delegated medical tasks, responding to minute-to-minute near-crisis situations, or doing the chores that must be done to keep the unit running smoothly. The nurse is responsible for doing bits of caring for large numbers of patients and for acting as a messenger and coordinator for other workers in the hospital.[12] Even when the unit is quiet, the patients are stable, and everyone scheduled to work actually shows up for their shift, there is *never* enough time. Formulating nursing diagnoses and designing treatment plans may very well be the last thing on the staff nurse's mind. In this very real scenario, the nursing process has gotten lost.

This brief discussion of the realities of nursing practice illustrates a critical paradox in the profession and practice of nursing. In schools of nursing, the professional literature, and the standards set by both professional and regulatory groups, there is a clear expectation that nursing care will be directed by the nursing process. Yet, examinations of nursing practice indicate that some very different patterns of behavior are in use. The notion that the nurse's primary responsibility is to follow physician's orders, the expectation that nurses will accept whatever tasks are given to them in the hospital, and the lack of authority in determining policies related to patient care and hospital operation seem to be more important than professional socialization in determining the behavior of nurses.[13]

The concept of culture is helpful in examining this phenomenon. Culture may be defined as the integrated pattern of human behavior that includes thought, speech, action, and artifacts. It depends upon man's capacity for learning and transmitting knowledge to succeeding generations. Anyone who has practiced as a staff nurse recalls the lessons of culture that are learned in that first job: what is really important (getting baths done before 10 A.M.!), sanctions for inappropriate behavior (complaints from other staff if time is spent "just talking" with a patient), what to complain about (time schedules and assignments), what is not discussed (unsafe staffing levels), and who *really* knows how to get things done (the clerk).

The culture in which nursing is practiced holds different values and expects different behaviors than those taught in schools of nursing. This fact has been described as the phenomenon of "reality shock,"[14] and many schools of nursing and hospitals have developed programs to assist the new nurse in coping with it. Only recently has serious attention been paid to changing the hospital culture and the nursing practice within that culture to be more consistent with the values and culture of a professional nursing practice.[15]

One of the most important determinants of culture is the environment in which the culture operates.[16] The environment in which health care organizations now find themselves is rapidly changing and constricting, particularly in the economic arena. Recent developments, such as diagnosis-related groups and prospective payment plans and the concern about the federal health care budget at all levels of the political structure, are major environmental factors that affect the health care organizational culture. The changing economic climate and greater political involvement in the health care industry are critical factors that affect the culture in which nursing is practiced.

Another issue that has directly affected the nursing practice culture is the increasing acuity level of hospitalized patients. According to one study, in 1969 42.3 percent of patients in a large acute-care hospital were ambulatory and able to care for most of their own needs; however, in 1985 only 18.5 percent of the patients were ambulatory and able to care for themselves.[17] With this increase in patient dependency on nursing care has come a concomitant change in the level of knowledge and sophistication required to practice nursing. This has also resulted in an increased number of registered nurses required to provide nursing care for these more acutely ill patients.[18] In the face of an on-again, off-again nursing shortage and the decreased length of stay mandated by the economic forces in health care, the practice culture in which nurses find themselves is bewildering and contradictory.

A major influence on the culture of an organization is the values of the culture. Values provide a sense of common direction for all employees and guidelines for their day-to-day behavior. It is very possible that organizations succeed because their employees can identify, embrace, and act on the values of the organization.[19] The values of nursing, such as individualized nursing care that is thoughtfully and professionally planned and dealing with the whole person and family, are also reflected in the accreditation standards and professional standards by which nursing practice is judged.[20]

The values of nurses that can be determined by actual observation of nursing practice are decidedly different from these professional values. In one study, 75 percent of the registered nurses in a large city's hospitals spent about 28 percent of their time on functions requiring no formal preparation and often little practical experience.[21] Is this situation the result of organizational values overriding the values of the profession? In that case, a way to merge these value sets is needed so that the goals of both cultures can be accomplished.

REASONS FOR IMPLEMENTING NURSING DIAGNOSIS

The reasons for implementing nursing diagnosis fall into two major categories. The first category includes the clinical benefits for the patient who receives this type of care and the nurse who is planning and providing diagnosis-based nursing care. The second category consists of those benefits to the institution that result from the use of nursing diagnosis. In order to define these benefits, it is first necessary to describe diagnosis-based nursing practice.

How would this diagnosis-based nursing practice culture look? While a number of aspects would appear very different from their present states, many of the needed attributes are present in the existing practice culture. The strong commitment to patient care and the needs of patients is a value of the practice culture that can be built upon and emphasized.

Another value that can be utilized is one that most nurses share, the value of getting things done. The professional values of nursing should not be overlooked in this analysis. By structuring the practice culture so that the differences between the values of the practice and professional cultures are minimized, frustration and confusion can be lessened, and the energy and productivity of nurses can be captured for the goals of both the profession and the organization.

Some aspects of diagnosis-based nursing practice would look very different. In practice environments that have not adopted a clearly defined model of nursing practice, this would be a major, essential, and initial change. The model would be a critical enabling force for the effective use of nursing diagnosis and the merging of the professional and organizational cultures. A variety of nursing practice models have been described, but the key factor for this discussion is the support of the model for the role of the professional registered nurse to carry out the major function of nursing: identifying nursing diagnoses, and designing and implementing nursing treatment plans.

Diagnosis-based nursing practice would also require that other components of nursing activity be defined and organized so that they can be accomplished effectively. Development of clinical protocols to define routine aspects of nursing care for groups of patients and the appropriate use of other levels of nursing personnel are two examples of strategies that can be employed in structuring the practice environment to support the registered nurse, making the practice situation more predictable and more supportive of the professional role. Another critical issue in this restructuring of nursing practice is the delegation of non-nursing tasks to non-nurses. Diagnosis-based nursing practice requires time, and the professional nurse's time must be spent diagnosing and treating the patient rather than performing tasks for other disciplines in the health care organization.

Clinical Benefits for Patients and Nurses

A number of benefits of diagnosis-based nursing practice are directed to the patients receiving nursing care and the nurses providing it. The ability of the nurse to provide effective and consistent nursing care depends on a number of factors; however, a critical one is a knowledge of the problems that the patient is experiencing and of the most beneficial nursing interventions. In the absence of clearly identified problems, time is required in each nurse–patient interaction to determine exactly what these problems are and what should be done about them. The use of nursing diagnosis to identify and communicate patient problems consistently and to convey the required nursing interventions would save time, energy, and, ultimately, money.

Consider the patient who has had a stroke, specifically a right middle cerebral artery infarction. The patient is easily arousable, converses with a somewhat euphoric affect, and is oriented to person, place, time, and circumstance. A left hemiparesis is present. One pressing problem that this patient is experiencing is difficulty swallowing, which includes drooling of saliva, coughing and choking on liquids, but the patient can effectively swallow solid and semi-solid foods. Furthermore, the patient has lost 25 pounds since admission to the hospital.

If the information that the staff nurse receives in report is that the patient has a right brain, left body stroke, and that the main nursing concern is to "encourage good nutrition," then each new nurse who encounters the patient will have to discover the swallowing problem independently. This will result in subjective distress to the patient, who is consistently being offered fluids to drink that elicit coughing, choking, and sputtering. This "nursing by discovery" will occupy more nursing time and energy as well. One possible negative result of this approach to the patient might be to forego oral feedings in favor of placing a nasogastic tube and feeding the patient "safely and easily" by that route.

Imagine a different scenario instead. In diagnosis-based nursing practice, one of this patient's nursing diagnoses would be Alteration in Nutrition: less than body requirements related to Impaired Swallowing. Accompanying this nursing diagnosis are the following interventions:

- Place patient in full, upright, sitting position with head flexed forward for meals. (Use a pillow.)
- Do not give any liquids! Patient coughs, chokes, and sputters, and this is uncomfortable and embarassing.
- Give only solid or semi-solid foods. Patient does particularly well with (and likes!) jello, pudding, crushed ice, and mashed potatoes. Eats regular solid food without any difficulty.
- Calorie count in progress, please save menus.

This brief nursing care plan would enable any nurse to feed the patient safely and effectively. Time and energy would be saved for application to other patient problems. And the patient would receive the individualized nursing care that is the nurse's goal. This is a very simple example, but there are many situations in day-to-day nursing practice that could be handled more easily and effectively if information about the precise problem and the best interventions for a particular patient were readily available.

As seen in the preceding example, the simplest reason for using nursing diagnosis is to identify those patient problems that nurses deal with in the practice of their profession. There is clarity and improved communication as a result of using consistent problem names. Another benefit is the focus that the diagnostic step provides in the nursing process. In order to solve problems, it is necessary to know what those problems are. A clearly identified problem gives guidance in selecting effective nursing interventions, and this is a significant benefit for both nursing practice and the patient who is the recipient of that practice.

Another reason for implementing nursing diagnosis is professional accountability. This is often a shared responsibility in many practice settings. Even when primary nursing is the practice model used, other nurses are responsible for carrying out the plan and evaluating its effectiveness. Yet, how can this be effective if the problems that the patient is experiencing are not named, or those names are not agreed upon by the nurses caring for the patient?

Consider the patient whose primary nurse has identified a need for emotional support on the nursing care plan, and nursing interventions have been specified to accomplish this. If the associate nurse sees the patient as demonstrating demanding, manipulative behavior rather than needing emotional support, the nursing care provided to the patient is likely to be inconsistent at best. When the problem is clearly identified, however, these types of differences can be minimized, or at least the discussion of differing opinions has a point from which to start.

In diagnosis-based nursing practice, a nursing diagnosis of Anxiety related to new diagnosis of lung cancer would make it clear *why* the emotional support was indicated. This nursing diagnosis would also serve as a basis for the primary nurse and the associate nurse to explore the differential diagnosis possibilities. While this example is presented within the context of primary nursing, disagreements about patient problems can and do occur in all types of nursing practice models. Often the fundamental cause is the lack of a clearly identified patient problem. Without that, nurses may find themselves treating their opinions about the patient rather than attempting to improve or address the human response that the patient is demonstrating.

Benefits for the Health Care Organization

A number of benefits also accrue to the institution as well. The first of these is the professional accountability that is inherent in the use of nursing diagnosis. By working with consistent problem names in the form of nursing diagnoses, the responsibility to make a nursing diagnosis and employ certain nursing interventions in specific situations becomes clearer. It must be acknowledged that much of the research to validate the problem names and associated interventions is yet to be done, but, even in its formative state, nursing diagnosis can be a powerful tool for nursing accountability.

One of the benefits of the implementation of nursing diagnosis is that it provides a mechanism for developing some congruence between the goals of the nursing profession and the organizational culture in which nursing is practiced. The goals of the nursing profession are to address patient problems through effective nursing care. The goals of the health care organization are to provide the services needed by their clients in an effective and efficient manner.

A common focus for both sets of goals is needed, and this is not that difficult to envision. As nursing attempts to define the problems that nurses treat, and health care organizations endeavor to define the services that they provide and the costs associated with these, some common ground begins to emerge. The use of standardized, consistent problem names is an integral component of both of these efforts. This common ground for the goals of the profession of nursing and the goals of the health care organization is one of the most compelling reasons for implementing nursing diagnosis and establishing diagnosis-based nursing practice.

A very practical benefit from the use of nursing diagnosis is that it provides a focus for nursing documentation systems. In view of the economic and legal concerns that affect health care institutions today, accurate and descriptive documentation of services to patients is essential. Many systems for documenting nursing care and evaluating nursing care have been proposed, and documentation issues will be discussed in chapter 7.

This issue of documentation of nursing care is a critical one, encompassing the administrative structures and objectives of the institution and the professional goals and philosophy of the nursing profession. The culture of the clinical practice environment is another important determinant of the approach to and compliance with documentation criteria. It is the clinical practice culture, through its unwritten values and norms, that decrees how important it is to "write all that stuff down" as opposed to the "real nursing work" of actually taking care of patients.

The successful incorporation of nursing diagnosis into the clinical and administrative systems of the organization must include strategies to deal with all of these driving forces. The outcome of such an endeavor can be a documentation system, grounded in practice reality, that accurately records patient problems and planned, organized strategies to solve or improve these problems. Surely this is another way to merge the goals of nurses and the goals of the health care organization, minimizing the discrepancies between the professional culture and the organizational culture that contributes to confusion and frustration for many nurses.

The lack of congruence between these cultures has manifested itself in high turnover rates for nurses, nursing shortages, and the brain drain in nursing, where nurses are leaving traditional areas of practice to pursue careers peripheral to or even unrelated to nursing. By redefining the culture of the nursing practice environment to include and support the professional practice of nursing, the distance between the culture of professional nursing and the culture of the health care organization can begin to close.

Nursing diagnosis can serve as the core of this effort. In fact it is the hook that everything else hangs on. The use of consistent problem names, which is what nursing diagnosis offers, fosters consistency in nursing care planning, delivery, and communication. This contributes to improved documentation and the subsequent evaluation of that care. Other results would include greater satisfaction for patients and nurses who are providing their care. Diagnosis-based nursing practice moves nursing care from a focus on tasks, chores, and routines toward a practice culture that contains values for both the profession of nursing and the health care organization.

CONCLUSION

The benefits of diagnosis-based practice will not be obtained, unless there is a genuine change in the clinical practice culture. The implementation of nursing diagnosis is not simply the use of some new terminology. It is an opportunity to structure the practice of nursing within the context of the health care organization so that the goals of both are congruent and achievable. The business of change is cultural transformation, and this is invariably risky, expensive, and time consuming.[22] The necessity for change in the nursing practice culture and the health care organization is being driven by forces from within and without: economic concerns, nurse satisfaction, the trend toward professionalism in nursing, and the changing resource pictures of nursing and health care. Let nursing take this opportunity to use the vehicle that nursing diagnosis offers to begin to make the needed changes to move toward diagnosis-based nursing practice.

REFERENCES

1. Gebbie, K.M. Nursing diagnosis: What is it and why does it exist? *Topics in Clinical Nursing*, 1984, *5*, 4, 1

2. American Nurses' Association. *Nursing: A social policy statement.* Kansas City: American Nurses' Association, 1980, p. 9

3. North American Nursing Diagnosis Association. *Nursing Diagnosis Newsletter*, 1988, *14*, 1, 3

4. Gordon, M. Nursing diagnosis and the diagnostic process, *American Journal of Nursing*, 1976, *76*, 8, 1298

5. Yura, H., & Walsh, M.B., Eds. *The nursing process* (1st ed.). Washington, DC: The Catholic University of America Press, 1967

6. Hersey, P., & Blanchard, K. *Management of organizational behavior: Utilizing human resources* (3rd ed.). Englewood Cliffs, NJ: Prentice-Hall, 1977

7. Massie, L., & Douglas, J. *Managing—A contemporary introduction*. Englewood Cliffs, NJ: Prentice-Hall, 1973

8. Lippitt, R. et al., *The dynamics of planned change*. New York: Harcourt, Brace, and World, 1958

9. Massie & Douglas

10. American Nurses' Association

11. Hughes, E.C. *Men and their work*. Glencoe, IL: The Free Press, 1958, p. 74

12. Jacox, A. Role restructuring in hospital nursing. In L.H. Aiken & S.R. Gortner (Eds.), *Nursing in the 1980s: Crises, opportunities, challenges*. Philadelphia: J.B. Lippincott, 1982

13. *Ibid.*

14. Kramer, M. *Reality shock: Why nurses leave nursing*. St. Louis: C.V. Mosby, 1974

15. Jacox

16. Deal, T.E., & Kennedy, A.A. *Corporate culture: The rites and rituals of corporate life*. Reading, MA: Addison-Wesley, 1982

17. Donovan, M.L., & Lewis, G. Increasing productivity and decreasing costs: The value of RNs. *Journal of Nursing Administration, 17*, 9, 16

18. McClure, M.L., & Nelson, M.J. Trends in hospital nursing. In L.H. Aiken & S.R. Gortner (Eds.), *Nursing in the 1980s: Crises, opportunities, challenges*. Philadelphia: J.B. Lippincott, 1982

19. Deal & Kennedy

20. American Nurses' Association

21. Goldstein, H. & Horowitz, M.A. *Utilization of health personnel: A five hospital study*. Germantown, MD: Aspen Systems Corp., 1978

22. Deal & Kennedy

CHAPTER 2

Nursing Diagnosis: What It Is, What It Is Not

Emmy Miller

In order to begin the implementation of nursing diagnosis, there must be a clearly defined statement of what nursing diagnosis is, why and when it will be used, where it will be documented, and who will be responsible for making it. This operational definition of nursing diagnosis is the foundation of an implementation plan and also serves as a touchstone against which evaluation of the implementation process can be made.

An important reason for developing an operational definition of nursing diagnosis is that there is a great deal of variability in the definitions that have been proposed. Many of these definitions describe the process by which a nurse arrives at a diagnosis, while others are efforts to define and name the patient problem identified by the nurse. Both of these are important arenas of discussion and exploration for the profession of nursing. Throughout this book, "diagnostic process" is used to refer to the thinking process whereby nurses arrive at the patient's problem; "nursing diagnosis" is used to refer to the problem names or labels.

Definitions of nursing diagnosis abound in the nursing literature; however, most of these are of an abstract and conceptual nature. It is essential that the operational definition chosen to guide the implementation process defines nursing diagnosis within the scope and context of nursing practice and the realities of the clinical practice culture, as well as considering the goals and mission of the organization, the values of the clinical practice culture, the available personnel and material resources, and the vision of the nursing leaders. In this chapter the historical development of nursing diagnosis is reviewed and various definitions are analyzed. This serves as the basis for the presentation of a model operational definition of nursing diagnosis that is used throughout this book.

Despite the variations in the proposed definitions of nursing diagnosis, there are a number of common themes that can be used to arrive at a useful, working definition. All of the definitions indicate that nursing diagnosis is concerned with matters relating to health; however, the emphasis is on the patient's response to a health condition and not the identification of the condition itself. There is also the expectation in all of the definitions that the nurse will do something about the identified problem. This focus on nursing treatment or intervention for the nursing diagnosis is a critical factor.

HISTORICAL DEVELOPMENT OF NURSING DIAGNOSIS

The concept of identifying specific patient problems that require nursing care is not a new one. (See Table 2–1.) A starting point for the historical perspective on the development of nursing diagnosis can be found in 1929 when Wilson attempted to separate the nursing problems from the medical problems experienced by patients.[1] There was also an effort to identify which of those problems were predictive of a need for nursing action. These lists were generated by student nurses and represented an early effort to discover the contribution of nursing care to the recovery of the patient.

Twenty years later the term diagnosis first appeared in the nursing literature as a responsibility of the professional nurse.[2] Diagnosis, in this usage, referred to the "identification or diagnosing of the nursing problem"; however, what type of problems this should include were not described. Three years later the qualifier "nursing" was added to the term "diagnosis,"[3] and the endeavor of problem identification and classification was begun.

TABLE 2–1.   NURSING DIAGNOSIS HISTORICAL DEVELOPMENT

1929	Attempts to separate the patient's nursing problems from their medical problems; no formal reference to diagnosis.[a]
1950	Description of the functions of the professional nurse as: 1. the identification or diagnosing of the nursing problem and the recognition of interrelated aspects. 2. the deciding upon a course of nursing action[b]
1953	Identification of five areas of patient needs composing the domain of nursing and the focus for nursing diagnosis, which were determined through a process of professional observation including reading, watching, and listening.[c]
1959	Nursing Problems Classification, identified from a survey of more than 40 schools of nursing, that were essentially therapeutic goals for nursing care.[d]
1963	Many nurses believed that they made nursing judgments, not nursing diagnoses.[e]
1963	The term "nursing diagnosis" was employed in a client evaluation instrument to predict the needs for nursing services in long-term care facilities.[f]
1965	The term "trophicognosis" is proposed as a solution to the problem of nurses using the word "diagnosis."[g]
1966	A list of 14 basic human needs that comprised the components or functions of nursing.[h]
1967	The nursing process was defined in four phases with the first phase as assessment and determination of the problem the patient was experiencing.[i]
1973	The second standard of nursing practice is the derivation of nursing diagnoses from health status data.[j]
1973	First National Conference on Nursing Diagnosis
1975	The nursing process expands to a five step model with diagnosis listed as the second phase[k]
1982	The formation of NANDA, the North American Nursing Diagnosis Association

[a]Wilson, *AJN, 29,* 245
[b]McManus, 1950, p. 54
[c]Fry, 1953
[d]Abdellah, 1959, p. 83
[e]Komorita, *AJN, 63,* 83
[f]Bonney and Rothberg, 1963
[g]Levine, ANA, 1965
[h]Henderson, 1966
[i]Yura and Walsh
[j]*Standards of Nursing Practice,* ANA, 1973
[k]Mundinger and Jauron, *Nursing Outlook, 23,* 94; Roy, *Nursing Outlook, 23,* 90

The concern about identifying those patient problems needing nursing care continued on through the 1950s and 1960s. Two classification systems for nursing problems were proposed for use by student and practicing nurses: the Nursing Problems Classification, better known as Abdellah's 21 Problems,[4] and the Basic Human Needs, a classification of 14 basic needs developed by Henderson.[5] During this time, there seemed to be great anxiety about the use of the term "diagnosis" for both professional and legal reasons. A number of other terms were coined, ranging from "nursing problem," "patient need," and "clinical judgment" to the ambitious, multisyllabic term "trophicognosis."[6] These were all attempts to avoid the controversy associated with the term diagnosis, while continuing the effort to identify patient problems that nurses encounter.

An important development in the 1960s was the introduction of the concept of deliberative nursing actions.[7] A clear distinction was made between the automatic or routine activities that constituted a great deal of nursing practice and those nursing actions designed to achieve a specified goal. This focus on the nurse's thinking process, based on careful observation and thoughtful analysis of the patient's situation, was an important precursor of the nursing process.

The issues of problem identification, deliberative nursing actions, and the nurse's thinking merged to become the nursing process. The four-step model of nurse problem-solving was introduced in the late 1960s, and it rapidly became the most popular method for nursing education, nursing practice, and nursing documentation. While most nurses could agree on the process of nursing, there still remained many questions and less agreement on the substance of nursing.

In the early 1970s a number of factors came together to begin to identify, describe, and classify nursing problems and to explore the thinking process of diagnosis. An important influence was the publication of the *Standards of Nursing Practice* by the American Nurses' Association (ANA). This document presents eight standards of nursing practice based on the nursing process. The second of these states that "Nursing diagnoses are derived from health status data."[8] by 1975 the diagnostic step had been incorporated into the nursing process by a number of authors.[9,10]

In the political arena in 1972 New York passed a Nurse Practice Act that contained the following statement:

> The practice of the profession of nursing as a registered professional nurse is defined as diagnosing and treating human responses to actual or potential health problems.[11]

Since that time 34 states have adopted language in their Nurse Practice Acts that describes nursing diagnosis as a key part of the practice of nursing.

The 1970s also saw efforts to examine the practice of nursing using the tools of research and theory development. Prior to this time most nursing research was about nurses and nursing education. The focus of nursing research shifted toward scientific discovery of patient problems and nursing interventions that are the substance of nursing practice. Availability of federal funding for research and increasing numbers of nurses with advanced preparation also contributed to this important professional trend.

The development of nursing theory has had a significant impact on the historical development of nursing diagnosis. In fact, the development of nursing diagnosis as the name given to a statement or conclusion about the nature or cause of some phenomenon has been described as the first level of theory development, factor-isolating theory.[12]

The use of computers in health care organizations also played a role in the development of nursing diagnosis. During the 1950s computers were used for data-processing functions such as payroll and accounting. The use of computers for business and financial applications and for hospital–medical applications that included documentation and frontline clinical support was first proposed in the early 1960s. The development of computerized nursing documentation systems was an outgrowth of these efforts.

As nurses worked with these systems, a need was perceived for a consistent way of naming problems for computerized nursing care planning. Nursing diagnosis provided a mechanism for this. Indeed, the need to store, access, and analyze nursing data in a fashion similar to the medical diagnosis-related groups may well be a major driving force for the implementation of nursing diagnosis.

The early 1970s also saw the birth of an organized national effort to identify and define the problems that nurses treat. The First National Conference on Nursing Diagnosis was held in 1973, and that group has continued its work with publication of an accepted list of nursing diagnoses and incorporation as a formal organization, the North American Nursing Diagnosis Association (NANDA), in 1982. The purpose of this group is to develop, refine, and promote a taxonomy on nursing diagnostic terminology of general use to professional nurses.[13]

NANDA began the work of determining those human responses to actual or potential health problems that nurses treat through an inductive process. Nurse experts from clinical practice, education, and research came together at the meetings of the National Conference Groups. Intensive work in small groups was the mechanism for the identification of an initial list of nursing diagnoses. Publication of the proceedings of these meetings and the nursing diagnoses generated there has been augmented by books, articles, and programs from individuals who applied these nursing diagnoses to various clinical practice issues.

The formal incorporation of the National Conference Groups in 1982 to form NANDA, and the development of a diagnosis review process by that group, has moved this process from an inductive one to a much larger and more representative mechanism. Now, any nurse may submit a diagnostic label to NANDA for consideration. This review process includes clinical review and debate by the membership of NANDA at its biannual meetings.

There were 21 new nursing diagnoses approved at the 1986 NANDA meeting. There are now 98 accepted nursing diagnoses, and these have been organized in a taxonomy.[14] This classification scheme, Taxonomy I, is important as a way to begin to show relationships among the nursing diagnoses and to identify areas where further diagnosis development is needed.

The forum for discussion and the exchange of ideas provided by this group has stimulated a great deal of activity: articles in nursing journals, books on nursing diagnosis, chapters in specialty nursing texts, and nursing diagnosis workshops and classes. Much of this has focused on defining the concept of nursing diagnosis. It sometimes seems that *everyone* has written a definition of nursing diagnosis. At first glance these definitions may seem different or confusing. Rather than adopting any one particular definition, it is helpful to analyze their development and to identify the common themes. There are a number of similarities and common themes that can be identified, and this examination will considerably lessen this confusion.

DEFINITIONS OF NURSING DIAGNOSIS

In 1953 Fry offered five categories for problem identification in nursing and described a process of observation the nurse should use to determine the problem.[15] Since then a number of definitions have been proposed to define the practice of nursing in terms of problem identification. (See Table 2–2.) Many of these definitions fall into one of two categories. Diagnosis is referred to as the *process* of determining the diagnosis, or it is described as the

TABLE 2–2. DEFINITIONS OF NURSING DIAGNOSIS HISTORICAL DEVELOPMENT

1957	*"The determination of the nature and extent of nursing problems presented by the individual patients or families receiving nursing care."*[a]
1962	*"Nursing diagnosis is a careful investigation of the facts to determine the nature of a nursing problem . . . a specific need of the patient that requires nursing action to meet the need.*[b]
1965	*"Nursing diagnosis is the identification of the patient's functional disabilities, or symptoms, as well as identification of his most important functional abilities."*[c]
1966	*"A statement of a conclusion resulting from a recognition of a pattern derived from a nursing investigation of the patient."*[d]
1975	*"The judgment or conclusion that occurs as the result of nursing assessment."*[e]
1975	*"An evaluation of the client's personal responses to his human experience through the life cycle, be they developmental or accidental crisis, or illness, hardships or other such stresses."*[f]
1975	*Nursing diagnosis is the statement of a patient's response that is actually or potentially unhealthful and that nursing interventions can help to change in the direction of health. It should also identify essential factors related to the unhealthful response.*[g]
1976	*"A process of clinical inference from observed changes in patient's physical or psychological condition; if it is arrived at accurately and intelligently, it will lead to the possible causes of synagogue."*[h]
1976	*"Actual or potential health problems which nurses, by virtue of their education and experience, are capable and licensed to treat."*[i]
1978	*"The process of inferring the nature and cause of an unwanted or undesirable state of affairs."*[j]
1982	*"It describes the client's health problem, the client's health needs, or both."*[k]
1983	*"Nursing's domain for diagnosis and management, as a distinct focus among the health-care disciplines, is daily living and health status. . . Nursing diagnoses link these two concerns."*[l]
1983	*"Nursing diagnosis is a statement that describes a health state or an actual or potential alteration in one's life processes (physiological, psychological, socio-cultural, developmental and spiritual). The nurse uses the nursing process to identify and synthesize clinical data and to order nursing interventions to reduce, eliminate, or prevent (health promotion) health alterations which are within the legal and educational domain of nursing."*[m]
1984	*"A clinical judgment about an individual, family, or community which is derived through a deliberate systematic process of data collection and analysis. It provides the basis for prescriptions for definitive therapy for which the nurse is accountable. It is expressed concisely and includes the etiology of the condition when known."*[n]
1985	*"Nursing diagnosis is the determination and statement of a clinical judgment in which a client's response to a change in health status is described in terms of the effect on routines or activities of daily living and lifestyle in an individual, group, or community."*[o]

[a]Abdellah, *Nursing Research, 57,* 4
[b]Chambers, *AJN, 62,* 102
[c]McCain, *AJN, 65,* 82
[d]Durand and Prince, *Nursing Forum, 5,* 50
[e]Gebbie and Lavin, *Proceedings of the Fifth Conference,* 1975
[f]Bircher, *Nursing Forum, 14,* 10
[g]Mundinger and Jauron, 1975
[h]Aspinall, *Nursing Outlook, 24,* 433
[i]Gordon, *AJN, 76,* 1298
[j]Mundinger, *Cancer Nursing, 1,* 221
[k]Bowers, 1982, p. 17
[l]Carnevali, p. 12
[m]Carpenito, 1983, p. 4
[n]Shoemaker, 1984, in Proceedings of the 5th conference
[o]Kelly, 1985, p. 17

name or *label* that is applied to the problem. A few of the more recent definitions include both of these aspects.

The definitions that focus on the diagnostic process are those by McManus,[16] Durand and Prince,[17] Aspinall,[18] and Mundinger.[19] Nursing diagnosis as an inference or clinical judgment is the important aspect of these definitions. A number of other definitions emphasize the importance of nursing assessment: the evaluation or investigation of patient problems without expanding that concept to the diagnostic process. These include definitions by Chambers,[20] McCain,[21] Gebbie and Lavin,[22] and Bircher.[23]

This emphasis of the process of diagnosis is important because the ability to analyze and organize information is a vital skill for making diagnoses. Diagnosis is both a process and a product. The purpose of the diagnostic process is to provide a sound, logical basis for treatment decisions for a particular patient at a particular time.[24] A number of factors affect the diagnostic process and the resulting diagnoses. These factors include intellect, theoretical knowledge, experience, intuition, competence in data-gathering skills, and the individual's philosophy and conceptual framework.[25]

By focusing on the diagnostic process, these definitions of nursing diagnosis provide a mechanism to direct clinical thinking in nursing practice. Diagnostic thinking requires that data is collected, clustered, and named in accordance with recognized patterns. The result of this process, the diagnostic label, can then be validated with subjective and objective data from the patient and from the professional literature; however, the relevant cue clusters and patterns must be available, and there is much work yet to be done in this area. The diagnostic process and its application to nursing diagnosis will be discussed in detail in Chapter 4.

Another group of definitions is concerned with defining the types of problems that nursing diagnoses describe. Some of the older definitions refer to nursing problems[26-28] or to patient needs.[29,30] These definitions represent an initial effort at describing patient problems that nurses treat; however, they tend to be somewhat circuitous.

Definitions by Bircher,[31] Gordon,[32] Bowers,[33] Carpenito,[34] Kelly,[35] and the American Nurses' Association refer to these problems as some type of response,[37-39] an actual or potential health problem,[40,41] or a change in health status.[42-44] These definitions represent attempts to define the type of patient problems where a nursing diagnosis should be made.

While terms such as "human response" or "health problem" may seem vague upon first exposure, they do offer guidance for distinguishing between the disease-based medical diagnostic framework that nurses have been using for years and nursing diagnoses. The clinical testing, both formal and informal, that is essential to determine exactly what these human responses and health problems are, and what labels should be used for them, is the work of the nursing profession for many years to come. Implementation of nursing diagnosis in clinical practice settings will provide a great deal of that testing.

FORMATS FOR NURSING DIAGNOSTIC STATEMENTS

There are a number of formats suggested for the writing of nursing diagnoses. Some authors recommend a concise, clear label. Others utilize a complex structure of several parts. There are a number of good reasons for both positions. On the side of brevity, a useful diagnostic label should be able to convey a constellation of characteristics that are the components of that label. This increases the ease with which one can communicate a large amount of data quickly and easily. For example, the medical diagnosis of urinary tract infection brings to mind a number of symptoms as well as therapeutic possibilities. This "shorthand" facilitates communication among care-givers and reduces the cognitive strain on their memories as well.

The advocates of a longer, more descriptive nursing diagnosis format take their position for a very important reason. They recognize that the foundation for concise, clear diagnostic labels that reliably convey consistent information is simply not yet available for nursing. The National Conference Groups, now NANDA, have begun this process with the development of 88 diagnostic labels; however, the work of validating these labels and the clinical research to further define other labels is only beginning.

The longer, more descriptive format is useful at this point in the development of nursing diagnosis. Because the current problem names have not been investigated in many cases, there is a need to specify exactly what the problem is, what is causing it, and on what symptoms that determination is based. This clarity is also important in view of the fact that the nursing diagnosis should direct the nurse in the selection of the most beneficial and effective nursing interventions. Again, the research base to support this is in its infancy, so there is a need for the nursing diagnosis to provide more information about the patient's problem than could be done with a true "shorthand" type of label.

One of the most popular formats for nursing diagnosis is the P–E–S format.[45,46] In this format the problem, the etiology, and the signs and symptoms that led to determination of the problem are listed. Consider the patient with a productive cough. If the nursing care plan simply reflects the presence of this symptom with direction for nursing intervention of suctioning, there is no clear indication of the patient's problem or why suctioning would be the most effective intervention. Using the P–E–S formation, however, gives a very different picture of the patient:

Problem: Ineffective Airway Clearance
(related to)
Etiology: general weakness and easy fatiguability
(as manifested by)
Signs and Symptoms: weak cough
       crackles and rhonchi bilaterally
       inspirometer volumes of 900–1000cc
       thick, greenish-yellow secretions
       subjective complaint of shortness of breath after coughing/
        deep breathing exercises
       subjective complaint of feeling too tired to eat if coughing/
        deep breathing exercises are done within 30 minutes of
        meal times
       medical diagnosis of chronic obstructive pulmonary disease

Here, instead of suctioning to remove the pulmonary secretions, the nurse would work with the patient on scheduling pulmonary toilet so that this did not conflict with other activities that required significant expenditure of energy, such as eating. Nursing interventions that would increase the patient's ability to clear secretions independently, such as positioning, splinting, or exercises to increase respiratory muscle strength, would also be useful for this patient. The major advantage of this type of format is that it leads to the identification of the most beneficial and effective nursing interventions for the identified problem.

In the preceding example, the medical diagnosis of chronic obstructive pulmonary disease (COPD) is included as a piece of data for making the diagnosis of Ineffective Airway Clearance. Carpenito[47] suggests another way to use the medical diagnosis: incorporate it into the diagnostic statement. A nursing diagnosis in this format would be:

Ineffective airway clearance related to generalized weakness and easy fatiguability secondary to COPD as manifested by . . .

The addition of specific contributing factors such as medical diagnosis makes the diagnostic label highly individualized. While the use of the medical diagnosis as the etiology statement is not advised, inclusion of this information can assist in determining the most effective interventions.[48]

A structure for diagnostic statements, similar to the P–E–S format is offered by Resler.[49] A two-part statement is recommended consisting of an "alteration phrase" and a "reason phrase" that are connected by an expression of relationship such as "associated with" or "related to." A nursing diagnosis in this format for the patient above would be:

Inability to keep lungs clear related to generalized weakness and easy fatiguability

While this example gives a clear description of the patient's situation, it is less helpful in assisting the nurse to determine specific nursing interventions.

An alternative view of nursing and a format for nursing diagnosis is presented by Lunney,[50] who focuses on wholeness and health as the primary concerns of nursing. In this context, the nurse is encouraged to make diagnoses only in those situations that need to be treated and to avoid labeling situations just because they are problems. Etiology as causation is seen as philosophically inconsistent with this focus; therefore, Lunney recommends that the second component of the diagnostic statement consist of indicators that further validate the problem rather than causes of it.

This approach's format to nursing diagnosis consists of two parts: a statement of the overall human response demonstrated by the patient related to a more specific indicator of that response. The first part indicates the nurse's focus on wholeness and health, and the second part indicates a more specific level of diagnosing. This format satisfies the goal of being specific as well as identifying the effect of that specific response on the overall response of the patient.[51] A nursing diagnosis in this format would be:

Alteration in Respiration related to inability to clear airway.

This diagnosis uses abstract and holistic concepts as the first component of the diagnostic statement in order to illustrate clearly the holistic nature of nursing work and nursing's focus on health.

A four-component structure for diagnostic labels has been presented by Carnevali.[52] The focus of nursing diagnoses in Carnevali's framework is those alterations in daily living that result from alterations in health status. An example of a nursing diagnosis in this format is:

target area	self care: activities of daily living
dysfunction	severe shortness of breath, creating deficits in strength and energy
cause	pneumonitis
time	acute[53]

This format also provides a great deal of information about the patient's situation; however, it is a somewhat clumsy and awkward way to convey information.

A structure to overcome the lack of precision in meaning of diagnostic titles has been proposed by Kelly.[54] This diagnostic label consists of the title of the diagnosis, the type, the status, and the stimulus. In this structure the title refers to the name of the patient's health problem. The addition of the type of problem helps narrow the focus of the problem. This may be a degree or level, or it may describe the different forms of the problem. Status refers to two characteristics; the developmental condition of the patient and the nurse's clinical judgment. This is usually indicated by the terms actual, potential, possible, acute, chronic, and intermittent. The identification of the stimulus involves the clinical judgment about cause, source, origin, or other related factors of the health problem.[55]

A nursing diagnosis stated in this format would be:

Title   Ineffective Airway Clearance
Type   excessive mucus
Status   actual
Stimulus   generalized weakness and easy fatiguability

Again, this format gives a great deal of information about the patient's human response. It also includes an important qualifier in the form of the problem status. This listing of the nursing diagnosis appears clumsy in the above example. It is less awkward if rearranged to:

actual Ineffective Airway Clearance: Excessive Mucus related to generalized weakness and easy fatiguability

All of these formats or structures for stating a nursing diagnosis have common features. Each requires a clear statement of the problem, and they include a statement as to the nurse's clinical judgment about the cause or contributing factor for the problem. While some formats require listing defining characteristics in the diagnostic label itself, others do not. All of these formats, however, are designed to name a cluster or group of signs and symptoms rather than simply identify a particular symptom. This clear identification of the patient's problem, its type, and the probable cause or contributing factor serve as the foundation for the development of a nursing treatment plan, including measurable patient outcomes and specific nursing interventions.

NURSING DIAGNOSIS AND THE NURSING CARE PLAN

Another major theme that appears in these definitions of nursing diagnosis is that of nursing care or intervention for the identified nursing diagnosis. The statement that nurses offer treatment directed toward the nursing diagnosis is included in definitions by McManus,[56] Chambers,[57] Gordon,[58] Shoemaker,[59] Carpenito,[60] and Carnevali.[61] These definitions allude to the nursing diagnosis as the basis of nursing intervention, and they utilize the capability of the nurse to treat the identified problem as a criterion for distinguishing the nursing diagnosis from other types of patient problems.

The linkage of nursing diagnosis and nursing intervention establishes the place of nursing diagnosis within the nursing process. The introduction of nursing diagnosis as a formal problem-naming step in the nursing process adds a clarity and focus that had been lacking. Now, planning and implementation of nursing care may be directed toward achieving measurable patient outcomes for clearly identified problems. It is impossible to solve a problem before it is identified.

One advantage in using consistent problem names, or nursing diagnoses, is that the determination of measurable patient outcomes is greatly facilitated. Traditionally in nursing practice, goals were established for patients. Ideally, these goals were established *with* the patient; however, in the absence of a precisely defined problem, these goals tended to be vague or ambiguous. To keep with the running example of the patient with the productive cough, a goal might be Improved Respiratory Function. While this is an admirable goal, determining if it has been achieved cannot be done with any degree of objectivity.

On the other hand, if the patient's problem has been clearly identified as Ineffective Airway Clearance related to generalized weakness and easy fatiguability (see example, p. 19), then the determination of objective, measurable patient outcomes is possible. These would include:

Breath sounds will be clear bilaterally.
Patient will perform 10 breaths on inspirometer without feeling of distress or shortness of breath.
Inspirometer volumes will exceed 1200 cc by next Thursday.

There is a clear relationship between the identified problem and the patient outcomes. The ability to accomplish this component of nursing care planning is greatly enhanced by an accurate, precise description of the problem.

Once the appropriate patient outcomes have been determined, the next step is to identify the most effective and beneficial nursing interventions. Nursing interventions may be defined as autonomous actions, based on scientific rationale, carried out to benefit the patient in a predicted way that is related to the nursing diagnosis and stated goals.[62] They are specific directives designed to be carried out by the nurse in order to improve, resolve, ameliorate, or compensate for the problem identified in the nursing diagnosis.

Nursing interventions have traditionally been divided into three categories. The first category of dependent nursing interventions does not meet the criteria listed in the preceding definition. Dependent nursing interventions are those delegated medical functions ordered by the physician, and they do not require the exercise of nursing judgment or discretion in their execution. The responsibility to monitor the patient's condition in relation to the progression of disease and the responses to medical treatment are also included in this category. This definition does not abrogate the nurse's professional responsibility to question inappropriate orders; rather it refers to situations where the order is appropriate, and the nurse follows it as directed.

At the other end of the spectrum are independent nursing interventions. These are therapeutic actions initiated by the nurse without consultation from other health care professionals, including physicians.[63] Nurses have independent functions in the areas of health problem interventions, wellness promotion, and development of knowledge.[64] Independent functions also include the observation and assessment of the patient to determine those human responses that may require nursing intervention, and the implementation of the indicated nursing care plan.

Interdependent nursing interventions fall somewhere in between these positions. (See Figure 2–1.) These are collaborative associations between nurses and other health care professionals. Nurses have interdependent relationships with patients, physicians, and other health professionals. Often the focus of interdependent nursing interventions is health problem intervention. Interdependent nursing interventions are therapeutic actions performed by the nurse with reciprocal dependence on a physician or another health care professional for the prescription or regulation of that action, including nursing judgments when carrying out a physician's orders.[65] This category of nursing interventions includes those activities carried out under standing medical orders or protocol when there is little or no variation of the

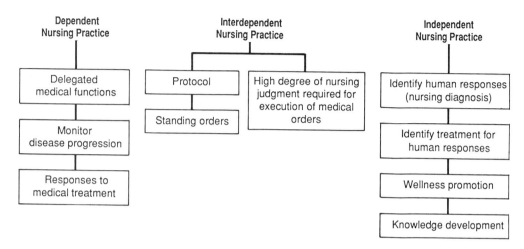

Figure 2–1. Three categories of nursing interventions.

treatment regime for individual patients, as well as those more individualized situations when execution of the medical order requires a great deal of judgment and discretion by the nurse in its implementation.

Interdependent nursing interventions under standing medical orders or clinical protocol do not meet the criteria in the definition of nursing interventions; however, when the execution of interdependent nursing interventions requires judgment and discretion by the nurse, as described in the paragraph above, then interdependent nursing interventions do fall within the scope of nursing practice.[66] Nursing diagnoses may require both independent and interdependent nursing interventions.[67]

This distinction about the types of nursing interventions is important in relation to the use and determination of nursing diagnoses. There is major debate about the question of whether nursing diagnoses should describe those patient problems that are treated with independent nursing interventions *only,*[68–70] or whether those patient problems that are treated with both independent and interdependent nursing interventions be included in a nursing diagnostic framework.[71–73]

For nurses practicing in acute and critical care settings, this capability to apply nursing diagnoses to physiologic problems that nurses often treat with interdependent interventions is essential. Many of the problems that these patients experience are related to physiologic alterations and require interdependent interventions. These nursing diagnoses are not medical diagnoses renamed, but rather they describe nursing issues that are not the exclusive concern of medicine.[74] Limiting the use of nursing diagnoses to only those problems treated with independent interventions would severely restrict the ability of nurses practicing in acute or critical care to make nursing diagnoses. The issues around physiologic nursing diagnoses that require interdependent nursing interventions are complex, and the answers to these questions will be found only in research and the examination of nursing practice.

An example of a patient problem that nurses treat with interdependent nursing interventions is postoperative pain, which will elicit a variety of human responses from patients. Here the physician orders a specific medication for pain relief. It is the nurse, however, who makes essential decisions as to the timing of the medication, coordinating the patient's activities with periods of maximum pain relief, and the use of adjunctive pain control measures such as positioning or relaxation. It would be possible to write a nursing diagnosis of Impaired Physical Mobility related to pain and design a nursing care plan without including the physician-ordered medication. This approach does keep nursing diagnosis focused on independent nursing care, but the total picture of the patient's situation is not reflected in the plan, and an important collaborative aspect of nursing practice is lost.

There are, however, a number of problems that nurses encounter that must be addressed through a physician's order or some type of medical protocol. In this situation, renaming the problem with a nursing diagnosis is awkward at best and confusing and misleading at worst. An example would be the patient in cardiac arrest. Nurses are educated to recognize and respond to this through the well-defined protocol of cardio-pulmonary resuscitation (CPR); labeling this scenario with a nursing diagnosis such as Decreased Cardiac Output or Alteration in Tissue Perfusion is not helpful or accurate.

Not all of the problems that nurses encounter in clinical practice can or should be described with a nursing diagnosis. Often a problem may be a medical one such as the detection of a critical symptom, a complication, or an important observation about the patient's progress in relation to the disease process. These observations should be described in medical terminology rather than attempting to rename them with a nursing diagnosis. The patient who is in shock, who is experiencing acute angina, or who is developing tentorial herniation needs a doctor and medical treatment, not a nursing diagnosis! The detection of these conditions constitutes an important part of nursing practice within the delegated, dependent nursing responsibilities. These problems however, must be referred to the physician for definitive treatment and, therefore, are not consistent with the definitions of nursing diagnosis.

This does not mean that the physiologic realm should be excluded from nursing diagnosis. Patients frequently demonstrate physiologic responses to health problems that are the concern of nursing and not the exclusive domain of medicine. There are a number of nursing diagnoses included in the NANDA Taxonomy I that address physiologic problems patients experience that nurses deal with every day in their practice. Some of these are:

Alteration in Nutrition
Potential for Infection
Ineffective Thermoregulation
Constipation
Reflex Incontinence
Fluid Volume Deficit
Ineffective Airway Clearance

More examination of nursing practice and nursing research is needed to identify other physiologic responses that constitute nursing diagnoses.

This book applies nursing diagnosis to those problems that require both independent and interdependent nursing interventions. This approach supports the collaborative, interdependent aspects of clinical practice, particularly in acute and critical care. The nursing diagnosis and nursing care plan are a part of the overall plan of care for the patient. All members of the health care team contribute to this overall plan by identifying discipline-specific patient problems and interventions for these problems. While this overall plan does not usually exist as a single document in the patient's record, it does exist. The nursing care plan describes and documents our contribution to this.

NURSING DIAGNOSIS AND MEDICAL DIAGNOSIS

Nurses are consistently called upon to recognize and identify medical problems that must be referred to the physician for definitive treatment, as well as other types of problems that may be referred to other health care professionals such as social workers or therapists. This responsibility to identify problems accurately in domains of practice other than the nursing domain is an important part of nursing practice, and its importance should not be minimized. It is critical, however, to distinguish this type of problem identification from the determination of nursing diagnoses.

This distinction is particularly important in relation to the determination of medical problems that the nurse "diagnoses" for purposes of referral to the physician for definitive treatment. Many nurses are very comfortable and very skilled with medical diagnostic terminology and identifying problems within that framework. Again, it should be emphasized that this is an important component of clinical nursing practice.

This responsibility for symptom detection, reporting, and recognition of medical/surgical conditions falls within the delegated, dependent intervention component of nursing activity. The purpose, however, of using nursing diagnosis in clinical practice, and its implementation at the institutional level, is for nurses to identify and treat problems amenable to nursing intervention, not to rename those patient problems resulting from disease processes or related complications. In diagnosis-based nursing practice, both the identification of nursing diagnoses and the detection of medical symptoms and complications occur with the nursing care component assuming an importance that nursing care planning and its implementation has not traditionally enjoyed.

The distinction between nursing diagnosis and medical diagnosis can be examined in a number of ways. It is helpful to begin by comparing the definitions of nursing diagnosis and medical diagnosis. Medical diagnosis may be defined as:

> the determination of what kind of disease the patient is suffering from, especially the art of distinguishing between several possibilities.[75]

Medical diagnoses, which are the names of actual diseases, disorders and syndromes, have been identified and described through many years of medical practice and research. Precise definitions of medical diagnostic labels promote quick and efficient communication. The medical diagnosis of congestive heart failure, for example, brings to mind a specific constellation of signs and symptoms. By using standardized names for diseases, a great deal of information can be readily conveyed and recognized.

The definitions of nursing diagnosis (Table 2–2), with its emphasis on human responses, health problems, or changes in health status, have a focus distinct from medical diagnosis, which is the naming of disease. Unfortunately, this distinction can become less clear when actual patient situations are analyzed. What are the human responses or health problems for the patient whose medical diagnosis is congestive heart failure? Shortness of breath, chest pain, or fatigue are certainly symptoms that many patients with this medical diagnosis experience, but are they nursing diagnoses? These pieces of information are all important, but they are not a label for a patient problem; they are simply specific symptoms that the patient experiences.

An important point about a diagnosis, whether medical or nursing, is that the diagnostic label should describe a cluster or pattern of signs and symptoms.[76–78] One symptom is not a nursing diagnosis, nor a medical one for that matter. Many nurses who are beginning to develop their diagnostic skills have difficulty with this because nurses traditionally have identified and responded to medical symptoms, reporting these to the physician when they are detected.

One helpful strategy to differentiate the nursing diagnosis and the medical diagnosis is to return to the concept of human response. By using this as a touchstone, the differences become clearer. Consider the following examples:

Medical Diagnosis:	Nursing Diagnoses Based on Possible Human Responses:
Diabetes Mellitis	Anxiety
	Knowledge Deficit
	Alteration in Health Maintenance
	Impaired Physical Mobility
	Fluid Volume Deficit
Peripheral Vascular Disease	Activity Intolerance
	Alteration in Comfort
	Impaired Skin Integrity
	Self-Concept Disturbance
Multiple Sclerosis	Self-Care Deficit
	Sensory-Perceptual Alteration
	Potential for Injury
	Reflex Incontinence

These examples demonstrate the distinction between the medical diagnosis that names the disease, disorder, or syndrome that the patient has, and the nursing diagnosis that names the individual human response to the disease that is being experienced by the patient.

NURSING DIAGNOSIS AND OTHER DIRECTIVES OF NURSING PRACTICE

The practice of nursing is directed, internally and externally, by directives from the institution, professional organizations, regulatory agencies, and the law. A number of types of directives have resulted from this, and they sometimes get confused with nursing diagnoses. These directives include standards of care, standards of practice, performance standards, policy, procedure, and protocol. Nursing diagnoses and care plans also direct nursing practice, but in a different fashion.

It is helpful to begin this discussion with some definitions. A standard is defined as "something set up as a rule for measuring or as a model to be followed."[79] This concept of measurement is a critical one. Standards of care or practice are designed as mechanisms for measuring the care that patients receive and the practice of nursing necessary to meet these. Standards of care will be examined first.

The legal definition of a standard of care for nursing refers to a standard of care expected of reasonably competent nurses. Evidence of the standard of care may be found in the regulations of state and federal government as well as in the standards of the Joint Commission on Accreditation of Health Care Organizations (JCAHO).[80] The standard of care is also determined by position statements of recognized professional groups, philosophies of nursing care, job descriptions, hospital bylaws and directives, and current nursing literature.[81] Often, these standards are operationalized for a specific institution in the form of institutional standards. These form the nucleus of that institution's Quality Assurance Program. An example of this type of standard, familiar to most nurses, is the JCAHO standard that every patient will have a nursing care plan and that this will be initiated within 24 hours of admission.

Standards of nursing practice are criteria for nursing performance, against which actual performance can be judged.[82] Many professional nursing organizations have developed and published nursing practice standards. The ANA has established a set of standards that describe the process of nursing and are applicable to all types of nursing practice.[83] Specialty organizations such as the American Association of Critical Care Nurses, the American Association of Neuroscience Nurses, and others have defined standards for nursing practice in those specialty areas. These standards reflect varying degrees of generality and specificity.

As with standards of care set by legal, regulatory, and professional groups, standards of nursing practice are often brought down to an institutional level by the development of policies, procedures, or other types of operational guidelines such as protocols or clinical guidelines. In this way the values, beliefs, and practices of the clinical practice culture are incorporated into national, professional standards. The relationship of standards, criteria, and documentation of these are discussed in detail in chapters 7 and 8.

Performance standards also provide a way to measure something, in this case the performance of an individual in relation to the job description. An effective performance appraisal system must have well-defined position descriptions that contain performance-oriented objectives that are measurable in quantitative terms. Performance standards will reflect the prevailing standards of care and practice, but their focus is on evaluating individual performance. This is another way for national standards to be incorporated into the institution's own culture.

All three types of standards are ways to measure the quality of care, although they take different approaches to this. An important factor in applying these standards is that they must be operationalized and individualized for a particular institution. One way to accomplish this is through the development of policies, procedures, protocols or guidelines.

A policy is a guide that clearly spells out responsibilities and prescribes actions to be taken in a given set of circumstances. Policies provide general direction for decision-making so that action can be taken within the framework of the organization's beliefs and principles. Written policies are useful because they direct uniformity of action, assist in the settlement of conflicts, establish a standard of performance, and generally assure consistent treatment of staff.[84] Policy, by and large, is concerned with staff behavior and the decisions that the staff must make.

Procedures describe the steps that should be followed, either to implement a policy or to perform a specific task. A procedure lists a series of functions established on a predetermined basis to provide for the accomplishment of a specific endeavor. Most institutions have both administrative procedures to guide the implementation of policy and clinical procedures to direct the nurse in the performance of clinical activities in a manner that complies with the institution's standards of care and practice.

A protocol or clinical guideline is a document that is developed by the staff in a given institution and it reflects the practice expectations for a given unit, department, or institution. Many times, this is the mechanism used to operationalize standards of practice. In this way the clinical practice culture can determine and organize how the standards of practice will be met and what is required to accomplish this.

How do all of these directives relate to the identification of human responses, that is, nursing diagnoses, and the determination of a nursing care plan for these? An example is helpful at this point. Consider Mr. Jones who is admitted to a medical unit at General Hospital with a medical diagnosis of pneumonia. There are medical orders for intravenous fluids and antibiotics. The following directives would direct his care:

Policy	Determines *who* may start IVs, change tubing and dressings, add medications, where certain types of IV catheters (large bore catheters, triple lumen catheters) can be used
	Determines *when* nursing care plans will be initiated, *who* may make nursing diagnoses, *what* type and *where* documentation will occur
Procedure	Directs *how* to perform IV insertion, tubing and dressing changes, adding medications
Performance Standard	Evaluates if the nurse carried out the responsibilities for IV therapy in accordance with hospital policy and procedure
	Evaluates if the nurse makes appropriate nursing diagnoses and nursing care plans
Standards of Care	Set at national and professional levels for IV therapy by organizations such as JCAHO, the Center for Disease Control, the National Intravenous Therapy Association
	Set at national and professional levels for nursing process by the ANA, NANDA, and specialty nursing organizations
Nursing Diagnosis	Ineffective Airway Clearance related to thick secretions and fatigue
Nursing Treatment	Chest physiotherapy q4h while awake, special attention to lower lobes bilaterally
	Place patient in sitting position, leaning forward, splinting with pillow across abdomen for coughing q2h
	Give oral fluids to 1,500 cc, patient likes orange juice, ginger ale, and iced tea

This example focuses on the medical treatment modality of IV fluids and antibiotics, and one nursing diagnosis. This patient would certainly have other medical and nursing concerns, but for purposes of this example these are not identified.

In this example some of the directives for nursing care have been applied. Policy, procedure, and standards are important directives for nurse activity; however, they do not describe individual patient responses or delineate specific nursing interventions for that problem. That is the role of nursing diagnosis within the context of nursing practice. There are other problems that nurses encounter in daily practice, however, that do not fit into any of the categories discussed so far.

Nurses may often encounter problems that are patient problems, but the treatment of these problems is consistent for all patients who have the problem. These situations may be dealt with through the mechanism of standing medical orders or clinical protocols that require little if any individualization. In this situation a nursing diagnosis is probably not required. An example of this would be standing admission orders for certain types of conditions or assessment guidelines.

The issue of assessment guidelines is a particularly important one. Consistent assessment of certain parameters is critical for many types of patients. In the steps of the nursing process, assessment of the patient precedes the determination of the problem. Guidelines for postoperative assessment, neurological assessment, or assessment of discharge needs are excellent vehicles for ensuring consistency of nursing care for groups of patients.

Nurses often identify these assessment interventions as part of the nursing care plan. It may often be useful to specify certain observations for the purpose of monitoring the patient's progress and responses to nursing treatments. This is decidedly different from those assessment activities that should be performed for a particular patient population or for all patients who have had a procedure.

Ensuring that these types of assessments are done properly and consistently is a responsibility of the professional nurses. These assessments are not based upon the patient's unique human response. A clinical guideline for assessment of specific patient groups is an ideal way to accomplish this.

Providing a smooth admission process or postoperative recovery routine is an important goal, and steps to accomplish this may be best organized through standing orders or clinical protocol. When the interventions required are consistent for the group of patients rather than individualized for specific patients, the situation is distinctly different from identifying individual human responses that should be named with a nursing diagnosis. Here again, a clinical guideline may be an excellent way to accomplish this.

The differentation between patient problems that should be described with nursing diagnosis, and those problems that are best addressed through a policy, procedure, protocol or clinical guideline can be based on a number of criteria. There are two questions that are helpful in this determination:

1. Is the problem a human response that this particular patient is experiencing?
2. Is the problem amenable to nursing interventions, and do these interventions fall into either the independent or interdependent categories?

If the answer to both of these questions is yes, then a nursing diagnosis and nursing care plan are indicated. If the answer to 1. is yes, and the answer to 2. is no, then the problem may need to be referred to another health care professional. If the answer to 1. is no, and the answer to 2. is yes, then a protocol or clinical guideline is the best way to address the problem. If the answer to both questions is no, then the problem is probably a nursing problem, not a patient problem. Policy, procedure, or protocol may be the best approach.

It is not the purpose of this discussion to deter the nurse from making nursing diagnoses. In diagnosis-based nursing practice, these consistent and routine aspects of nursing care are an important part of nursing practice that is organized and effectively completed. This removes a number of routine concerns from the nurse's workload so that there is time and energy for patient assessment and determination of nursing diagnoses and care plans. The purpose of the nursing care directives discussed in this section is to standardize and organize aspects of nursing care so that standards of nursing practice will be met. The determination of nursing diagnosis-based care plans adds another, exciting, professional dimension to nursing practice.

CONCLUSION

Components of an Operational Definition of Nursing Diagnosis

The operational definition of nursing diagnosis provides a vehicle for the institution or agency to bridge the gaps between abstract, conceptual descriptions of nursing diagnosis and the realities of the clinical practice culture. This definition should contain two components that address the current issues with nursing diagnosis and that reflect the philosophy and mission of the institution or agency. The first component of an operational definition of nursing diagnosis should be a conceptual statement. This should define the reasons for and uses of nursing diagnosis.

A key aspect of this conceptual statement is the differentation of the nursing interventions based on nursing diagnosis from other types of nursing activities. The distinction between nursing and medical diagnosis, the direction of nursing care by procedures, protocols or guidelines, and the role of standards of care set by regulatory agencies and professional organizations must be made.

The second component of the operational definition should address the logistics of nursing diagnosis. This refers to the practical realities of who will make nursing diagnoses, when these should or should not be made, where the nursing diagnoses and related nursing interventions will be documented, and against which criteria they will be evaluated. Many of the logistical decisions will be based on the mandates of regulatory agencies, such as the JCAHO requirement that a nursing care plan will be initiated within a 24 hour period.

The logistical statement about the use of nursing diagnosis should be concise, but it must also be clear and descriptive enough to direct the formulation of supporting policy, procedure, and protocol. The policies and other directives of the institution need to outline in detail how these logistical decisions will be carried out. If the logistical statement ascribes the responsibility for making nursing diagnoses to the registered nurse, then the performance standards, the model of nursing practice, and the unit assignment guidelines must reflect and support this.

The characteristics of the institution are another aspect to consider in developing this component, and this may need to be further delineated at sub-levels within the organization. For example, the use of nursing diagnoses in the critical care areas require a different set of guidelines than in the ambulatory care setting.

The clinical practice culture must also be considered in developing these operational guidelines for the use of nursing diagnosis. If the values of the culture are supportive of nursing care planning and focused on patient problems, then the logistical statement can build upon those values. On the other hand, if the culture strongly values "doing" over "thinking and writing," then the logistical component of the operational definition will, of necessity, reflect this value. The implementation plan however, will require strategies to shift the values of the practice culture to ones that are more consistent with those of the profession and the organization.

In reality nurses often tend to emphasize the actual doing of nursing care because there is rarely time for anything else. It should be recognized from the beginning of the implementation process that formulating, documenting, and evaluating nursing diagnoses takes time. The logistical component of the operational definition must take the realities of the clinical practice environment into account. An unrealistic or utopian requirement for the use of nursing diagnosis is the surest way to sabotage its use. On the other hand, the implementation of nursing diagnosis requires that nurses at all levels change, adapt, and improve their practice. This cannot be accomplished without some striving for higher goals.

The following operational definition of nursing diagnosis is proposed as a model for guiding an implementation process. In this model definition, references are made to various policies, guidelines, and standards. This is in keeping with the purpose of an operational definition, which is not only to guide the implementation process but also to direct the formulation of policy, procedure, and protocol. These various components of the implementation process are discussed in detail in the chapters of Part II.

Operational Definition of Nursing Diagnosis

This operational definition of nursing diagnosis has been developed to guide its implementation and use. It is based on the work of a number of authors and the American Nurses' Association. This definition consists of two components: a conceptual statement about nursing diagnosis and a logistical guideline describing the use of nursing diagnosis here at General Hospital.

I. Nursing Diagnosis

It is our belief that the delivery of high quality, professional nursing care is dependent upon careful patient assessment, accurate identification of the patient's problem, precise determination and implementation of nursing intervention, and thoughtful evaluation of their effectiveness. Problem identification is a critical juncture in this process. Only if problems are clearly and accurately defined will strategies to solve them be effective. It is for this purpose that nursing diagnosis has been added as a step in our model of nursing care planning.

Nursing diagnosis may be defined as a way for nurses to name the patient problems that they are capable and licensed to treat by virtue of their education and experience. While a medical diagnosis describes an actual disease, disorder, or syndrome, the nursing diagnosis describes the patient's response to that. Nursing diagnosis describes the unique responses of a particular patient. These responses may be actual or potential health problems, changes in health status, or conditions that interfere with the patient's ability to perform activities necessary for daily living.

The NANDA list of nursing diagnoses will be the starting point for identifying diagnostic labels; however, it is recognized that this list is still developing and incomplete. When a patient problem is identified and there is no diagnosis on the NANDA list for this, a diagnostic label in keeping with the format described in the operational definitions may be used. Consultation with clinical experts such as Clinical Nurse Specialists is recommended in this situation.

A nursing diagnosis is a label for a cluster or group of signs and symptoms. This label consists of two parts, the problem statement and the etiology. This second component may be the cause of the problem, if known, a contributing factor, or a specific aspect of the problem. This information is important in determining nursing interventions for the nursing diagnosis.

The nursing diagnosis and nursing care plan direct the nursing care for an individual patient. Nursing care is also directed by standards of care and standards of practice developed by regulatory, legal, and professional groups. These direct nursing care for groups of patients in order to assure that standards for quality of care are met. Policy, procedure, protocol and clinical guidelines are means by which the institution assures that these standards are carried out. These things are distinctly different from the nursing diagnosis and nursing care plan and should not be repeated in it.

II. Logistical Considerations for Nursing Diagnosis

It is the responsibility of the Registered Nurse to assess patients, formulate nursing diagnoses, design and implement the nursing care plan, and evaluate its effectiveness. (Refer to the Performance Standards for Nursing Personnel.)

The initial assessment of the patient, performed within 24 hours of admission, will be recorded on the Nursing History form. Data from this form will be clustered and analyzed to determine the nursing diagnosis for the patient. (Refer to the Documentation Policy.)

The nursing diagnosis and care plan will be recorded on the Nursing Care Plan form, and this will serve as the basis for nursing care delivery for each patient. The progress notes will reflect the implementation and evaluation of the nursing care plan.

Nursing assessment of patients is a continuous process. This will be directed by appropriate assessment guidelines for the unit or specialty patient population (Post-Op Assessment Guideline, Neuro Assessment Guideline, etc.), and recorded on the bedside flow sheet. (See Documentation Policy.) Narrative, descriptive data will be recorded in the progress notes. The defining characteristics for nursing diagnoses will be recorded here when the nursing diagnosis is added to the nursing care plan. (Refer to Policy on the Development of Clinical Guidelines, Documentation Policy, and Performance Standards.)

The nursing care plan describes the contribution of nursing to the overall plan of care for the patient while hospitalized. Recognizing that many patient problems require a multidisciplinary approach, the nursing care plan may include interdependent interventions that reflect collaboration with physicians, therapists, or other members of the health care team. Medical orders should not be repeated on the nursing care plan, but nursing directives for carrying out those interdependent interventions are often an important part of the plan.

REFERENCES

1. Wilson, F. Nursing medical patients: An analysis of problems encountered by student nurses in caring for them. *American Journal of Nursing.* 1928, *29,* 245
2. McManus, R.F. Assumptions of the functions of nursing. In *Regional planning for nursing and nursing education.* New York: Bureau of Publications, Teachers College, Columbia University, 1950
3. Fry, V.S. The creative approach to nursing. *American Journal of Nursing,* 1953, *53,* 301
4. Abdellah, F., Beland, L., Martin, A., & Matheney, R. *Patient centered approaches to nursing.* New York: Macmillan, 1960
5. Henderson, V. *The nature of nursing.* New York: MacMillan, 1966
6. Levine, M. Trophicognosis: An alternative to nursing diagnosis. In *exploring progress in medical-surgical nursing, ANA regional clinical conferences* (vol. 2). New York: American Nurses' Association, 1965
7. Orlando, I.J. *The dynamic nurse-patient relationship.* New York: G.P. Putnam's Sons, 1961
8. American Nurses' Association. *Standards of nursing practice.* Kansas City: American Nurses' Association, 1973
9. Roy C. A diagnostic classification system for nursing. *Nursing Outlook,* 1975, *23,* 90
10. Mundinger, M. & Jauron, G. Developing a nursing diagnosis. *Nursing Outlook,* 1975, *23,* 94
11. Kelly, L.Y. Nursing practice acts. *American Journal of Nursing,* 1974, *74,* 7, 1310
12. Kritek, P.B. The generation and classification of nursing diagnoses: Toward a theory of nursing. *Image,* 1978, *10,* 2, 33
13. North American Nursing Diagnosis Association. *Taxonomy I.* Saint Louis: 1986
14. North American Nursing Diagnosis Association
15. Fry
16. McManus

17. Durand, M. & Prince, R. Nursing diagnosis: Process and decision. *Nursing Forum,* 1966, *5,* 50
18. Aspinall, M.J. Nursing diagnosis: The weak link. *Nursing Outlook,* 1976, *24,* 433
19. Mundinger, M. Nursing diagnosis for cancer patients. *Cancer Nursing,* 1978, *1,* 221
20. Chambers, W. Nursing diagnosis. *American Journal of Nursing,* 1962, *62,* 102
21. McCain, R.F. Nursing by assessment—not intuition. *American Journal of Nursing,* 1965, *65,* 82–84
22. Gebbie, K.M. & Lavin, M.A., eds. *Classification of nursing diagnoses: Proceedings of the first national conference.* Saint Louis: C.V. Mosby, 1975
23. Bircher, A. On the development and classification of diagnoses. *Nursing Forum,* 1975, *14,* 10
24. Carnevali, D.L. *Nursing care planning: Diagnosis and management.* Philadelphia: J.B. Lippincott, 1983
25. Edel, M. The nature of nursing diagnosis. In J.H. Carlson, C.A. Craft, & A.D. McGuire (Eds.), *Nursing diagnosis.* Philadelphia: W. B. Saunders, 1982
26. McManus
27. Chambers
28. Yura, H. & Walsh, M.B., Eds. *The nursing process* (1st ed.). Washington, DC: The Catholic University of America Press, 1967
29. Fry
30. Henderson
31. Bircher
32. Gordon, M. Nursing diagnosis and the diagnostic process. *American Journal of Nursing,* 1976, *76,* 8, 1298
33. Bower, F.L. *The process of planning nursing care* (3rd ed.), Saint Louis: C. V. Mosby, 1982
34. Carpenito, L.J. *Nursing diagnosis: Application to clinical practice.* Philadelphia: J.B. Lippincott, 1983
35. Kelly, M.A. *Nursing diagnosis source book: Guidelines for clinical application.* Norwalk, CT: Appleton-Century-Crofts, 1985
36. American Nurses' Association. *Nursing: A social policy statement.* Kansas City: American Nurses' Association, 1980
37. *Ibid.*
38. Bircher
39. Kelly, M.A.
40. Gordon. The diagnostic process
41. Bower
42. Mundinger
43. Carnevali
44. Carpenito. *Application to Clinical Practice*
45. Gordon
46. Gordon, M. *Nursing diagnosis: process and application.* New York: McGraw-Hill, 1982
47. Carpenito. *Application to Clinical Practice*
48. Carpenito, L. J. Nursing diagnosis: Selected dilemmas in practice. *Occupational Health Nursing,* 1985, 397
49. Resler, M.M. Formulation of a nursing diagnosis. In J.H. Carlson, C.A. Craft, & A.D. McGuire (Eds.), *Nursing diagnosis.* Philadelphia: W.B. Saunders, 1982
50. Lunney, M. The PES system: A time for change. In M.E. Hurley (Ed.), *Classification of nursing diagnoses: Proceedings of the sixth conference.* Saint Louis: C. V. Mosby, 1986
51. *Ibid.*
52. Carnevali
53. *Ibid.*
54. Kelly, M.A.
55. *Ibid.*
56. McManus
57. Chambers
58. Gordon. The diagnostic process
59. Shoemaker, J.K. Essential features of a nursing diagnosis. In M.J. Kim, G.K. McFarland, & A.M. McLane (Eds.), *Classification of nursing diagnoses: Proceedings of the fifth national conference.* Saint Louis: C. V. Mosby, 1984
60. Carpenito. *Application to Clinical Practice*
61. Carnevali
62. Bulechek, G.M., & McCloskey, J.C. (Eds.). *Nursing interventions: Treatments for nursing diagnoses.* Philadelphia: W. B. Saunders, 1985
63. American Nurses' Association. *Social policy statement*
64. Kelly, M.A.
65. American Nurses' Association. *Social policy statement*
66. *Ibid.*
67. Hubalik, K. & Kim, M.J. Nursing diagnoses associated with heart failure in critical care nursing. In M.J. Kim, G.K. McFarland, & A. M. McLane (Eds.), *Classification of nursing diagnoses: Proceedings of the fifth national conference.* Saint Louis: C. V. Mosby, 1984
68. Gordon. *Process and Application*
69. Carpenito. *Application to Clinical Practice*
70. Carnevali
71. Kim, M.J. Physiologic nursing diagnosis: Its role and place in nursing taxonomy. In M.J. Kim, G.K. McFarland, & A.M. McLane (Eds.). *Classification of nursing diagnoses: proceedings of the fifth national conference.* Saint Louis: C. V. Mosby, 1984
72. Guzzetta, C.E., & Dossey, B.M. Nursing diagnosis: Framework, process, and problems. *Heart & Lung,* 1983, *12,* 3, 281
73. Jacoby, M.K. The dilemma of physiological problems: Eliminating the double standard. *American Journal of Nursing,* 85, 3, 281
74. Kim, M.J. Without collaboration, what's left? *American Journal of Nursing,* 1985, *85,* 3, 281
75. Schmidt, J.E. *The attorney's dictionary and word finder.* Albany, NY: M. Bender, 1962
76. Carnevali
77. Gordon. *Process and Application*
78. Kelly, M.A.
79. *The Merriam-Webster dictionary.* New York: Pocket Books, 1974

80. Cazalas, M.W. *Nursing & the law* (3rd ed.). Germantown, MD: Aspen Systems Corporation, 1978
81. Cushing, M. Critical care nursing: Applied legal principles. In C.M. Hudak, T. Lohr, & B.M. Gallo (Eds.), *Critical care nursing* (3rd ed.). Philadelphia: J.B. Lippincott, 1982
82. Bloch, D. Criteria, standards and norms: Crucial terms in quality assurance. *Journal of Nursing Administration,* 1977, *7,* 20
83. American Nurses' Association. *Standards of Nursing Practice*
84. Bennett, A. Departmental policies—Guides to action. *Hospital Topics,* 1967, *45,* 44

CHAPTER 3

Etiology: Making Nursing Diagnoses Descriptive and Prescriptive

Emmy Miller

Most of the formats for writing nursing diagnoses include a statement about the cause or etiology of the problem. The P–E–S format[1] requires listing those causal factors that can be changed and are predicted to have an effect on the problem. The two-part format presented by Resler[2] consists of an alteration phrase and a reason phrase. Other formats have included the etiological component as a contributing factor,[3] antecedent or current events,[4] response stimulus,[5] or specific human response.[6]

Despite this repeated reference, the actual role of etiology and its use in the application of nursing diagnoses to clinical situations has received little attention. The author listed above describe the etiology as a critical component of the diagnostic statement, the purpose of which is to direct nursing interventions. Yet, many of the nursing texts that utilize nursing diagnosis either do not list etiologies, or the etiologies are lumped together into one group and the nursing interventions for the problem are lumped into another.[7–12]

Discussions with practicing nurses lead to a very different interpretation of the importance of etiology. In actual practice situations, information about the cause of the patient's condition can be vital, and its usefulness in directing nursing interventions is undisputed. This does not mitigate the difficulties of determining *what* the etiology or contributing factor is, but it does seem to make the effort worthwhile.

Consider the patient with a nursing diagnosis of Anxiety. As a concept, anxiety and the wide range of nursing interventions available to address this problem are well covered in most schools of nursing. In clinical nursing practice, however, the question becomes: Which of the possible nursing interventions are most likely to do this particular patient some good?

Adding a statement about a possible cause or contributing factor to the nursing diagnosis Anxiety can offer some direction for answering this question. This direction can be seen in the following nursing diagnoses:

Anxiety related to new diagnosis of lung cancer
Anxiety related to repeated painful procedures (weekly bone marrow tests)
Anxiety related to physical dependency

The three patients who are experiencing anxiety in this example require distinctly different nursing interventions.

The first patient would benefit from some information about this new diagnosis, if the level of anxiety was not too high; validation of the feeling of anxiety, supportive presence, and active listening would be other appropriate nursing interventions. The second patient requires more focused nursing interventions. This patient might benefit from learning relaxation or imagery techniques for use during procedures. Advocacy for the patient, in the form of obtaining appropriate procedure pain medication, would be another useful nursing intervention. The third patient's anxiety could best be approached through the development of trusting relationships between patient and care givers, the establishment of a consistent daily routine, and identification and support of effective coping mechanisms.

In these examples, the addition of a statement about the situation giving rise to the problem is a critical determinant for the selection of the most appropriate and beneficial nursing interventions. It must be pointed out, however, that none of the etiologies presented in this example can be construed as direct, single causes for the patient's subjective sense of anxiety. This question of causation is one of the major concerns about the use of etiology, both the term itself and the concept.

Two issues are pertinent in the discussion of etiology for nursing diagnosis. One is the concept of causation. Another concern is the present developmental state of the nursing diagnostic framework. Both are important reasons that the concept and the application of the etiology component of nursing diagnosis are still relatively unformed.

ETIOLOGY AS CAUSATION

The issue of etiology has been described as "troublesome" in the efforts to identify, classify, and standardize nursing diagnoses.[13] From a practical point of view, knowledge of a problem's cause is usually helpful in solving that problem. The approach to etiology from the perspective of nursing diagnosis is based on two assumptions: factors that cause nursing problems do exist and study of these causes will be useful to nursing practice.[14]

Concern about the causes of nursing diagnoses, when the diagnoses themselves are not clearly or completely defined, may seem somewhat premature, but the concept of causality seems implicit in human thinking. There is an observable link between action and outcome that produces the notion of cause and effect.

The medical view of causation is a familiar one to nurses. The etiology of disease is an important factor in determining treatment, and the approach to this is often one of single, direct causation. Consider the patient who comes to the physician with cough, fever, and pulmonary congestion. A medical diagnosis of pneumonia is made, and the treatment decisions will depend upon what type of pneumonia is present, such as bacterial, viral, or aspiration.

Other things may also have an important bearing on why this patient developed pneumonia, such as malnutrition, smoking, or environmental factors. These issues, however, will probably receive less attention in the treatment of this patient's pneumonia. While the concept of multicausation is becoming more prevalent in medical science, particularly in relation to diseases such as cancer, arteriosclerosis, and lung disease, clinical practice situations often address disease through a single-cause approach. In contrast, nurses often recognize that problems patients experience are the result of complex, multiple-factor chains of events.[15,16]

The concept of causation can also be examined by considering other issues of causality. The sequence of the cause and the problem is an approach that focuses on the chronology of the events in order to establish a causal relationship. The definition of etiology offered by

Carnevali[17] is consistent with this approach. Another strategy to determine causation is logic; however, the use of logic to justify cause-and-effect relationships is fraught with pitfalls, leading to invalid, inferential conclusions about the relationships between events.[18]

The concept of sufficient cause implies that *all* the conditions necessary for the occurrence of an event are present; necessary cause is that which *must* be present for the event to occur. These are rigorous requirements for causation, and it may be that the concept of probable cause is of most use in the formulation of etiology statements for nursing diagnoses. In this case etiological factors are treated as hypotheses, not facts, but this information can serve to direct nursing intervention. If the interventions are not successful in accomplishing the desired patient outcomes, it may be that the causal hypothesis or etiology was incorrect.[19]

In order to use etiology statements effectively within the context of nursing diagnosis, it is necessary to know those situations or conditions that are frequently associated with the problem and how they affect the progression of it. Much of this knowledge is still to be discovered. Examination of clinical nursing practice and research in this area are greatly needed.

ETIOLOGY AND NURSING DIAGNOSES

Many of the authors who have proposed definitions of nursing diagnosis have used the term "etiology" in their definitions. A number of statements about or definitions of etiology are presented in Table 3–1. The concept of causation is present in many of these statements. Alfaro,[20] Carpenito,[21] Gettrust et al,[22] Gordon,[23] Guzzetta and Dossey,[24] and Kelly[25] use the word "cause" in their discussion of etiology. Other approaches to causation taken in several of these statements are that the etiology is a contributing factor to the problem,[26] a factor that maintains the problem,[27] or a basis or reason for the problem.[28] There seems to be a common-sense, practical recognition of the causation of problems that nurses treat, and this supports the assumptions, mentioned earlier, that factors that cause nursing problems do exist and that their study is useful to nursing practice.[29]

Some of these same authors, however, offer disclaimers about causation as well. Gordon states that:

> "Identifying the etiology is not always easy to do, because cause and effect relationships are usually complex and contain an element of uncertainty".[30]

Carpenito suggests caution in linking the parts of the diagnostic statement with "words implying cause and effect, because such a relationship can result in legal or professional difficulty."[31] Concerns about legal responsibility and implications of blame are also raised by Mundinger and Jauron, who recommend against legally inadvisable statements.[32] One result of these concerns is the use of the term "related to" rather than "caused by" or "due to," as the connecting phrase for the nursing diagnostic statement.

Another approach to etiology is offered by Forsyth,[33] who wonders if the use of etiology in nursing diagnosis statements reflects concern for validity rather than causality. In this view, the etiologic factor is another indicator of the concept described in the nursing diagnosis, and the validity of the nursing diagnosis is recognized only through the combination of the diagnostic label and supporting indicator.[34] This is based upon beliefs that the multidimensional nature of nursing does not lend itself to drawing conclusions about causation, and actual identification of the cause of the problem may be impossible.[35]

TABLE 3–1. DEFINITIONS OF ETIOLOGY

Author	Approach to Etiology
Alfaro, 1986	The cause of, or factors that contribute to a problem, nursing diagnosis, or disease
Bulechek and McCloskey, 1985	The intent is to direct the interventions toward altering the etiological factors associated with the diagnosis
Carnevali, 1983	Antecedent or current events, factors in the environment, changes or predicted changes in internal or external resources that preceed the occurance of the problem
Carpenito, 1983	The etiological and contributing factors are those physiological, situational, and maturational factors that can cause the problem or influence its development
Gettrust, Ryan, and Engelman, 1985	Etiologies are underlying or related causes of the problem. They "suggest" interventions and help direct care
Forsyth, 1984	Causality for all theoretic and practical purposes of nursing is multifactorial. Etiology is a possibility when all possible information is gathered and analyzed, when the cause of an effect is isolated and can be stated with certainty. It is a final stage in the conceptualization and reasoning process
Gordon, 1982	. . .causal factors that can be changed and are predicted to have an effect on the problem
Guzzetta and Dossey, 1983	The etiology is the probable cause of the actual or potential health problem. . .The etiology should be easily understood and useful at the bedside. It helps to identify what is maintaining the problem and what is preventing an improvement in health. It guides the plan of care because it conveys what the nurse and patient must change in order to achieve a state of health
Kelly, 1985	The clarity and at times the individuality, of diagnostic statements are enhanced by the addition of a phrase indicating the nurse's judgment about the situation giving rise to the problem (p. 13) Identification of the response stimulus involves clinical judgment about cause, source, origin, or other related factors of the health problem (p. 66)
Lunney, 1986	Specific problems are understood in the context of how they affect the whole person's achievement of health. . . the second part of the diagnostic statement indicates a more specific level of diagnosing
Mundinger and Jauron, 1975	In the second part of the diagnosis, the nurse identifies factors which are maintaining the undesired response and preventing the desired change. By this statement, she also indiciates in a general way the areas in which she will plan to change the contributing factors' influence on patient response
Resler, 1982	The diagnostic statement usually consists of two main phrases: the first describes the alteration and the second suggests a basis or reason for the alteration

In a similar vein, Lunney questions the P–E–S format for its negative focus on problems and causation.[36] This approach of problem and cause is not consistent with the major concerns of nursing; wholeness and health.[37] Furthermore, common sense approaches to etiology have resulted in a lack of definition and consensus for this term in nursing practice. Some definitions identify factors that existed prior to the problem, others identify factors present at the same time as the alteration, while some recommend identifying only those factors that the nurse can alter or manipulate.[38] (See Table 3–1.)

It is useful to decide which aspects, factors, or dimensions of the problem *can* be treated for improvement of the problem. Although the scientific base may not be known, clinical experience and judgment often indicate that treating a particular aspect or part of the problem has a beneficial effect on the patient's situation. This approach is probably consistent with Forsyth's idea that it is not etiology-as-cause that nurses are identifying but further indicators of the diagnosis that increase the validity of it.[39]

Despite these reservations about causation, a consistent and repeated theme in statements about etiology is its role in directing nursing interventions, the importance of which is acknowledged by Bulechek and McCloskey,[40] Carpenito,[41] Gettrust et al,[42] Guzzetta and Dossey,[43] Kelly,[44] Mundinger and Jauron,[45] and Resler.[46] There must be a reason for this emphasis on etiology directing nursing intervention in the face of concerns about causation and the incomplete state of our diagnostic framework.

THE CLINICAL USE OF ETIOLOGY

The reasons for the recurring attention to etiology can be found in clinical nursing practice based on both approaches to etiology: etiology as a probable cause and etiology as a supporting indicator for the diagnosis. Employing this combined approach, etiology is useful for two reasons: etiology can make diagnostic labels clinically precise and etiology can direct nursing interventions. The current nursing diagnoses tend to be broad and abstract labels, and the addition of an etiological statement is very helpful in making these diagnoses useful for practicing nurses. Etiology is also valuable in clinical practice because it allows the application of standardized problem names for a variety of patients in an individualized or specialized manner.

The most important reason for using etiology in clinical practice, however, is the direction it provides in determining the most effective and beneficial nursing interventions for the identified situation. This linkage of the nursing diagnosis and nursing interventions is essential. In the clinical practice culture, there is little time and less interest in activities that do not directly affect patient care. Clinically precise nursing diagnostic labels can help focus nursing time and energy on patient problems that require nursing care. The goal of using etiology in clinical nursing practice is to make nursing diagnostic statements descriptive of the patient and prescriptive of the nursing interventions that the patient requires.

It is helpful to begin a discussion of the use of etiology in clinical nursing practice with an examination of the nursing diagnostic labels themselves. There are 98 nursing diagnoses that have been accepted by the North American Nursing Diagnosis Association (NANDA). While other labels have been proposed in the literature and are in use in many clinical practice settings, the NANDA list is a practical place to begin. Indeed, this is where many nurses begin their work with nursing diagnosis.

In 1986 the nursing diagnoses approved by NANDA were organized into a taxonomy that replaced the previous alphabetical listing. Nine human response patterns are used as the horizontal headings of a matrix of phenomena; the vertical organization is by levels of abstraction. The nine patterns constitute the first level of Taxonomy I. (See Table 3–2.) These human response patterns are very abstract, conceptual labels, such as exchanging, communicating, and valuing, and, as such, are not clinically useful for identifying patient problems.

The next level is Alteration in Human Responses. Labels at this level of abstraction are

TABLE 3–2. NINE HUMAN RESPONSE PATTERNS

Exchanging:	*Mutual giving and receiving*
Communicating:	*Sending messages*
Relating:	*Establishing bonds*
Valuing:	*Assigning relative worth*
Choosing:	*Selection of alternatives*
Moving:	*Activity*
Perceiving:	*Reception of information*
Knowing:	*Meaning associated with information*
Feeling:	*Subjective awareness of information*

subcategories of human response patterns. The use of the term "alteration" refers to "the process or state of becoming or being made different without changing into something else," and it is essentially a neutral term, indicating neither a positive or negative change.[47] These Level II concepts include Alteration in Nutrition, Alteration in Communication, Alteration in Coping, Alteration in Thought Process, and Alteration in Self Concept, to name a few. While these are important concepts for nursing practice, they are somewhat vague and lack the specificity necessary to describe an individual patient's problem.

The diagnostic labels in Level III describe Phenomena of Concern Categories and appear to be more useful for clinical practice. Nursing diagnoses such as Potential for Injury, Ineffective Family Coping, Impaired Physical Mobility, Sleep Pattern Disturbance, Disturbance in Body Image, Anxiety, and Grieving are found at Level III. Nursing diagnoses at Level IV are even more specific and descriptive. At this level are Ineffective Airway Clearance, Stress Incontinence, Rape Trauma Syndrome, Activity Intolerance, Impaired Swallowing, and Chronic Pain. These nursing diagnostic labels describe very real phenomena that practicing nurses deal with every day.

Taxonomy I has been endorsed by the membership of NANDA as a framework to be tested, refined, revised, and expanded.[48] While its developmental state is recognized, one strength of the taxonomy is that diagnostic labels with the most clinical utility are more apparent. When confronted with the alphabetical list, many nurses found it difficult to see how abstract labels such as Alteration in Comfort or Sensory/Perceptual Alteration could be applied to the care of patients in a meaningful or effective way.

ETIOLOGY AS A TOOL FOR CLINICAL ACCURACY AND SPECIALIZATION OF NURSING DIAGNOSES

The use of etiology provides clinical relevance and a degree of diagnostic accuracy that is not available with the current diagnostic labels. Consider the difference between the following nursing diagnoses:

Alteration in Elimination: Constipation
Constipation related to lack of fiber in diet

This second statement is more precise and it is also consistent with the way that nurses actually talk about patient problems. It also gives direction about the best way to address the problem.

Clinical accuracy of nursing diagnoses can be enhanced through the use of etiology in another way. Including an etiology statement in the diagnostic label allows the use of standardized problem names for a variety of patients in many different settings. In this way the same diagnostic label can be applied to a broad spectrum of patients experiencing the problem, and the clinical specialization can be added through the etiology statement.

The nursing diagnosis Ineffective Airway Clearance is a useful one for a number of patients. For Mr. Jones, who has chronic obstructive pulmonary disease, fatigues easily, and has large quantities of thick, tenacious, pulmonary secretions, the addition of the etiology statement "related to thick secretions and fatigue," tells the nurse which aspects of the situation require nursing intervention. Across the hall is Mr. Smith who has sustained a spine fracture at the sixth cervical vertebrae. He, too, has Ineffective Airway Clearance, but the important factor in this situation is the paralysis of intercostal musculature, preventing effective coughing or deep breathing. The addition of an etiology statement "related to respiratory muscle paralysis" would direct the nurse to a different set of interventions such as assisted coughing and diaphragmatic strengthening exercises.

In these examples the same diagnostic label, Ineffective Airway Clearance, is used for patients who have very different causes for their respiratory alteration and require different types of nursing interventions. The addition of an etiology statement provides individualization for two different patients; moreover, the specialty aspects of nursing care can be included as well. The same diagnostic label could be applied to a pulmonary patient and a neurosurgical patient; both the unique requirements of the specialty focus and the individual response of the patient can be addressed. This clinical precision and relevance provided by the etiology statement is a key point to the successful use of nursing diagnosis in clinical practice.

Diagnosing Patient Problems Versus Labeling Phenomena

In clinical practice, nurses make nursing diagnoses because the clear identification of the patient's condition is helpful in deciding when nursing treatment is needed and which strategies will be most useful. Here theoretical or academic issues of labeling phenomena are perceived as less important than solving or improving existing patient problems. In the clinical setting, a nursing diagnosis must do more than simply label a phenomenon; it should describe the patient's condition in such a way that approaches and solutions to it are readily seen. The use of etiology statements plays a key role in this. If nursing diagnosis is to be the tool that nurses use to think about, talk about, and write about patient problems, then the nursing diagnosis itself must be clinically functional.

Consider the difference between labeling a phenomenon and diagnosing a situation that needs nursing treatment. A young woman with multiple sclerosis is admitted to the hospital with an exacerbation of her disease. During the medical history and physical examination procedure, it is determined that the patient has a spastic bladder. In the nursing history and physical examination procedure, the patient confides that her incontinence has adversely affected her sexual relationship with her husband, and the nurse observes that the patient's perineal area and inner thighs are red and chafed.

It would be possible to label this patient's situation with a nursing diagnosis of Reflex Incontinence. This is a very concrete label from Level IV of Taxonomy I. While this approach does label the phenomenon precisely, it does not identify the patient's response to the incontinence or give any insight into the best intervention for the situation. If the American Nurses' Association (ANA) definition of nursing as the diagnosis and treatment of human responses to actual or potential health problems is followed, then the nurse's diagnostic question is: What is this patient's response to the incontinence, and how should I treat it?

This line of thinking could lead to the following nursing diagnostic possibilities:

Sexual Dysfunction related to Reflex Incontinence
Potential Impaired Skin Integrity related to Reflex Incontinence

Nursing diagnoses should focus on those patient situations which need to be treated and avoid labeling things just because they are problems.[49] Describing the patient's response, rather than simply naming phenomena, is more descriptive and prescriptive, identifying important nursing care issues that would not be addressed with a nursing diagnosis of Reflex Incontinence alone.

This argument in favor of using etiology in nursing diagnostic statements does not ignore the importance of accurate labeling of phenomena or the necessity for continued efforts in that direction. Identifying human responses and subcategories that are nursing diagnoses will be the work of the nursing profession for years to come. Today's practicing nurse, however, must be able to work with currently available labels in a way that describes the patient's response and gives direction for nursing treatment.

The addition of etiology statements that identify either a probable cause or a critical supporting indicator makes the nursing diagnosis a tool for solving patient problems rather than "something else to do" in the busy day of the practicing nurse. The enhanced diagnostic accuracy and the strong link with nursing interventions are tremendous benefits that can result from the inclusion of an etiology statement in the nursing diagnosis.

Etiology as a Tool for Directing Nursing Interventions

When a nurse identifies a patient situation, two questions come to mind: Why is this condition present? What should I do about it? These questions are linked in that oftentimes the treatment of the problem is to do something about what is causing it.

In the context of the nursing process, the nursing diagnosis is identified after assessment of the patient and prior to the planning of nursing interventions. Nursing interventions are based on the factors that cause or maintain the problem as well as the health problem itself.[50] The accurate determination of a probable cause, contributing factor, or supporting indicator is critical in selecting those nursing interventions that will be most effective for the patient's problem.

This use draws from both approaches to etiology: the probable cause of the problem, and the supporting indicator that gives the problem validity. While the determination of causation in clinical practice may be impossible, the association of events often supports a common-sense criterion for causation, and this can be helpful in planning nursing care.

By including a statement of the probable cause, a contributing factor, or simply a clinical judgment about the problem, the nurse is guided in selecting nursing interventions. Instead of feeling obligated to deal with *all* possible nursing interventions for the problem, the scope of the problem is focused on the particular aspects manifested by this patient, and the selection of nursing interventions can be focused as well. This moves the formulation of nursing diagnoses from the academic or theoretical realm to a practical, useful tool for nursing practice. Making nursing diagnoses *real*, by using diagnostic labels that are both descriptive and prescriptive, is essential for nursing diagnosis to be accepted and incorporated into the clinical practice culture.

Sometimes, in the effort to identify a probable cause or contributing factor for the nursing diagnosis, the medical diagnosis appears as the most obvious or important factor. This results in diagnostic statements such as Ineffective Airway Clearance related to pneumonia or Decreased Cardiac Output related to congestive heart failure. While the pneumonia and the congestive heart failure are indeed important contributing factors to the Ineffective Airway

Clearance and Decreased Cardiac Output, use of the medical diagnosis as an etiology statement does not meet the goals of a diagnostic label, that of being both descriptive of the patient and prescriptive of nursing interventions. There are a number of legal and professional concerns that are also important.

The definition of nursing diagnosis excludes those health problems for which the accepted mode of therapy is prescription drugs, surgery, radiation, and other treatments that are legally defined as the practice of medicine.[51] From a legal perspective, nurses are educated in and licensed to practice nursing, not medicine; therefore, the diagnosis of medical diseases is not within the scope of nursing practice. While this does not alter the nurse's responsibility to monitor disease conditions and to make pertinent observations as well as to respond to certain medical situations, the actual determination a patient's disease is a medical responsibility. This is certainly one reason not to use medical diagnoses as etiology statements.

Another reason is that the etiology statement should direct nursing interventions.[52–56] By stating the etiology as a medical diagnosis, the nurse appears to be treating medical disease. While nursing care certainly includes the implementation of physician orders for disease treatment, this is very different than determining that treatment.

The most important reason for not using the medical diagnosis as an etiology statement is that it does not provide either the descriptive or prescriptive accuracy that is desirable in a nursing diagnostic statement. In the preceding example, the use of the medical diagnosis, pneumonia, gives no insight into the patient's response to the disease process or suggestions for nursing care. Furthermore, when the medical diagnosis is used as an etiology for the nursing diagnosis, there is a tendency for nurses to practice medicine at the expense of nursing.[57]

The intent of using nursing diagnosis is to identify those patient conditions that benefit from nursing care, and to direct the nurse in selecting the most beneficial nursing interventions. Medical diagnosis as an etiology does not support or encourage this goal. Yet nurses often want to use the medical diagnosis as an etiology statement, especially when first learning to work with nursing diagnosis.

One possible explanation for this is that the use of medical diagnoses as etiology statements reflects a developmental stage of diagnostic conceptualization and clinical reality. It may be a strategy to bridge the adjustment from working with the medical diagnosis to working with a nursing diagnosis.[58] While this might possibly be a useful interim strategy, it is essential to begin identifying etiology statements that can be treated with nursing interventions; failure to do so is a problem with using the medical diagnosis as etiology.

Etiology, within the context of the nursing diagnostic statement, may refer to either a probable cause of the patient's situation, or it may describe an additional indicator of the situation, where the combination of indicators indicates a need for nursing treatment. Using the second part of the diagnostic statement to identify a supporting indicator for the nursing diagnosis is an alternative to listing the probable cause of the problem. This use of etiology does not attempt to describe the cause of the patient's condition; rather, it is the combination of factors that constitutes a situation requiring nursing care.

This approach to etiology requires careful attention to nursing diagnosis and etiology as two factors that in combination describe the patient's response. A danger here would be that the nursing diagnosis and the etiology were the same. This type of statement is a tautology. Examples would be Alteration in Urinary Elimination related to incontinence or Self Care Deficit related to inability to care for self. The nursing diagnoses and the etiology are the same thing rather than two related indicators of the state of the patient.

This approach covers those diagnostic statements when additional information is important, but the problem or its cause cannot be changed. In this case, nursing intervention is directed toward the signs or symptoms of the problem,[59] or the nurse attempts to compensate for the problem through nursing interventions.

Consider the nursing diagnosis of Impaired Physical Mobility. This Level IV diagnostic label could be used to describe many patients; however, there is no precise delineation of how or why mobility is impaired. Including a second statement that describes the scope or the type of mobility impairment makes this a more useful label for clinical nursing practice. This use of etiology is seen in the following examples:

> Impaired Physical Mobility related to left hemiparesis
> Impaired Physical Mobility related to post-op pain
> Impaired Physical Mobility related to fatigue

These nursing diagnoses describe the patient's response (Impaired Physical Mobility) and give specific indicators (post-op pain) or supporting data (left hemiparesis, fatigue) for the response. In each of these cases, the nurse cannot "fix" or otherwise resolve the etiologies. It is very helpful to know the type (left hemiparesis) or extent (post-op) of the factor contributing to the Impaired Mobility, and there are many nursing interventions to compensate for the immobility in order to ameliorate the negative effects of it. This additional indicator makes these diagnostic labels more useful in clinical practice than Impaired Physical Mobility alone.

The inclusion of an etiology statement to the nursing diagnosis provides improved accuracy of the diagnostic label, the ability to apply standardized nursing diagnoses to individual patients and to specialty patient populations, and direction for selecting the best nursing interventions for the particular patient's problem. This approach also focuses diagnostic thinking on the identification of situations that need nursing treatment rather than just labeling problems because they are there. Making nursing diagnosis a tool for clinical problem-solving is a critical step in successful implementation of nursing diagnosis and the establishment of diagnosis-based nursing practice.

CONCLUSION

Suggestions for Using Etiology in Clinical Practice

In order to get the most benefit from the use of etiology statements in the diagnostic label, it is helpful to have an operational definition of what etiology is and what it is not. The following is proposed as a useful, working definition:

> The etiology statement is the second part of a nursing diagnosis. There are two approaches to etiology. One is to identify a probable cause or contributing factor for the patient's problem. Another approach is to describe a supporting indicator for the patient's condition; in this case, it is the combination of the problem and indicator that constitutes a situation that requires nursing treatment. The etiology statement should be as specific as possible in order to make the nursing diagnosis descriptive of the patient's situation and prescriptive of the nursing care required by the patient.

This definition focuses on making the nursing diagnosis as accurate and precise as possible. This also supports the usefulness of the nursing diagnosis in directing nursing interventions.

Attention to etiology can be an effective tool for clinical accuracy and precision in nursing practice. Directing clinical thinking toward etiology, as defined above, moves diagnosing from simply labeling phenomena to identifying patient situations that need nursing treatment. The following suggestions are offered to help practicing nurses use etiology statements to make nursing diagnoses useful and precise.

Define Etiology Broadly. The concept of etiology as causation *only* is too narrow and lacks the supporting clinical research base at this point. A broad definition of etiology, as a probable cause, contributing factor, or supporting indicator, allows the nurse to utilize clinical judgments about the patient's particular situation and to communicate those in the diagnostic statement.

Focus on Etiology for Diagnostic Accuracy and Precision. The addition of an etiology statement makes the nursing diagnosis individual and specific. It can also incorporate areas of specialization in nursing care. This moves the identification of nursing diagnoses from an academic or theoretical effort of labeling phenomena to a tool for the practicing nurse to treat the problems of individual patients. Just because two patients have Impaired Physical Mobility does not mean that their situations are exactly the same or that the same nursing interventions will be effective. Including an etiology statement that describes each patient's unique contributing factor or supporting indicator makes the diagnostic label useful and *real*.

Use Etiology to Direct Nursing Intervention. Just as an etiology statement can make a nursing diagnosis more useful in describing a patient's situation, it also can make it more useful in prescribing the nursing interventions. The number of possible nursing interventions for the patient with Impaired Physical Mobility is large. With the addition of a probable cause, contributing factor, or supporting indicator, however, the spectrum of possible nursing interventions can be narrowed to focus on those interventions most likely to do this particular patient some good. For both the busy staff nurse and the patient who needs nursing assistance, this focus and direction is a significant benefit.

The nursing diagnosis should be a statement that describes the patient's situation and gives prescriptive direction for nursing intervention. The current state of nursing diagnostic labels does not yet offer this direction, and it will probably be many years before the examination and study of clinical nursing practice can provide concise labels that do. For the nurse who wants to work with nursing diagnosis *now,* the use of etiology, as described in this chapter, is a way to make nursing diagnoses a precise and accurate tool for nursing practice.

REFERENCES

1. Gordon, M. *Nursing diagnosis: Process and application.* New York: McGraw-Hill, 1982
2. Resler, M.M. Formulation of a nursing Diagnosis. In J.H. Carlson, C.A. Craft, & A.D. McGuire (Eds.), *Nursing diagnosis.* Philadelphia: W.B. Saunders, 1982
3. Carpenito, L.J. *Nursing diagnosis: Application to clinical practice.* Philadelphia: J.B. Lippincott, 1983
4. Carnevali, D.L. *Nursing care planning: Diagnosis and management.* Philadelphia: J.B. Lippincott, 1983
5. Kelly, M.A. *Nursing diagnosis source book: Guidelines for clinical application.* Norwalk, CT: Appleton-Century-Crofts, 1985
6. Lunney, M. The PES system: A time for change. In M.E. Hurley (Ed.), *Classification of nursing diagnoses: Proceedings of the sixth conference.* Saint Louis: C. V. Mosby, 1986
7. Thompson, J.M., McFarland, G.K., Hirsch, J.E., et al. *Clinical Nursing.* St. Louis: C.V. Mosby, 1986
8. Carpenito
9. Kim, M.J., McFarland, G.K., & McLane, A.M. (Eds.). *Pocket guide to nursing diagnosis.* Saint Louis: C. V. Mosby, 1984
10. Bulechek, G.M., & McCloskey, J.C. (Eds.). *Nursing interventions: Treatments for nursing diagnoses.* Philadelphia: W. B. Saunders, 1985
11. Kelly

12. Gettrust, K.V., Ryan, S.C., & Engelman, D.S. (Eds.). *Applied nursing diagnosis: Guidelines for comprehensive care planning.* New York: John Wiley & Sons, 1985

13. Forsyth, G.L. Etiology: In what sense and of what value? In M.J. Kim, G.K. McFarland, & A.M. McLane (Eds.), *Classification of nursing diagnoses: Proceedings of the fifth national Conference.* Saint Louis: C.V. Mosby, 1984

14. Derdiarian, A.K. Etiology: Practical relevance. In A. M. McLane (Ed.), *Classification of nursing diagnoses: Proceedings of the seventh conference.* St. Louis: C.V. Mosby, 1987

15. Gordon. *Process and Application*

16. Forsyth

17. Carnevali

18. Gordon. *Process and Application*

19. *Ibid.*

20. Alfaro, R. *Application of nursing process: A step-by-step guide.* Philadelphia: J. B. Lippincott, 1986

21. Carpenito

22. Gettrust et al.

23. Gordon. *Process and Application*

24. Guzzetta, C.E., & Dossey, B.M. Nursing diagnosis: Framework, process, and problems. *Heart & Lung,* 1983, *12,* 3, 281

25. Kelly

26. Carpenito

27. Mundinger, M., & Jauron, G. Developing a nursing diagnosis. *Nursing Outlook,* 1975, *23,* 94

28. Resler

29. Derdiarian

30. Gordon. *Process and Application*

31. Carpenito

32. Mundinger & Jauron

33. Forsyth

34. *Ibid.*

35. *Ibid.*

36. Lunney

37. *Ibid.*

38. *Ibid.*

39. Forsyth

40. Bulechek & McCloskey

41. Carpenito

42. Gettrust et al.

43. Guzzetta & Dossey

44. Kelly

45. Mundinger & Jauron

46. Resler

47. North American Nursing Diagnosis Association. *Taxonomy I.*

48. *Ibid.*

49. Lunney

50. Gordon. *Process and Application*

51. Gordon, M. Nursing diagnosis and the diagnostic process. *American Journal of Nursing,* 1976, *76,* 8, 1298

52. Kim, M.J., Amoroso-Seritella, R., & Gulanick, M., et al. Clinical validation of cardiovascular nursing diagnosis. In M.J. Kim, G.K. McFarland, & A.M. McLane (Eds.), *Classification of nursing diagnoses: Proceedings of the fifth national conference.* Saint Louis: C.V. Mosby, 1984, p. 136

53. Bulechek & McCloskey

54. Kelly

55. Gordon. *Process and Application*

56. Carpenito

57. Kelly

58. Kim, Amoroso-Seritella, & Gulanick, et al.

59. Bulechek & McCloskey

CHAPTER 4

Clinical Thinking in Diagnosis-based Nursing Practice

Emmy Miller

Clinical thinking in nursing practice is concerned with two closely related areas: diagnostic decisions and treatment decisions. A nursing diagnosis is the diagnostic decision, and it directs the subsequent treatment decisions. An understanding of what a nursing diagnosis is and what it is not is essential in order to use nursing diagnosis in the clinical thinking process. In the preceding chapters the foundations, definitions, and formats for nursing diagnosis were examined. Next, this information must be put to work.

Clinical thinking is the foundation of nursing practice. How a nurse thinks about patient situations and available strategies to address these situations will ultimately determine the type, variety, and eventual success of nursing care for that patient. Nursing diagnosis can be a powerful tool to direct clinical thinking in nursing practice.

The approach to clinical thinking in nursing practice that has received the most attention is the nursing process. This model of assessment, nursing diagnosis, planning, intervention, and evaluation [1-5] is the one most commonly seen in nursing education and nursing practice. It is also reflected in many of the professional and regulatory standards for nursing practice.

Clinical thinking in nursing practice encompasses a number of cognitive processes, such as diagnostic reasoning, problem-solving, clinical judgment, and decision-making. The diagnostic reasoning process focuses on how nurses use data from patient assessment and clinical knowledge to arrive at a nursing diagnosis. The diagnostic reasoning process in nursing has been described by a number of authors, and there are similarities between this process and the steps of the nursing process. (See Table 4–1.)

THE NURSING PROCESS

The recognized thinking model of the nursing profession is the nursing process. It was originally described as a four-step model of assessing, planning, implementing the plan, and evaluation of the plan's effectiveness.[6] Inserting the diagnostic step between assessment and

TABLE 4–1. DIAGNOSTIC REASONING AND THE NURSING PROCESS

Nursing Process	Kelly	Gordon	Carnevali
Assessment	*Data collection*	*Collecting information*	*Pre-encounter data*
			Entry to the data search field
	Data analysis	*Interpreting the information*	
		Clustering the information	*Developing cue clusters*
Nursing Diagnosis	*Naming*	*Naming the cluster*	*Activating diagnostic hypotheses*
			Guided search
			Evaluation of diagnostic hypotheses
			Assignment of the diagnostic label
Planning			
Intervention			
Evaluation			

planning provides a critical link between these components for only if the patient's problem is clearly and accurately identified can planning to solve it be effective.

The nursing process is a problem-solving model, but for years nurses have been solving problems without ever stating just what these problems actually were. Although some authors included problem identification as a part of the assessment process,[7-9] there was little or no emphasis on carefully describing the condition that had been identified or naming it in such a way as to indicate the need for nursing treatment. The lack of such names has been a major stumbling block in the evolution of nursing as a professional entity and as a theory-based science.

Nursing diagnosis provides this focus for the nursing process. It is both a product and a process. The product is a label that is clinically functional. In nursing practice its function is to describe the patient's situation clearly and accurately and to do this is a way that is prescriptive of nursing treatment. The product of nursing diagnosis is also the second step in the nursing process. By concluding the assessment of the patient with a name for the condition or problem that requires nursing treatment, the remaining steps of the nursing process, planning, intervention, and evaluation, are founded on the nursing diagnosis.

The process of nursing diagnosis is the thinking process that nurses use to access patients, evaluate and organize the data collected, and determine the nursing diagnosis. In order for nursing diagnosis to be a meaningful tool for nursing practice, nurses must be able to perform the requisite cognitive processes, including recognition and collection of data, organization of data in terms of particular knowledge, and the classification and labeling of the phenomena encountered.[10] This thinking process is a means, however, not an end.

To achieve the desired end of a nursing diagnosis that is both descriptive and prescriptive, the diagnostic reasoning process must be carried out in an effective manner. Each nurse in the practice culture must be able to make nursing diagnoses. Skill in the diagnostic process is an essential component for the development of a diagnosis-based nursing practice.

BASIC CONCEPTS: INFORMATION AND DECISION MAKING

In its simplest form, the nursing process is founded on two basic concepts: information and decisions about that information. Only if the nurse has adequate, appropriate, and valid information about the patient's situation can diagnostic and treatment decisions be made. To make these decisions, the nurse must determine which information about the patient is important and which is not, what relationships exist between data, and what clinical information from the nurses's memory should be used to interpret the patient data.

Information

What constitutes adequate, appropriate information? This can be examined in two categories. The first consists of information obtained from the patient through interview, observation, and other physical examination techniques. Data from laboratory tests, X-rays, and other diagnostic tests also fits into this category as patient information.

The second category of information that the nurse must have is clinical information about the *meaning* of the data thus obtained. The significance of certain symptoms, the usual progression of the disease process, or the expected responses to medications or treatments are critical pieces of information that the nurse must know before the decision-making component of clinical thinking can begin.

This clinical information about the meaning of patient data must also include information about defining characteristics of various nursing diagnoses and the appropriate nursing treatments. Those critical indicators that distinguish when the situation should be referred to other health care professionals, most commonly the physician, must also be known. The identification of these defining characteristics, effective nursing treatments, and the framework for nursing diagnoses has begun, and this information is available for clinical use. Taxonomy I, nursing research of nursing diagnoses, and various clinical references provide the current state of the art in nursing diagnoses.

The debate about what nurses need to know is still occurring in nursing schools and in the nursing practice arena. There is agreement that nursing education should include content from the physical, biological, and psychosocial sciences; however, exactly what this content should be remains unclear. There is also agreement that nursing preparation should include content in nursing arts and science. There is even more controversy and confusion about this. The identification of a knowledge base for nursing is one of the major tasks that faces the profession.[11]

Even when the focus of this discussion is narrowed to that information the nurse needs in order to formulate nursing diagnoses, these larger issues still play a role. The essential information needed to formulate a nursing diagnosis can be examined in the following categories:

1. Data from the patient (physical examination, interview, lab and diagnostic tests)
2. Clinical information about the *meaning* of the data obtained from the patient
3. Knowledge of nursing practice, including the cues and cue patterns and the nursing treatment options associated with various nursing diagnoses

These three categories of information do not simplify the question of a knowledge base for nursing; instead, they expand it.

Leaving the clinical information question for a moment, it is helpful to examine certain basic skills that will assist in making nursing diagnoses and nursing treatment decisions. A skill is the ability to use knowledge effectively to do something. In this sense skills reflect a body of knowledge or information that can be applied to patient situations.

One of the most basic skills that the nurse must possess in order to make nursing diagnoses is the ability to examine and interview patients effectively. A nurse who does not know what abnormal breath sounds are will have a difficult time making the nursing diagnosis, Ineffective Airway Clearance. In the same way the nurse who cannot establish rapport or conduct an effective interview with the patient will have difficulty obtaining the necessary information for making nursing diagnoses that deal with psychosocial conditions.

The nurse must also possess the skills necessary to carry out the nursing treatments that are indicated for the nursing diagnosis. Once the nursing diagnosis Ineffective Airway Clearance is made, the available treatment options might include postural drainage and chest physiotherapy; however, in the absence of the ability to perform these skills, this nurse will be unable to offer treatment for this nursing diagnosis. Another example might be the nurse who makes a nursing diagnosis of severe or panic-level Anxiety but lacks the crisis-interventions skills to assist the patient.

Another set of skills that is essential for making nursing diagnoses are critical thinking skills. These thinking strategies include logic and reasoning, judgment, problem-solving, and decision-making. These critical thinking skills play an important role in the diagnostic reasoning process, and they are important skills that the nurse must possess in order to make diagnostic and treatment decisions.

Judgment is an important aspect of clinical nursing practice. "Good judgment" is one of the highest accolades in the clinical practice culture, although it may mean different things in different settings and to different individuals. The nurse who detects early warning signals of impending deterioration in a critical patient is demonstrating a characteristic of expert practice called "future think."[12] This is a type of judgment that permits the nurse to anticipate changes in the patient's condition, and it is highly valued in practice cultures where physiologic instability is common. Other clinical practice cultures may place more value on those judgments that support the administrative practices of the organization such as prompt and appropriate notification of supervisors.

Judgment may be defined as the process of forming an opinion by discerning or comparing.[13] Many types of judgment are a part of clinical nursing practice, and a schema of four types of judgment had been described by Doona.[14] These four types are common sense, speculative judgment, pragmatic judgment, and ideal judgment. These types of judgment reflect differing uses of information in order to arrive at an opinion.

In practice, judgment is often instantaneous, and the clinician may not be able to identify the reasons for arriving at a certain conclusion. Oftentimes it is helpful to analyze judgments retrospectively in order to restructure the process and the information used; however, this may not always be possible. Four methods of arriving at judgments have been described by Berne.[15] The conscious, logical derivation of conclusions is one method; however, preconscious, subconscious, and unknown processes also take place. With the exception of preconscious judgments, where observations may be identified retrospectively, these methods of making judgments cannot be tapped by the individual for analysis.

An important aspect of judgment is intuition. While intuition has not always enjoyed a sense of scientific legitimacy, a recent examination of the nursing practice and the expertise within that practice shows a different picture. In a description of levels of competency in clinical nursing practice, it appears that a "gut feeling" or vague hunch is the beginning of the perceptual awareness which is central to good nursing judgment.[16] Intuition can be defined as understanding without a rationale, and intuitive judgment distinguishes expert human judgment from the decisions or computations that might be made by a machine or a beginner.[17]

Decision Making

Decision making involves making choices. Clinical decision making involves making choices about patient conditions, the meaning and importance of clinical findings, and the treatment options best suited to the situation at hand.

Two approaches that have been used to describe clinical decision making are the information processing theory and the behavioral model of decision making. Both of these perspectives are based on an assumption that decisions result from an orderly, sequential analysis of the situation. Experienced clinicians, however, make many decisions without having conscious awareness of which cues were used, how they were clustered, or what weight each cue held.[18]

The information processing model is an effort to characterize the sequence of cognitive processes used in particular problem-solving tasks and to explain those processes in terms of psychological concepts and principles. This approach likens the human mind to a computer and concerns itself with the interaction between the person processing the information and the requirements of the task.[19,20]

One contribution of research based on this model is the identification of cognitive strategies that humans use to adapt to our limited information-processing capabilities. The major limitations are the structure and capacity of our two main memory systems: short-term and long-term memory. Strategies such as serial information processing, careful data selection, and simplified problem representation are examples of strategies to cope with these limitations.[21,22]

The behavioral decision model deals with the question of what decisions should be made rather than the processes of how they are made. This model describes four major components of decision making: (1) a set of possible actions, (2) consequences of those actions, (3) judgments concerning the likelihood that those consequences will occur if the action is taken, and (4) judgments concerning the value of the consequences to the decision maker. An assumption of this model is that a rational person chooses the alternative with the highest expected value and the best consequences.[23]

The terms judgment and decision are often used interchangeably, although judgment tends to be seen as a process of arriving at an opinion or conclusion,[24] while decisions are viewed as a product, the choice that results from the decision-making process. Diagnostic reasoning is a type of decision-making process.

The diagnostic reasoning process can be defined as:

A complex, sometimes unconscious, integration of critical-thinking, and data-collecting processes that clinicians use to identify and classify phenomena in presenting clinical situations.[25]

The diagnostic process is comprised of many decisions. A nurse must decide which information and observations are important in a patient situation. Decisions must be made about what additional information would be helpful and whether to act upon any of that information. In the latter case, decisions must be made about which nursing interventions would be most beneficial and then evaluating their effectiveness.

Judgment, intuition, problem-solving skills, and patient-assessment skills are all required in order to make appropriate and effective diagnostic decisions. The decision-making process involved in making treatment decisions has not been investigated to the same degree. There are a number of decision points in making diagnostic and treatment decisions. These decision points are influenced by a number of factors, and examination of these can be helpful in working with nursing diagnosis, as well as improving skill and ability to make diagnostic and treatment decisions.

DECISION POINTS IN THE NURSING PROCESS

The decision-making requirements of the nursing process are presented in Table 4–2. These decision points have been identified from a number of models of clinical thinking and decision making, including Gordon,[26] Carnevali,[27,28] and Kelly.[29] In nursing practice these decisions may be guided by clinical knowledge and experience, tradition and ritual, theoretical frameworks, clinical protocol, and personal preference. Nursing diagnosis can play a crucial role in all of the decision points in the nursing process, by providing a focus for diagnostic and treatment decisions and a common language for nurses to use in discussing and communicating these decisions.

Decisions about Data

The first five decisions listed in Table 4–2 have to do with obtaining data about the patient and making decisions about that data, based on clinical information from knowledge and experience. Having accurate, valid data about the patient is an essential part of these decisions. Another critical component is the clinical information used to evaluate and attribute significance to the patient data.

   The result of these decisions is a statement of the patient's condition. The relationship of data to diagnosis has been described as:

TABLE 4–2. DECISION POINTS IN THE NURSING PROCESS

Decisions about Data:

To notice *a piece of patient data (sign, symptom, observable finding)*

To attend *to a piece of patient data, that is to attribute some importance to it*

To attribute clinical significance *to a piece of patient data, based on clinical knowledge or experience*

To recognize relationships *between pieces of data*

To recall experiences *with other patients who had the same or similar signs, symptoms, or observable findings*

Decisions about Naming:

To label *the cluster or pattern of patient data*

To test *this label as a diagnostic hypothesis*

To accept or reject *the diagnostic label; if accepted as the best judgment at the time, to assign a nursing diagnosis*

Decisions about Treatment:

To project expected outcomes *based on the identified patient state or situation*

To determine the need *for treatment,*

To identify treatment options/interventions, *including nursing treatments and referral to other health care professionals*

To prioritize *which treatment options should be implemented in order of importance*

To evaluate *the effects of the treatment on the identified patient situation*

---

that of the raw ingredients for a cake to the finished product. The cake has neither the appearance nor the taste of the individual raw ingredients, yet it could not exist as a finished product without the presence of all of them. Similarly, the diagnosis does not look like the data, yet a valid diagnosis is a skilled mixing and processing, a distillation of all the related data to create a concise statement and the essence of the situation.[30]

Patient data and clinical information about the meaning of that data are the ingredients, and knowledge of nursing diagnosis is the recipe for the making of a nursing diagnosis.

Data Collection. The process of collecting data about the patient is the assessment step of the nursing process. Some authors use the term assessment to refer to all of the steps of the diagnostic process, including the determination of the nursing diagnosis.[31,32] Other authors identify two distinct phases within the assessment step: data collection and identification of the nursing diagnosis.[33,34] In recent years the determination of the nursing diagnosis from assessment data has become a separate step in the nursing process. Assessment and diagnosis overlap, and together they constitute the diagnostic process.[35]

It is helpful to examine these overlapping processes separately. Assessment refers to the data collection procedure; diagnosis refers to the interpretation of that information, including both analysis of the information and naming the cluster or pattern of data. While data collection is the first step in the assessment process, the first decision that must be made in the nursing process is the decision to notice a piece of data. If the patient's pallor or labored breathing is not noticed or attended to, the nurse cannot use that data in the decision-making process. Student nurses who memorize long lists of symptoms for observation are learning what patient data requires notice and attention.

Errors in data collection can influence the entire decision-making process for diagnosis and treatment. Errors can be in the failure to collect adequate or appropriate data as well as the collection of irrelevant or overwhelming amounts of data. Data may be neglected because of distraction, lack of organization, or insufficient clinical knowledge.[36]

Cue Identification. The terms "cue identification" and "inferencing" are used to describe the skills that relate to the perception and accurate identification of information in the environment and the assigning of valid meanings to the situations.[37] A cue can be defined as a unit of sensory input, a single message that is noticed and usually named. The noticing of cues is an outgrowth of both experiential and theoretical knowledge.[38] Cues are information that influence decisions; these decisions may be to collect more data or to make a diagnostic or treatment decision.[39]

For example, during an admission interview the nurse may notice that Mr. Jones does not make eye contact when questioned about his low-salt diet. This cue could have a number of meanings: that he does not understand the question, that he has not been following his diet, or that he is unsettled by the hospital admission process, to name a few possibilities. Unless the nurse notices this cue, there can be no thinking about its possible meanings.

Inference. Thinking about cues is the process of inferencing. Inferences are subjective, personal meanings assigned to a situation, usually to a group of cues. This means that the original input, in this case the patient data, has been screened and processed by the nurse. In this way the data is subject to modification by the experience, the knowledge, the language available to describe the inference, and the value system of the individual making the inference.[40]

Returning to Mr. Jones and his low-salt diet, suppose that the nurse infers from his lack of eye contact that he has not been following his diet. If his blood pressure is also up, then this inference would have some support. The inference, however, has not been validated with the patient. It might be that Mr. Jones has been following the prescribed low-salt diet, and his lack of eye contact is because he is frightened about being admitted to the hospital.

Errors in diagnostic reasoning can occur if inferences about cues are not carefully checked and validated with the patient and with other data. In the case of Mr. Jones, if the nurse's inference is that he is not following his diet, then the subsequent treatment decision might be to review principles of nutrition, including avoidance of high-sodium foods and the use of alternative seasonings. This would be well and good but would not do a thing for his anxiety related to hospitalization.

Diagnostic errors can result if the interpretation of the data is faulty. Another diagnostic error is overgeneralization from one observation of patient behavior. For example, one episode of anxiety about undergoing a procedure does not mean that the patient has Ineffective Coping. Attributing the same inference to every patient with the same symptom is another way of overgeneralizing.

Once a cue has been noticed, the next decision is to evaluate the cue and derive some meaning from it, an inference. Cues are evaluated by comparing them with expected values such as normal values, population norms, research, the patient's baseline, or past clinical experiences.[41] Cues may also be evaluated and validated by discussion with the patient (You look upset, Mr. Jones), looking for other supporting cues (poor eye contact when asked about low-salt diet, blood pressure is up), or consulting with colleagues (I wonder if Mr. Jones' lack of eye contact when we were talking about his low-salt diet means he has not been following it. What do you think?).

Cues may be relevant or irrelevant. The relevance of the cue depends upon the purpose of collecting the information. This is another decision that must be made in thinking about patient data. Attention to irrelevant cues can overload short-term memory, making decisions about patient data much more difficult. The advantage to focusing on relevant data is that less time and energy are required in the assessment process.[42]

Certain cues may be highly significant in certain situations, and the situation may determine what data are relevant to collect. The context in which cues are seen tends to influence whether they are noticed and how they are labeled. In many cases the meaning of the cue is context-dependent, in that the cue assumes significance only in light of the patient's past history and current situation.[43]

Consider the following example. Mrs. Smith is admitted to the obstetrical unit after vaginal delivery of her third child, a healthy eight-pound boy. On the day after delivery she is independent in her self-care activities, walking in the halls comfortably, and has assumed care of her new son. The nursing staff agrees that Mrs. Smith is doing well and will be able to go home in the morning.

On the medical unit is Mrs. Williams, who was admitted with a medical diagnosis of unstable angina. The evening shift nurse has twice caught Mrs. Williams walking to the bathroom, even though she was instructed to use the bedside commode. Furthermore, Mrs. Williams took a shower. In report, Mrs. Williams is described as willful and non-compliant. While both of these patients are independent in their self-care activities, the meaning of these behaviors within the context of the clinical situation is very different.

In the above example the cue was independent self-care behaviors. For Mrs. Smith, the post partum patient, the inference or meaning of this cue is that she is doing well and is ready for discharge. This cue results in a different inferential conclusion for Mrs. Williams whose independent activity, viewed within the context of her unstable angina and specific instructions not to walk to the bathroom, is interpreted as willful, non-compliant behavior.

If the nurse confuses the cue, independent behavior, with the inference, willfulness and non-compliance, there is the distinct possibility that diagnostic and treatment decisions will be inaccurate. When cues and inferences are not clearly distinguished, decisions are made based on the subjective, personal meanings assigned to the cue rather than on patient data. Carnevali suggests that "The difficulty arises when the nurse's judgment *about* the situation is used as if it *were* the actual situation."[44] If Mrs. Williams is treated as if she is indeed willful and non-compliant without validating her perceptions of her behavior, then the nurse will have confused inference and the cues on which that inference was based. This could result in a frustrated patient and nurse if the treatment does not alter the behavior.

Only if cues are noticed, attended to, and interpreted with appropriate inferential conclusions can accurate nursing diagnoses be determined. These decisions require assessment skills, clinical knowledge and experience, and a degree of curiosity. The next step is to examine the cues and inferences for clusters or patterns.

Cue Clustering and Pattern Recognition. Many times a nurse may believe that a diagnostic decision was based on a single cue. Often, this is a highly significant cue such as pain, a change in vital signs, or a behavior like crying. It is very likely that this diagnostic decision is reached in response to a cluster or pattern of cues, although this pattern is not consciously known by the nurse.

The coalescing of cues into clusters or patterns is a phenomenon that is known to occur, but it is not well understood. In short-term memory, cues cluster according to previously encountered patterns or learned diagnostic syndromes.[45] This putting together of information obtained from assessment is a critical activity in the diagnostic process, and it probably occurs as soon as information is perceived and inference or meaning is determined. In fact the inference of meaning of the cue may very well determine how that cue should be grouped with other data. This information clustering is a continuous activity throughout diagnostic decision making.[46] Pattern recognition is a perceptual ability to recognize relationships without prespecifying the components of the situation. Like cue recognition, pattern recognition is context-dependent.[47]

As an example of cue clustering and pattern recognition, consider a 23-year-old male patient who is admitted from the emergency room with a spinal cord injury from a motor vehicle accident. He is alert, looking about with a worried expression, and asking questions. Gardener-Wells tongs have been placed to reduce the subluxation of the fifth and sixth cervical vertebrea. No spontaneous motor function is present, other than facial movement, shoulder shrugging, and diaphragm function. His vital signs are within normal limits, and arterial blood gas sampling in the emergency room was also normal.

While admitting this patient to the neuro unit, the nurse learns that the patient is a two pack-a-day cigarette smoker. This piece of data about the patient immediately triggers a diagnostic decision: this patient will have Ineffective Airway Clearance related to respiratory muscle weakness! The smoking history acted as a high-significance cue to alert the nurse to the pattern of cues that indicate potential respiratory problems for this patient. (See Table 4–3.) In reporting on this patient to the next shift of nurses, the patient is described: "He's a smoker and a quad—look out for trouble."

What happened here? The nurse reacted to a pattern of cues within the context of the situation, but what really got attention was the smoking history. That was the high-significance cue that focused attention on this patient's respiratory status. The experienced nurse does not consider all observations of the patient equally pertinent, and certain perceptions leap out as the most important within the context of the situation. This sense of salience helps the nurse to make skilled complex observations based on a particular patient's condi-

TABLE 4–3. CUES AND INFERENCES

Cues	Inferences
Alert, looking around, asking questions	Anxious, shaken up after being in a car wreck
Spinal cord injury, paralysis, Gardner Well tongs	At risk for immobility complications
Diaphragm function but paralyzed intercostal muscles	Spontaneous respirations but inability to cough effectively or to deep breathe
Two pack-a-day smoker	Increased pulmonary secretions and ciliary paralysis
Cue Cluster/Pattern *(including inferences)*	**Nursing Diagnosis**
Immobility Inability to effectively clear airway by coughing or deep breathing smoker	Ineffective Airway Clearance related to respiratory muscle weakness

tion.[48] No single cue or piece of data, however, can be considered in isolation. A great deal of clinical knowledge and past experience with quadriplegic patients was used to recognize the risks of this clinical situation.

The recognition of pertinent cue clusters or patterns can be triggered by three situations. The first of these is a change in the patient's usual pattern that cannot be explained by expected norms for growth and development. A second situation that should receive attention is deviation from an appropriate population norm. When a cue cluster indicates behavior that is nonproductive within the context of the whole person, this is a third area for diagnostic decision making.

Errors in data clustering and pattern recognition tend to occur in three categories. There is premature closure when the nurse identifies the cluster or pattern before all the critical information has been considered. Incorrect clustering of data and the failure to cluster appropriate data so that the pattern can be determined are also ways that can result in diagnostic error.[49]

Decisions About the Nursing Diagnosis

Cue identification, inferencing, cue clustering, and pattern recognition are decisions that must be made about patient data and clinical information. The next series of decisions involves naming the cluster or pattern, testing this label as a diagnostic hypothesis, and assigning a nursing diagnosis which can be used to guide treatment decisions.

Naming. The first step in this series is to name the cluster or pattern. Nurses have traditionally used a variety of names for the situations that require nursing treatment. These have included medical diagnoses, nursing problems, symptoms, clinical judgments, and labels from other disciplines such as psychology or social work. With the advent of nursing diagnosis, names for the patient problems that nurses treat have become available. While it is recognized that this framework is not as yet complete, the nursing diagnoses that have been approved by the North American Nursing Diagnosis Association (NANDA) are a place to begin.

One of the first decisions about naming a cluster or pattern is deciding whether this situation falls within the domain of nursing. If the cluster or pattern falls within the domain of another health care profession, the choice of a name should reflect this. Nurses are often required to identify and name conditions outside the domain of nursing practice.

As the health care provider with the patient 24 hours a day, nurses are often the first to notice changes in the patient's condition. Nurses are consistently called upon to recognize medical problems that must be referred to the physician for definitive treatment. These judgments are an important part of nursing practice, but they are not nursing diagnoses and should not be named in nursing diagnosis language.

If the cluster or pattern seen in the patient information is consistent with a pulmonary embolus, that is what it should be called. Naming it as such clearly indicates the seriousness of the problem and that it should be referred to a physician. If this situation were named with a nursing diagnosis such as Decreased Cardiac Output, the impression is given that nursing treatment is adequate for the problem and the referral to the physician is just one part of the required treatment.

This decision to name the cluster or pattern with a nursing diagnosis instead of medical terminology can be very tricky. Part of the difficulty rests in the debate about physiologic nursing diagnoses (see Chapter 2) and in the developing state of the nursing diagnosis framework. A few suggestions are offered in Figure 4–1 to help with this decision.

Once the decision to name the problem with a nursing diagnosis has been made, several other questions arise. These include stating the nursing diagnosis in a concise and appropriate format, identifyinig the etiology of the problem, and determining the status of the patient's condition. (For a complete discussion of nursing diagnosis formats, see Chapter 2.)

Naming the State of the Patient. In developing a nursing diagnosis the focus should be on describing the patient's response. The tendency to use nursing problems as diagnostic labels may have become ingrained into nursing thinking processes. Certain questions can help shift thinking patterns from the problems about providing nursing care to the patient's responses that require nursing treatment. The first question is:

What is the patient's response to _____ ?

Answering this question focuses attention on the state of the patient and away from a particular symptom, medical diagnosis, or other situation. It will give some direction toward identifying and naming those human responses that nurses diagnose and treat.

A second question to help focus on the patient's response is to ask:

If this problem is treated, who will get better?

This question helps to sort out who has the problem. Consider the nurse who says, "This bladder irrigation is a real problem. I don't think it's working properly." In this situation Mr. Jones certainly needs for the bladder irrigation procedure to be effective; however, it may be the nurses' anxiety about the proper performance of the procedure is the issue here.

A similar example of this type of thinking is seen with statements such as "We need to encourage good nutrition," or "He really needs emotional support." These statements are indicative of therapeutic needs that nursing care should provide for the patient. They do not describe patient responses. It is the nurse's responsibility to provide the good nutrition or the emotional support. Therapeutic needs focus on what the nurse should do; rather, it is the patient's response that should provide the foundation for determining nursing care needs.

Maintaining the patient's response, or the state of the patient, as the focus of the nursing diagnosis will help to avoid some of these pitfalls. After this response has been identified, the next step is to determine the etiology. This second part of the diagnostic statement can be a cause of the problem, a contributing factor, or a more specific aspect of the response. (See Chapter 3 for a complete discussion of etiology.)

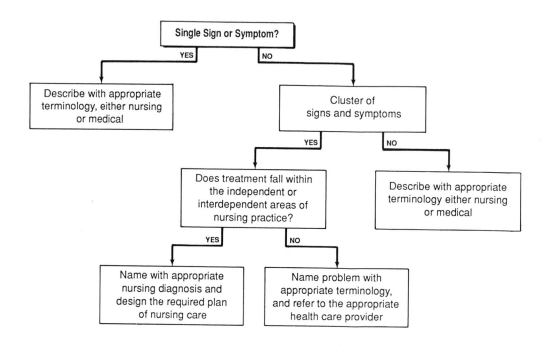

Figure 4–1. Decision Process for Nursing vs. Medical Diagnosis

Naming the Etiology. The distinction between the state of the patient and the etiology can be one of the most perplexing problems in using nursing diagnosis. A chicken-and-egg decision process can sometimes result. Consider the patient who had his gall bladder removed two days ago. He is experiencing post-operative pain, fear that if he coughs his incision will split open, hesitation to ambulate because of his fear about the incision, and pulmonary congestion. The nursing diagnostic possibilities include:

Should all four of these nursing diagnoses be made? Can a response, such as pain or fear, be used as both the state of the patient and the etiology? Which of these nursing diagnoses gives the best "sense of the patient?"

Alteration in Comfort: Acute, related to surgical incision
Ineffective Airway Clearance related to fear about surgical incision
Impaired Physical Mobility related to fear about surgical incision
Fear related to surgical incision opening during coughing, deep breathing, and ambulation

One way out of this dilemma is to ask: What really needs treatment here? In this case it is the patient's fear. Fear is a very distressing state, and it is having important effects on the patient's pulmonary toilet and mobility. The next question to ask is:

If this problem is treated, what will get better?

In this example if the fear is successfully treated, then the patient will be better able to perform coughing and deep breathing, and his airway clearance will be improved. His mobility status would also be improved if the fear of opening his surgical wound was removed and ambulation became a less frightening activity.

The determination of etiology is important because etiology directs nursing treatment. Nursing interventions are directed toward the etiology in order to solve, improve, or compensate for the state of the patient. Based on the answers to the two questions above, the following nursing diagnoses would be used for this patient.

State of the Patient	Etiology
Ineffective Airway Clearance	Fear about incision
Impaired Physical Mobility	Fear about incision

Fear is designated as the etiology because that is what needs to be treated in order to improve the status of the patient. Using this approach to determine the patient response and the etiology focuses the nursing diagnosis on the realities of the clinical situation and gives very specific direction for making treatment decisions. Nursing treatment for both of these nursing diagnoses would include strategies to reassure the patient and alleviate his fears during pulmonary toilet activities and ambulation.

Would the following nursing diagnosis accomplish the same thing?

Fear related to surgical incision opening during coughing, deep breathing, and ambulation

While this nursing diagnosis does convey essentially the same clinical information, the emphasis here is different. This diagnosis places greater importance on the fear as the state of the patient. The earlier diagnoses are more concerned with the effects of the fear, resulting in ineffective airway clearance and impaired physical mobility.

The decision about which approach to take will be based on contextual considerations. In the example, an important consideration is that the patient is only two days post-op. In that context, airway clearance and mobility are high-priority issues, and the choice of nursing diagnoses would be Ineffective Airway Clearance related to fear of incision opening and Imparied Mobility related to fear of incision opening.

On the other hand, if this patient was further into his convalescence and wound healing was progressing well, the second diagnostic statement might be more accurate. If the patient still expressed fear about the incision with coughing or ambulation two weeks after surgery, the fear related to surgical incision opening during coughing or ambulation would better describe the state of this patient.

A question arises when the etiology is unknown. Should a nursing diagnosis be made without an etiology statement or with the statement "etiology unknown?" In the example in the preceding paragraph, the actual cause of the patient's fears about his incision is not indicated. In the diagnostic statement, Fear related to surgical incision opening with coughing or ambulation, the etiology statement serves as a supporting indicator to describe the event that frightens the patient—the consequence of ambulation and coughing, specifically, the opening of the incision. A diagnostic statement of Fear related to unknown etiology would probably be more technically accurate; however, it would also be much less descriptive of the state of the patient.

Another way to address the issue of the unknown etiology is to ask:

What really needs treatment?

The answer to that question is probably the etiology, and that leaves the identification of the patient response as the next question. As the example of the patient who had gall bladder surgery showed, an important consideration in deciding which response is the problem and which is the etiology is the context in which the responses are occurring. In the event that a patient response seems to require nursing treatment, and there is not enough information to identify an etiology, then the diagnostic decision may have to be deferred until more information is available.

Status of the Nursing Diagnosis. Another decision that must be made in naming a patient situation or condition with a nursing diagnosis is the designation of the status of the problem. The status of the nursing diagnosis indicates a time course or developmental state of the condition. Status has two characteristics: the state of development of the condition and its duration. Six statuses have been identified for nursing diagnostic statements; these are actual, potential, possible, acute, chronic, and intermittent.[50]

The designations, actual, potential, and possible, refer to the developmental state of the condition. Oftentimes, when a nursing diagnosis is made, the word "actual" is not included; the actual existence of the problem is implicit in the label itself. Nursing diagnoses such as Anxiety, Constipation, Activity Intolerance, and Sleep Pattern Disturbance describe currently existing situations. Actual nursing diagnoses are based on the presence of a cluster or pattern of cues that indicate that the condition is present at this point in time. The existence of the nursing diagnosis can be validated by identifiable defining characteristics.[51]

A nursing diagnosis is designated as a potential state when there are risk factors for the condition, but the condition itself has not yet developed. An unconscious, undernourished patient would be at risk for skin breakdown, and a nursing diagnosis of Potential for Impaired Skin Integrity related to immobility and malnutrition would be appropriate for this patient. In this situation the etiology statement identifies the risk factors of the potential problem.

Potential nursing diagnoses direct nursing treatment toward preventive interventions and health promotion activities.[52] For the patient described in the preceding paragraph, this nursing diagnosis would direct the nurse toward nursing interventions to compensate for the immobility and to provide adequate nutrition in order to prevent skin breakdown. In the event that these interventions were unsuccessful, the problem could progress to an actual status.

Three accepted nursing diagnoses are described as potential problems: Potential for Injury, Potential for Infection, and Potential Alteration of Body Temperature.[53] These diagnoses identify the presence of high-risk states rather than actual conditions. Many other nursing diagnoses that describe actual conditions are associated with risk factors that would make their diagnosis as potential problems a useful strategy to guide diagnostic and treatment decisions in certain situations.

The possible status indicates that a condition or problem may be present, but more data is required to confirm or rule out the diagnosis.[54] The identification of possible diagnoses has been recommended as a way to preserve initial impressions and to serve diagnostic hypotheses to be investigated further.[55] It is essential that possible diagnoses that have not been validated or supported with adequate patient data be used in this fashion. Otherwise, these possible diagnoses may act as misleading labels and treatment decisions may be misdirected.

The acute, chronic, and intermittent status designations are familiar terms, and they indicate the duration of the condition or problem. An acute condition generally has a sudden onset and a short course. An acute condition may develop into a chronic or intermittent condition if the treatment is only partially successful or if the patient fails to follow the treatment recommendations.

A chronic condition is diagnosed on the basis of both the existence of defining characteristics to validate the nursing diagnosis and on the presence of risk factors that indicate that the condition will not resolve within a set timeframe. This differs from the potential problem where risk factors are present, but the defining characteristics of the diagnosis are not.[56]

When the course of the condition is one of periodic remission and recurrence, then a status designation of intermittent is indicated. In an intermittent condition, the defining characteristics will be present during the recurrences and absent during the remissions. An example of this type of nursing diagnosis would be Potential for Injury related to confusion at night, made for the elderly patient who becomes confused and disoriented only at night and is at risk to fall because of this. The intermittent designation is identified by specifying that the problem is present only at night.

Testing the Diagnostic Hypothesis.   After the cluster or pattern is named with an appropriate diagnostic label and etiology statement and the status of the condition is indicated, the next step is to test the name as a diagnostic hypothesis. This stage is concerned with refining the diagnostic possibilities. Other terms that describe this stage of diagnostic decision making are "working diagnosis" or "differential diagnosis." All three indicate that the diagnosis must be confirmed, and that this must occur through the consideration of alternative diagnoses and further evaluation of patient data.

Consider the spinal cord injury patient discussed earlier. The cluster of data about his respiratory status leads the nurse to a diagnostic hypothesis of Ineffective Airway Clearance related to respiratory muscle weakness. To confirm this nursing diagnosis, however, alternative diagnoses should be excluded and patient data that specifically supports this diagnostic label should be identified.

The alternative nursing diagnoses that should be examined for this patient are Impaired Gas Exchange and Ineffective Breathing Pattern. Along with Ineffective Airway Clearance, these three labels are the repertoire of respiratory nursing diagnoses. The defining characteristics of each can be compared with patient data in order to determine which has the best diagnostic fit.

This process of searching for confirming data for a particular diagnosis is called directed search because the assessment process at this point is directed by the diagnostic hypothesis.[59] Now the nurse is looking for patient data to support the diagnosis of Ineffective Airway Clearance. The presence of a weak cough, low inspiratory and expiratory pressures, and bilateral rhonchi would be findings that are consistent with difficulty clearing the airway.

The nursing diagnosis of Impaired Gas Exchange can be excluded based on the normal arterial blood gas results that were obtained in the emergency room. Furthermore, the patient's color is good, mucous membranes are pink, and nailbed capillary refill is brisk. This nursing diagnosis, however, should be kept in mind in the event that the patient's condition worsens. If measures to assist the patient with airway clearance are not effective, then oxygenation might be affected and this nursing diagnosis would be a more accurate description of the patient.

Ineffective Breathing Pattern should be seriously considered for this patient. After cervical spinal cord injury, paralysis of the intercostal muscles makes the patient dependent on the diaphragm for respiratory movement. Evaluation of this patient's breathing pattern shows a respiratory rate of 18 breaths per minute, which are quiet and unlabored. Accessory muscles are not in use. At this point there is no abnormality of the breathing pattern itself, although the mechanics of respiration have been changed. Therefore this nursing diagnosis is not supported.

In this example the original diagnostic hypothesis was confirmed. The nurse can make the nursing diagnosis of Ineffective Airway Clearance related to respiratory muscle weakness with a fair degree of confidence. Alternative diagnoses have been considered and excluded, and there is additional data to support the diagnosis of Ineffective Airway Clearance.

Decisions About Treatment

Once the nursing diagnosis has been decided upon, the focus of clinical thinking moves from diagnostic decisions to treatment decisions. This portion of clinical thinking is concerned with decisions about what is to be accomplished through nursing treatment, what treatments should be used, and evaluating how effective the treatment was in achieving the desired outcomes. These decisions are all based on the nursing diagnosis; goals cannot be formulated and nursing interventions cannot be derived without the nursing diagnosis.[58]

Decisions About Patient Outcomes. The first decision that must be made is to determine what is to be accomplished by treating the nursing diagnosis. Outcomes of care are projected as a means of predicting what should result from treatment of the diagnosis and of measuring the effectiveness of treatment.[59] They are similar to behavioral objectives and goals. Outcomes and behavioral objectives are synonymous in that both specify observable patient behaviors or measurable clinical data. Goals are usually broader statements. In order to achieve the goal of adequate oxygenation, the expected outcome of clear breath sounds bilaterally must be accomplished.

The determination of expected outcomes must be done before nursing care is planned or implemented. There are two reasons for this. The first is that the nursing diagnosis describes the patient's present health state. The expected outcomes describe the desired health state. The expected outcomes describe the desired health state. The difference between the two provides direction and focus for nursing treatment. Clarity of both the diagnostic statement and the expected outcomes is essential if this guidance for nursing intervention is to be realized. A second reason for projecting outcomes of patient behavior at this point is so that these outcomes can be used during the delivery of nursing care to evaluate daily progress toward their achievement.[60]

Expected outcomes describe the change that is anticipated in the state of the patient if nursing treatment is effective. They relate to the first portion of the diagnostic label. In the example of the spinal cord injury patient with Ineffective Airway Clearance related to respiratory muscle weakness, the expected outcomes would be:

Breath sounds will be clear bilaterally
Breath sounds will improve after assisted coughing

These expected outcomes identify the desired state of the patient, a clear airway. They are measurable, observable indicators about the condition of concern. Notice also that, in this example, the expected outcomes are the opposite of the nursing diagnosis. The nursing diagnosis is Ineffective Airway Clearance; the expected outcome is the reverse of that—a clear airway.

Expected outcomes should be written as specific, measurable, and observable behaviors or clinical findings. If "improved respiratory status," "optimal ventilation," or even "good breath sounds" had been listed as expected outcomes, these could not be measured to determine if nursing treatment had been effective. Vague statements or abstract concepts such as these are not helpful in evaluating nursing care, although many nurses have learned to speak this type of jargon fluently.

It is important that expected outcomes be realistic as well as specific. Expected outcomes should also be consistent with the health goals of the patient. Consider the nursing diagnosis of Anticipatory Grieving related to impending death, made for the patient with cancer and his wife. To identify expected outcomes that are simply the opposite of the nursing diagnosis, as in the last example, would be inappropriate. In this situation, establishing with the patient and his wife expected outcomes that are meaningful and realistic would be critical for the success of nursing intervention in this situation.

Expected outcomes should be evaluated within specified time frames and assigned evaluation dates when they are developed.[61] These evaluation dates must reflect the realities of the clinical situation. Professional judgment and discretion will be an important factor for determining this.

Decisions About Nursing Interventions. Decisions about nursing interventions can be divided into three categories: identifying treatment options, determining the priority of treatment, and evaluating the effectiveness of treatment. These decisions are directly linked with the nursing diagnosis and the outcomes that can reasonably be expected with treatment.

Determining Treatment Options. The first group of decisions about nursing interventions has to do with the identification of treatment options. These options include:

- assisting the patient to continue with self-care activities, including providing information, recommendations, and support;
- offering specific independent or interdependent nursing interventions for a particular nursing diagnosis; and
- referring the patient to another health care provider, usually the physician, for treatment, and assisting with the implementation of that care plan.[62]

The first two options are nursing diagnosis-based treatment options, and the third option may include patient conditions that can be effectively treated with interdependent nursing interventions.

Consider the patient with diabetes who has been managing well at home. She follows an appropriate diabetic diet without difficulty, performs home blood glucose monitoring and insulin injection accurately, and appears to be doing well with her health maintenence. In the clinic, the nurse may review the patient's regime with her and decide on the first treatment option listed above: that the patient continue with self-care.

In the course of the discussion between the clinic nurse and this patient, it emerges that the patient has been having some incontinence. The episodes occur when the patient has waited long periods between emptying her bladder, and a small amount of urine is expelled at these times. Immediately after these episodes, the patient has gone to the bathroom and voided large volumes of urine. She denies feeling an urge to empty her bladder, and the incontinence is the first indication to her that her bladder is full.

Based on this cluster of data, the nurse diagnoses Functional Incontinence related to decreased sensation. This is consistent with the definition of functional incontinence as the involuntary, unpredictable passage of urine,[63] and it is consistent with neuropathy that can occur with diabetes. The nurse treats this problem by developing a fluid intake regimen and toileting schedule with the patient that will prevent rapid overfilling of her bladder, with subsequent episodes of incontinence. Suggestions for preventing skin irritation are also included as a part of the care plan for the nursing diagnosis Potential for Impaired Skin Integrity related to incontinence. These diagnosis-based treatments fall within the second category of treatment options.

The nurse would also utilize the third treatment option for this patient: a referral to the physician to evaluate the incontinence. Urodynamic testing and treatment with medications are treatment options that must come from the physician, and this is an important component of the patient's management.

An important aspect of identifying treatment options is the ability to generate alternative interventions. One suggestion is to keep the problem in mind, but focus on the etiology.[64] In the example of the diabetic patient above, the problem was incontinence, but the interventions focused on the etiology, decreased sensation, and offered strategies to compensate for this. The nurse was generating other possible treatment options through the referral to the physician, as a way to obtain treatment options outside the scope of nursing practice.

During this process of generating alternative interventions, the care plan can be made specific for the needs of that particular patient. Factors that influence the decision of which nursing interventions would be most effective include characteristics of the patient, the patient's perception of the problem and treatment options, the degree to which the patient has already begun to compensate for the condition, the magnitude and urgency of the situation, and the cost-benefit considerations.[65]

The predicted effectiveness of the nursing care should also influence the choice of treatment options. The predicted effectiveness of an intervention is the probability that it will lead to the expected outcome, and this decision must take all of the factors listed above into account, as well as the clinical effectiveness of the intervention. The final decision about nursing interventions should reflect clinical necessity, the needs of the particular patient, and the effectiveness of the interventions.

Determining the Priority of Nursing Treatment. Making decisions about nursing interventions from a single nursing diagnosis can be challenging; when there are multiple diagnoses, the decision must also be made as to the priority of treatment. The priority decisions are guided by the urgency of the problem, the nature of the treatment required, and the interaction among diagnoses.[66]

Immediate life-threatening situations and conditions that could result in harm to the patient if left untreated, must have the first priority in determining nursing interventions and require immediate nursing action. When the nurse makes a diagnostic hypothesis about the medical condition of the patient, this judgment is made for the purposes of referral, and this type of judgment is made continuously in nursing, especially in critical and acute care settings.

Nursing intervention based on medical judgments falls into one of the following categories: to notify the physician, to record the information in the patient's record, to carry out or withold treatments designated by existing physician's orders, to carry out palliative treatments based on nursing judgment, or a combination of these.[67] This type of nursing intervention is based on the medical condition of the patient, and problems identified within this domain should be named with appropriate medical terminology.

There are also conditions that can result in harm to the patient if left untreated that can be identified with a nursing diagnosis. Potential for Violence, Potential for Injury, Impaired Gas Exchange, or panic-level Anxiety are a few examples of these conditions. After life-threatening situations, these would be next in priority for determining nursing intervention.

The nature of the treatment will also direct the decision for prioritizing nursing interventions. Those nursing interventions that require a certain amount of physical or intellectual participation might not be a high priority for very ill, weak, or debilitated patients. It would be inappropriate to focus on nursing interventions that required these patients to participate beyond their strength or endurance. On the other hand, patients with nursing diagnoses such as Self Care Deficit or Powerlessness should participate in both the selection and execution of nursing interventions for their conditions.

The interaction between diagnoses also influences the decision about priority of nursing treatment. Consider the patient who is sitting straight up in bed, holding her chest. Her respiratory rate is 38 breaths per minute and her respirations are audible at a distance. The admitting medical diagnosis is asthma, and the nursing diagnoses are Anxiety related to dyspnea, Ineffective Breathing Pattern related to anxiety, and Activity Intolerance related to imbalance between oxygen supply and demand. What are the treatment priorities here?

The medical priorities would address ordering the appropriate medications for this patient, and a nursing priority would be to ensure that they were administered properly and promptly. The nursing priorities would be:

1. Exclude the existence of a life-threatening situation
2. Offer immediate, short-term nursing treatment for the Anxiety as this is a problem in itself and is a contributing factor for another problem
3. Defer nursing treatment of Activity Intolerance.

This treatment scenario follows the guidelines of addressing life-threatening situations first, dealing with conditions that could cause harm to the patient next, and those interventions that require patient participation after the first two situations have been resolved. For this patient there was not a life-threatening crisis; however, the anxiety and increased respiratory rate might progress to one if not treated. Deferment of treatment for Activity Intolerance is appropriate at this point because successful treatment requires patient participation.

Decisions about which nursing interventions should be used must be guided by the expected outcomes of treatment, the clinical context of the situation, the characteristics of the patient, the available treatment options, and the treatment priorities. The next step is to carry out the indicated treatment options and to evaluate their effectiveness.

Determining the Effectiveness of Nursing Treatment. Evaluation is the fifth step in the nursing process of assessment, diagnosis, planning, implementation of the plan, and evaluation. It is concurrent and recurrent, as are the other steps.[68] This set of activities is always in mind and decisions made at any point can influence other decisions.[69]

While there is an evaluative component to decision making at each step in the nursing process, the formal step of evaluation after nursing treatment is an important one. It indicates the degree to which the nursing diagnosis and interventions have been correct and demonstrates the nurse's acceptance of responsibility for this.[70] The evaluation process also returns our thinking to the start of the nursing process. As data is collected for evaluation, the diagnostic and treatment decisions begin again.

According to Carnevali the evaluation process consists of three sequential steps:

1. Review of the nursing diagnosis and expected outcomes
2. Collection of data as indicated by the projected outcomes in a way that permits qualitative and quantitative measurement with some degree of reliability
3. Judgment of the progress of the patient in moving from the existing condition, the nursing diagnosis, to the desired health state, the expected outcomes[71]

Although this process is similar to the assessment and diagnosis steps of the nursing process, there are fundamental differences in the sequence and intent of the decision making.

For purposes of evaluation, the decisions about which data to collect are specified by the expected outcomes. This direction is decidedly different than data collection during the diagnostic phase of the nursing process; there data collection is influenced by a number of clinical, informational, and situational factors.

At its simplest level, the process of evaluation is one where the present state of the patient, the nursing diagnosis, is compared with the desired state of the patient, the expected outcomes.[72] The ability to do this is dependent on the clarity and precision with which the nursing diagnosis and expected outcomes are presented. Consider the patient with a nursing diagnosis of Ineffective Airway Clearance related to respiratory muscle weakness. The expected outcomes are that the breath sounds will be clear bilaterally and that breath sounds will improve after assisted coughing. The comparison of the patient's actual breath sounds and the expected outcomes can be made easily.

If the statement of the patient's condition was compromised respiratory status, rather than Ineffective Airway Clearance, making a comparison between the state of the patient and the desired outcomes would be much more difficult. The term "compromised respiratory status" lacks clarity and precision. *How* is respiratory status compromised? *What* effects does this compromise have on the patient? *What* component of respiration is involved: ventilation, perfusion, or gas exchange? When the patient's condition is described in general or vague terms, the identification of expected outcomes and the comparison of patient data with these is impossible.

Once the nursing diagnosis and expected outcomes are clearly described, and the necessary data for comparison has been collected and compared, the next decision is whether the patient is moving from the state identified in the nursing diagnosis to the desired state specified in the expected outcomes. This decision may take four different forms. These are (1) problem resolution, (2) resolution of the problem in the short term but remaining issues for intermediate or long-term consideration, (3) no resolution of the problem, and (4) the emergence of new or different problems that must be incorporated into the care plan.[73]

TABLE 4–4. TIPS FOR COLLECTING AND ANALYZING DATA

Remember that cues are indicators, not the diagnosis
Separate fact from inference: do not jump to conclusions!
Never settle for the first explanation: always consider alternative diagnoses
Validate both cues and inferences with the patient
Avoid premature closure: wonder what you might have forgotten to examine, ask about, or consider
Keep an open mind; be tentative in the diagnosis and make changes in the diagnosis when the patient's condition or the available data changes
Have confidence in your observational and clinical skills

IMPROVING DIAGNOSTIC AND TREATMENT DECISION MAKING

Making diagnostic and treatment decisions is not new to nursing; using nursing diagnosis as a focus for these decisions is. While the intuitive influences in these decisions is important, using models and flow diagrams to analyze these decision-making activities can be useful in examining our thinking processes and learning more effective ways to approach these decisions.

One of the best predictors of diagnostic accuracy is the thoroughness of data collection.[74] This is true for any diagnostician. One of the questions for nurse diagnosticians is what constitutes thorough data collection, and what framework can be used to assist in collecting that information. If data collection is done with a medical model, then diagnostic decisions will most likely be medical rather than nursing; therefore, a critical aid for making nursing diagnoses is to work from a nursing focus for data collection.

There are a number of frameworks that have been proposed for use by nurses. Some of these are not nursing frameworks per se, such as Maslow's hierarchy of needs, but have been found to be useful in nursing practice. Other frameworks such as Gordon's Functional Health Patterns[75] have been designed specifically to collect data in a manner that assists with identifying nursing diagnoses. A group of speciality assessment tools based on NANDA's Unitary Person Framework have been developed to provide appropriate assessment data for the formulation of nursing diagnoses.[76]

In addition to using a nursing focus for data collection, suggestions are offered in Table 4–4 to assist in collecting and analyzing data in a way that facilitates diagnostic decisions. These suggestions can help in the development of diagnostic thinking skills and also, retrospectively, in the analysis of diagnostic decisions.

Two strategies have been identified for self-monitoring of diagnostic reasoning: concurrent observation as the diagnostic reasoning process is occurring and retrospective analysis.[77] In concurrent observation the diagnostician has two tasks: the diagnostic task and the evaluation of the thinking processes used in that task.

Some questions that can be used for this evaluation process are:

- What influence does my specialty background have on what I *expect* to see in patients?
- What do I notice about patients *first*?
- How do I respond to initial data from the patient?
- What is the focus or pattern of early data collection? Is it medical, nursing, or a combination?
- How many problems do I identify in my first impressions of the patient?
- Is there a hierarchial arrangement to these problems, that is a general problem, then a more specific manifestation of the problem?

- Do I generate competing diagnoses? Do I fall in love with my first diagnostic hypothesis?
- Is further data collection guided by my diagnostic hypotheses?
- How well does the diagnostic hypothesis *fit* the patient's situation? How precise is the diagnostic label that I assign to this?[78]

These questions can help diagnosticians monitor their own thinking. After strengths and competencies are identified, the next step is to discover areas where the diagnostician is less skillful and to focus energy on improving those areas.

While these suggestions focus on diagnostic decisions, similar ones can be identified for treatment decisions. Some of these questions would be:

- How will this treatment option help to accomplish the expected outcomes?
- Do these treatment options consider the unique characteristics of this patient?
- Is this treatment option the most effective one for this nursing diagnosis?
- Is there an interaction between nursing diagnoses and expected outcomes that should influence the choice of treatment options?

Another useful strategy to improve diagnostic and treatment decision-making skills is retrospective analysis. Ask yourself why a diagnosis seemed "right," what data was presented to support inferences or conclusions, and what other possibilities were present in the situation. This retrospective analysis can be done in patient care conferences, instructional programs, or over lunch or breaks with colleagues. It is a highly effective way to fine tune your own clinical thinking skills and to develop insights and ideas from others.

The pairing of clinicians is another useful strategy for skill development in making diagnostic and treatment decisions. In this strategy, clinicians can observe and critique each other's diagnostic and treatment decisions, both concurrently and retrospectively. These pairings may be done formally or informally. Changing the pairs periodically will offer fresh perspectives on clinical thinking. Pairing clinicians across specialty areas, such as a critical care nurse with a surgical unit nurse or a rehabilitation nurse with a psychiatric nurse, would be another way to broaden exposure to clinical thinking strategies.

CONCLUSION

Clinical thinking in nursing practice encompasses both diagnostic and treatment decisions. These decisions are linked through the nursing diagnosis. The nursing diagnosis is the product of the diagnostic thinking process, and it guides the treatment decision-making process. The use of nursing diagnosis gives a focus to this activity that had been missing. Like any new skill, practice is required in these new thinking strategies for successful use of nursing diagnosis. Only when nursing diagnosis is the foundation for diagnostic and treatment decisions can diagnosis-based nursing practice become a reality.

The decision-making requirements of the evaluation component of the nursing process depend upon careful, accurate nursing diagnoses and expected outcomes that are stated with clarity and precision. Decision making at every point of the nursing process should be directed toward the identification of nursing diagnoses that clearly describe the state of the patient. The nursing diagnosis then becomes the foundation of the treatment and evaluation components of the nursing process. This is diagnosis-based nursing practice.

REFERENCES

1. American Nurses' Association. *Nursing: A social policy statement.* Kansas City: American Nurses' Association, 1980
2. Roy, C. A diagnostic classification system for nursing. *Nursing Outlook,* 1975, *23,* 90
3. Mundinger, J. & Jauron, G. Developing a nursing diagnosis. *Nursing Outlook,* 1975, *23,* 94
4. Alfaro, R. *Application of nursing process: A step-by-step guide.* Philadelphia: J. B. Lippincott, 1986
5. Yura, H. & Walsh, M.B., Eds. *The nursing process* (4th ed.). Norwalk, CT: Appleton-Century-Crofts, 1983
6. Yura, H. & Walsh, M.B., Eds. *The nursing process* (1st ed.). Washington, DC: The Catholic University of American Press, 1967
7. Carpenito, L.J. *Nursing diagnosis: Application to clinical practice.* Philadelphia: J.B. Lippincott, 1983
8. Yura & Walsh, (4th ed.)
9. Block, D. Some crucial terms in nursing—What do they really mean? *Nursing Outlook,* 1974, *22,* 689
10. Carnevali, D.L. *Nursing care planning: Diagnosis and management.* Philadelphia: J.B. Lippincott, 1983
11. Kelly, M.A. *Nursing diagnosis source book: Guidelines for clinical application* Norwalk, CT: Appleton-Century-Crofts, 1985
12. Benner, P. *From novice to expert: Excellence and power in clinical nursing practice.* Menlo Park, CA: Addison-Wesley, 1984
13. *The Merriam-Webster dictionary.* New York: Pocket Books, 1974
14. Doona, M.E. The judgment process in nursing. *Image,* 1976, *8,* 27
15. Berne, E. *Intuition and ego states.* San Francisco: Transactional Publications, 1977
16. Benner
17. Benner, P., & Tanner, C. Clinical judgment: How expert nurses use intuition. *American Journal of Nursing,* 1987, *87,* 1, 23
19. Carnevali, D.L., Mitchell, P.H., Woods, N.F., & Tanner, C.A. *Diagnostic reasoning in nursing.* Philadelphia: J.B. Lippincott, 1984
19. Newell, A., & Simon, H. *Human problem solving.* Englewood Cliffs, NJ: Prentice-Hall, 1972
20. Simon, H. Information processing models of cognition. *Annual Review of Psychology,* 1979, 363
21. Elstein, A., & Bordage, G. Psychology of clinical reasoning. In G. Stone, F. Cohen, and N. Adler (Eds.), *Health psychology.* San Francisco: Jossey-Bass, 1979, 333
22. Newell, & Simon
23. Elstein & Bordage
24. Doona
25. Carnevali, et al.
26. Gordon, M. *Nursing diagnosis: Process and application.* New York: McGraw-Hill, 1982
27. Carnevali
28. Carnevali, et al.
29. Kelly
30. Carnevali
31. Yura & Walsh, (4th ed.)
32. Little, D., & Carnevali, D. *Nursing care planning.* Philadelphia: J.B. Lippincott, 1969
33. Carpenito
34. Bloch
35. Gordon
36. *Ibid.*
37. Carnevali
38. *Ibid.*
39. Gordon
40. Carnevali
41. Gordon
42. *Ibid.*
43. Benner
44. Carnevali
45. *Ibid.*
46. Gordon
47. Benner
48. *Ibid.*
49. Gordon
50. Kelly
51. Carpenito
52. *Ibid.*
53. North American Nursing Diagnosis Association. *Nursing Diagnosis Newsletter,* 1986, *12,* 4, 4
54. Carpenito
55. Kelly
56. *Ibid.*
57. Putzier, D. & Padrick, K.P. Nursing diagnosis: A component of nursing process and decision making. *Topics in Clinical Nursing,* 1984, *5,* 4, 21
58. Gordon
59. *Ibid.*
60. Gettrust, K.V., Ryan, S.C., & Engelman, D.S., Eds. *Applied nursing diagnosis: Guidelines for comprehensive care planning.* New York: John Wiley & Sons, 1985
61. *Ibid.*
62. Carnevali et al.
63. North American Nursing Diagnosis Association
64. Gordon
65. *Ibid.*
66. *Ibid.*
67. *Ibid.*
68. Yura & Walsh (4th ed.)
69. Gordon
70. Yura & Walsh (4th ed.)
71. Carnevali
72. *Ibid.*
73. Gordon
74. Tanner, C. Factors influencing the diagnostic process. In D. Carnevali, P. Mitchell, N. Woods, &

C. Tanner *Diagnostic reasoning in nursing.* Philadelphia: J.B. Lippincott, 1984

75. Gordon
76. Guzzetta, C.E., Bunton, S.D., Prinkley, L.A., et

al. *Clinical assessment tools for use with nursing diagnosis.* St. Louis: C.V. Mosby, 1989

77. Tanner
78. Carnevali et al.

Planning and Preparing for the Implementation of Nursing Diagnosis and Diagnosis—based Nursing Practice

CHAPTER 5

Implementation Issues: An Overview

Emmy Miller

"Serious and massive effort is required to make the hospital a place where nurses are willing and able to do what they are prepared and want to do—provide good nursing care."[1]

Changing from a task-based nursing practice to a diagnosis-based nursing practice is a major step toward the goal of making the hospital a place where nurses can use their clinical thinking skills to deliver nursing care and receive the recognition and respect that those skills deserve. The implementation of nursing diagnoses as the focus of nursing practice, within the context of the nursing process, is the first step in establishing diagnosis-based nursing practice.

Implementation is a term familiar to all nurses. It is the fourth step of the nursing process, when the nursing care activities planned for the patient are put into practice. Implementation is the action phase of the nursing process as compared with the other phases that are more cerebral in nature.

Providing the implements or tools for professional nursing practice is another way to describe the implementation of nursing diagnosis. The implements required for diagnosis-based nursing practice are presented in Table 5–1. These implements are a philosophical commitment to professional nursing practice, an ability to use nursing diagnosis within the context of the nursing process, and a clinical nursing practice structure that enables the professional nurse to practice in a diagnosis-based manner.

The implementation of nursing diagnosis involves more than using some new terminology on care-planning forms, and it is more than a trend or a fad. It is the foundation of nursing practice. The decision to implement nursing diagnosis is a commitment by administrative and clinical leaders to the role of the professional nurse. This role must be founded in nursing practice that is diagnosis-based, rather than task-based or one that simply reacts to the situation of the moment. This philosophical commitment must be evident in the job descriptions and evaluation criteria for registered nurses, in the policies and procedures of the organization, and in the administrative practice of nurse managers at all levels.

A genuine commitment is required, and it goes far beyond the concept of administrative support. Adding the current jargon to administrative documents or mentioning nursing pro-

TABLE 5–1.   REQUIREMENTS FOR DIAGNOSIS-BASED NURSING PRACTICE

1. *A philosophical commitment to professional nursing practice*
2. *An ability to use nursing diagnosis within the context of the nursing process*
3. *A clinical practice structure that enables the professional nurse to practice in a diagnosis-based manner*

cess in orientation and never utilizing it does not present an "implement" for nursing diagnosis. A desire to implement nursing diagnosis because it is new, because "everyone is doing it," or because a visit is expected from the Joint Commission on Accreditation of Health Care Organizations (JCAHO) does not constitute a philosophical commitment. There must be a firm belief that nursing practice is based in careful patient assessment, accurate identification of nursing diagnoses, realistic planning, consistent implementation, and deliberative evaluation. Only if this belief is used as a basis for decision making will the implementation of nursing diagnosis be successful and lead to a diagnosis-based nursing practice.

The next implement or tool that is needed is the ability to use nursing diagnosis in clinical nursing practice. Nurses must have both the ability and the time to make nursing diagnoses. Determining nursing diagnoses from patient data, identifying and carrying out appropriate nursing treatment based on these, and evaluating the success of this treatment *is* nursing practice in diagnosis-based nursing practice; however, the present reality of the clinical practice environment shows a different picture. Despite the use of nursing process as the primary teaching methodology in nursing education and its place in regulatory evaluations of nursing practice, nursing process is rarely a driving force in clinical nursing practice.

Consider the busy day of the staff nurse. The focus of activity often is on tasks and chores rather than on patients and their problems. There are baths to be given, medications to be administered, and IVs to be started. In addition are the many phone calls to be answered and dealt with, the traffic of patients traveling to and from the operating room or diagnostic testing, charts to review, medical orders to process, and other personnel to assist and supervise. Furthermore, the rewards and sanctions of this culture are based on getting these tasks and chores done rather than on activities directed by the nursing process.

In this fast-paced environment, nursing process may be perceived as something "extra," unrelated to providing nursing care. Many nurses confuse nursing process with paperwork because it is only in the written format that the nurse is called upon to use nursing process; taking care of patients can be done without it. In fact, written care plans are viewed by many practicing nurses as impractical to use and difficult to write and maintain.[2]

In task-based nursing practice, nurses might or might not possess the skill and knowledge necessary to provide nursing care based on nursing diagnosis and nursing process; moreover, there is little call for those abilities. Nurses have developed a number of skills unrelated to the nursing process to cope effectively with the demands of the clinical practice environment. Some of these competencies have been identified by Benner[3] and include setting priorities, team building, contingency planning, anticipating periods of extreme workload, maintaining a caring attitude toward patients even in the absence of close and frequent contact, and maintaining flexibility in dealing with patients, technology, and bureaucracy.[4]

The implementation of nursing diagnosis must occur within the context of the clinical practice environment; it cannot occur in isolation. The necessity to incorporate nursing diagnostic and treatment activity into the existing clinical practice situation is both challenging and overwhelming. Yet, unless nursing diagnosis and nursing process are woven into the fabric of clinical activity in the health care organization, the benefits of diagnosis-based nursing practice will not be realized. Instead, nursing diagnosis will be just another task added into the busy day of the staff nurse, and it will probably be last on the list in importance.

The third requirement or implement for diagnosis-based nursing practice is a clinical nursing practice environment that supports this type of practice. A structure such as this includes the model of nursing practice, the documentation and information systems, the job descriptions and evaluation criteria, the physical structure and materials resources, the orientation and educational programs, and the norms and values of the culture, both stated and unstated. An examination of the clinical nursing practice structure must consider each of these factors, with attention to its relationship to and impact upon professional nursing practice.

For diagnosis-based nursing practice, there must be mechanisms for dealing with both the pragmatic realities of getting the tasks and chores done and the professional responsibility of nurses to diagnose and treat those human responses that are nursing diagnoses. The structure of the clinical practice environment must address both of these aspects. This chapter will present the foundations for this type of clinical practice environment. Examination of the existing nursing practice environment and ways of moving toward diagnosis-based practice will be discussed within the context of planned change theory. More detailed discussions of models of nursing practice, nursing documentation, information systems, quality assurance, legal concerns, and educational issues will be presented in their respective chapters in Part II.

THE CHANGE PROCESS AND THE IMPLEMENTATION OF NURSING DIAGNOSIS

The implementation of nursing diagnosis means more than using new categories for documentation, just as primary nursing is more than a different method of assignment. The implementation of nursing diagnosis demands careful examination and analysis of the existing clinical nursing practice structure. In some cases, significant changes will be required in order to implement nursing diagnosis within the context of nursing process. These changes can be exciting, stimulating, and challenging; however, they also can be fraught with frustration and anxiety.

Change invariably evokes strong feelings in individuals. The strength and effects of these feelings often cannot be predicted, and this adds an unknown factor to the change process. The concept of deliberative, planned change has been suggested as a way to approach change in a thoughtful, purposeful, and analytical manner so that these unpredictable responses and results can be minimized. The foundation of deliberate, planned change is a careful and realistic appraisal of the entity or system to be changed.

Change is an important and ever-present part of organizational life. It may be defined as:

> to alter by substituting something else for, or by giving up for something else; to put or take another or others in place of; to make different or convert; to exchange, alter, vary, or modify.[5]

The implementation of nursing diagnosis involves making clinical nursing practice different by altering certain behaviors, systems, and structures so that nursing practice becomes diagnosis-based, instead of task-based.

For the implementation of nursing diagnosis, it is helpful to take an eclectic approach to change that can provide the necessary flexibility for making a number of critical decisions about the specific strategies to be used in the change process. These decisions must be based upon the unique characteristics of the organization, the availability of resources, and the goals for the implementation project. In order to begin making decisions and analyzing requirements of a change project of this magnitude, it is helpful to identify the level of change that must occur.

Levels of Change

The approach to the implementation of nursing diagnosis recommended here means that it will affect attitudes, values, beliefs, and behavior at all levels of nursing within the organization. There will also be ramifications of this change for other groups and systems such as physicians, therapists, support services, and administrators. The level of change required for a project of this magnitude is organizational change.

Organizational change includes those changes in knowledge, the first level; attitudes, the second level; individual behavior, the third level, which must take place before the organizational change, the fourth level, can occur.[6] The presentation of new information about nursing diagnosis (the diagnostic labels and the thinking process) provides a basis for the first two levels of change.

For the purpose of implementing nursing diagnosis, these first two levels must be viewed within the context of individual behavioral change, the third level of change. These first two levels must be directed by consideration of those factors that will support, enable, and encourage nurses to act on diagnostic and treatment decisions. These factors include the necessary knowledge of nursing diagnosis, the attitudes that support diagnosis-based nursing practice, and the individual behaviors necessary for that practice.

Additionally, two conditions must be present for the fourth level of organizational change to be accomplished in the implementation of nursing diagnosis. The first is that there must be a sufficient number of individual registered nurses who are capable of diagnosis-based nursing practice. This depends upon the successful accomplishment of the required changes in knowledge, attitudes, and behavior; furthermore, these changes must occur in the majority of the nursing staff at all levels of the nursing organization.

The second condition is the restructuring of the clinical nursing practice environment to permit diagnosis-based nursing practice. The changes in individual behaviors of nurses must be supported by structural changes in the organization. One approach to changing organizational behavior is to alter the organizational structure and relationships.[7] The most important structure for the implementation of nursing diagnosis is the model of nursing practice at the unit level. The model of nursing practice must be supported within the context of the organizational structure as well. (See Chapter 6 for a complete discussion of nursing practice models.)

Changes in Knowledge. Knowledge is often used interchangeably with information; however, other definitions of knowledge include a clear perception of the truth, something learned or kept in mind, or an understanding gained by actual experience.[8] A review of these definitions offers some insight into the first level of change, change in knowledge.

If the giving of information is the *only* strategy used to effect a change in knowledge, this may or may not be successful in changing behavior. Only if that information is converted into a perception of truth or is combined with actual experience will it have an effect on behavior, thereby accomplishing change. How many times has one nurse been overheard to say about another "Why does that nurse keep doing that! And after having been told . . ." In this situation, information was conveyed, but it did not change subsequent behavior. On the other hand, everyone has had the experience of learning a piece of information that resulted in a "Eureka!" response, and that information was an important determinant of later behavior.

While knowledge itself may or may not result in a change in behavior, the lack of knowledge is instrumental in resistance to change.[9] This includes both the extent and the quality of knowledge about the particular issue or situation. Determining the amount, type, and quality of knowledge that nurses possess about nursing diagnosis will be an important part of the initial appraisal of the clinical practice culture. Providing information about the change process and soliciting information from nursing staff for the change process will be important strategies during implementation to avoid or minimize resistance.

Changes in Attitudes. The effects of knowledge on behavior are influenced by the individual's attitudes. A change in attitude is the second level of change, and this involves alterations in belief or value systems.[10] The relationship between knowledge and attitudes is complex and not always clear. Attitudes serve to guide thoughts, behavior, and feelings toward objects or people, and they play a significant role in the response to change. Many times attitudes may be based on incomplete, distorted, or erroneous information.[11]

One major process through which attitudes are changed is persuasion, which may be accomplished through personal influence or life circumstances.[12] Membership in a group and the resulting peer pressure is a critical life circumstance that persuades an individual to embrace certain attitudes. Many attitudes such as social behaviors and professional values are learned within groups. The attitudes of the registered nurse peer group, the nurse manager peer groups, and other groups such as physicians or therapists will be important factors in the implementation of nursing diagnosis. Strategies to influence these attitudes will be a critical part of the implementation plan.

Another strategy for changing attitudes is reeducation. Reeducation is indicated when the original educational process has resulted in certain behaviors that must be altered in order for the individual to change behavior.[13] Persuasion and reeducative strategies are used to help people recognize the need for change, which is a critical step in the change process.[14]

Reeducative strategies will be a substantial part of the implementation plan when major changes in the clinical practice structure are a part of the change to diagnosis-based nursing practice. Restructuring the clinical practice environment and then helping the nursing staff develop skills to work within the restructured clinical systems is a reeducative strategy. This is useful when extensive information or skills must be learned and incorporated into behavior before the change actually can occur.[15]

Changes in Individual Behavior. Knowledge and attitudes are powerful determinants of behavior and, as such, play an important role in achieving the third level of change, which is change in individual behavior. Only when knowledge is used to formulate nursing diagnoses and related care plans will nursing diagnosis have an effect on nursing practice. Only when the the majority of nurses in the clinical practice culture value nursing diagnoses and nursing care plans for the delivery of nursing care will attitudes be congruent with diagnosis-based nursing practice.

Changes in Organizational Behavior. In order to accomplish the implementation of nursing diagnosis as an organizational change, three major areas must be addressed. These areas are:

1. The introduction of nursing diagnosis and development of skill in the use of the language and the diagnostic thinking process
2. Building nursing diagnosis and nursing process into the structure of the clinical practice environment
3. Strategies for maintaining and continuing the use of nursing diagnosis after the formal implementation process is completed

These components are based on the levels of change that must first occur if true organizational change is to be accomplished. For example, if the nursing documentation system is revised to include nursing diagnosis but individual staff nurses are unable to formulate appropriate nursing diagnoses, then the change will not be successful.

STEPS IN THE IMPLEMENTATION OF NURSING DIAGNOSIS

Moving through these levels of change for each of the components in the implementation of nursing diagnosis will take time, energy, and commitment. In order to accomplish this, and to reap the rewards of diagnosis-based nursing practice, the following seven steps can be used as a framework for implementing nursing diagnosis. Each of these steps, as outlined in Table 5–2, will be discussed separately. These steps follow the phases in the process of change identified by Lewin: unfreezing, moving or changing, and refreezing.[16]

The first phase is a period of unfreezing, when the individuals and systems are prepared for change. This may occur because of dissatisfaction with existing conditions, from conflict between individuals or groups, or from a desire for growth. Unfreezing is a vital step in preparing individuals to accept new alternatives. Steps 1–5 are concerned with unfreezing the clinical nursing practice environment for the successful change to nursing diagnosis. The initial work of a change agent and the development of the change plan can often occur concurrently and within the context of the unfreezing phase, and this is seen in steps 3–5 in Table 5–2.

The second phase of the change process is the actual moving from one set of existing behaviors or conditions to a new set. The success of this phase is highly dependent on the unfreezing phase and a plan for change that reflects specific strategies to deal with the realities of the situation. The specific strategies and tactics for the change process must be chosen based on the unique characteristics and needs of each organization. Moving, or implementation, of the change plan is Step 6.

The last phase of the change process is refreezing, Step 7 in table 5–2. Refreezing has taken place when the new behaviors or conditions become firmly fixed within individual behavior and organizational culture. In order to accomplish this phase of change, there must be an effective mechanism for reinforcing the new behaviors and conditions. This is why the restructuring of the clinical nursing practice environment is such a critical component of the implementation of nursing diagnosis. Only if the use of nursing diagnosis becomes the way that

TABLE 5–2. STEPS FOR IMPLEMENTING NURSING DIAGNOSIS

Unfreezing	1. *Determine/establish the existence of a philosophical commitment to diagnosis-based nursing practice within the nursing leadership group*
	2. *Examine the clinical nursing practice structure and culture*
(Planning)	3. *Develop an operational definition of nursing diagnosis to guide the implementation process*
	4. *Identify outcomes for the implementation program, including broad goals and specific, measurable objectives*
	5. *Select specific implementation strategies, including the identification of change agent(s)*
Moving	6. *Carry out implementation strategies*
Refreezing	7. *Evaluate clinical practice structure against the predetermined goals at appropriate time intervals*

nurses actually practice nursing can it survive; otherwise there is too much competition in the health care organizational culture.

Two major problems tend to occur in the refreezing phase. The first problem is that refreezing simply does not occur. A new idea is presented, everyone loves it and agrees to try it, but it never becomes part of individual behavior or organizational culture because the reinforcement is not there. This is often seen when nurses attend workshops where specific skills or techniques are taught. On their return to the clinical nursing practice environment, however, these skills disappear; either they do not fit into the existing culture or there is no reward for them.

A second problem with refreezing it that the wrong thing may be refrozen. This is particularly true when the change is a large or complex one. Often there may be interim steps or strategies that are used during the change process. If these interim strategies are refrozen, rather than the desired end behaviors, then the change process may well be less successful, and decidedly different goals may result.

Recognizing certain responses or behaviors as interim strategies in the change process is an important part of the monitoring of the change. Care should be taken to avoid refreezing interim strategies, although this may be difficult at times. In a large and complex change, any movement toward the goals of the program is gratifying. The temptation may be to settle for progress toward identified outcomes rather than the outcomes themselves. The clinical and administrative leadership for the implementation of nursing diagnosis will need flexibility, tolerance for the developing state of nursing diagnosis, and determination to reach the goals of the program.

Refreezing the desired outcomes rather than interim strategies can be accomplished through precisely stated outcomes for the change process and careful monitoring. This evaluation of what is happening during the implementation process is critical to the success of the program. One of the pitfalls in the implementation of nursing diagnosis is inadequate evaluation methodology, reflecting both a lack of accurate assessment of the existence of valid nursing diagnoses in a unit or department and an unawareness of the state of the art of nursing diagnosis.[17] Monitoring of the actual use of nursing diagnoses by staff nurses is an important part of the implementation process. It will provide both useful evaluative data about the progress and success of the change process as well as a mechanism for reinforcement and reward of diagnosis-based nursing practice.

In order to progress through these seven steps for the implementation of nursing diagnosis, many choices must be made. These choices must be guided by the philosophical commitment to diagnosis-based nursing practice. In fact, the determination or establishment of this philosophical commitment is the first step in the implementation process.

Step 1: Determine/Establish a Philosophical Base for Diagnosis-Based Nursing Practice

The decisions that must be made in planning for each of these components must be based on a genuine philosophical commitment to professional nursing practice. This commitment must be supported by a realistic sense of confidence that professional nursing practice *can* happen. The choices made during the planning and implementation of nursing diagnosis must be firmly grounded in nursing practice reality, tempered with an optimistic view of what nursing practice can be.

If the guiding premise for these decisions is medical model-based thinking or a sense that diagnosis-based nursing practice really is *not* possible, success in moving from a task-based nursing practice to diagnosis-based nursing practice is not likely. In fact, the decision to implement nursing diagnosis should *not* be made without a thorough analysis of personal philosophy and attitudes about nursing practice, what it is and what it could be. Only if the philosophical base is present and genuine in the nursing leadership can the benefits of implementing nursing diagnosis and diagnosis-based practice be realized.

A useful approach to this step is the strategy of values clarification. A value is an affective disposition towards a person, object, or idea; values clarification is a process of self-discovery that allows the individual to analyze behavior choices.[18] The process of values clarification can be used within the nursing unit to identify those values that are supportive of diagnosis-based practice.

Values are also the foundation of the culture of the organization. They provide a sense of common direction and guidelines for day-to-day behavior. In fact, it may be that organizations are successful because individuals can identify, embrace, and act on the values of the organization.[19] For these reasons, values about nursing practice, professionalism, and nursing process play a critical role in the implementation of nursing diagnosis.

Although many nurses will indicate that they value nursing process, their behavior may not reflect this, and task-based nursing practice is the result. Observation of an individual nurse or the clinical practice on a particular nursing unit can give some insight into values. Does a nurse actually develop nursing care plans, communicate these plans to other staff and hold colleagues responsible for those plans? If this behavior can be observed, that nurse values diagnosis-based nursing practice. Even though the nursing diagnosis may not be in "approved" terminology and the plan may be verbal rather than written, the valuing is there.

Consider a nursing unit change of shift report. Does the information about patients focus *only* on medical orders, diagnostic tests, and technical information such as "bed in low position, side rails up, there's 300 ccs left in the IV?" This is task-based nursing practice. On the other hand, is this task and technical information integrated into a description of the patient that includes nursing care issues as well? The second unit values professional nursing practice, and this staff may be ready to implement nursing diagnosis.

The importance of the administrative and clinical leaders valuing and acting upon their value of nursing diagnosis and nursing process cannot be emphasized strongly enough. These nurses must lead the implementation process. The values and beliefs of an organization indicate which matters and information are treated seriously and which people are most respected. Shared values also affect organizational performance. Attention is focused on valued concerns, midlevel managers make better decisions, and people work a little harder because they are dedicated to the values of the organization.[20]

If the valuing of nursing process by nurse managers and clinical leaders is superficial or lacks active support, their leadership will lack conviction and will be less effective as a result. Those nurse managers who include clinical nursing practice issues, especially nursing care planning and its organizational supports, in their regular working meetings and conferences demonstrate they value the nursing process. When administrative or clinical meetings do not include these issues in the activities of the group, this lack of valuing will be discernible in the nursing practice areas.

The values clarification process attempts to bring to conscious awareness the values and underlying motivation that guide nurses' actions; values clarification involves choosing, prizing, and acting.[21] The administrative and clinical leaders in today's clinical practice culture are confronted with issues that make acting on values difficult: massive increases in patient acuity, pressing economic concerns, burgeoning technology, and nurses who assert their rights as professional employees. Values clarification is useful to resolve conflict rather than to find absolute answers of right or wrong.[22] Discovering which values are strongest provides guidance in sorting out these conflicting demands.

A number of values clarification exercises that deal with nursing are available.[23] Listing and ranking values, comparing organizational and personal values, and determining the amount of time actually spent in valued activities are a few exercises that can provide insight for individuals and groups of nurses. Particular areas to explore in relation to the implementation of nursing diagnosis are presented in Table 5–3.

The first step of the implementation process concludes with the firm commitment of the clinical and administrative leadership to the concept of diagnosis-based nursing practice. An appraisal of the existing systems and culture in the next step provides the information for making a decision to proceed with implementation and the specific aspects of the implementation plan.

Step 2. Examination and Analysis of the Clinical Practice Systems and Culture

Change is the process of moving from the current state or condition to a different, desired state or condition. In order to formulate a plan for the change process and to evaluate the effectiveness of the plan in moving toward the desired state, a careful and realistic appraisal of the existing situation must be made. Only if this information is accurate and unbiased, can it be used effectively. Planning based on fantasy, misperceptions, or incorrect information cannot succeed.

Seven areas of assessment have been identified by Lancour[24] as important for the implementation of nursing diagnosis. These are:

1. Philosophy
2. Staff
3. Standards of nursing practice
4. Resources
5. Job descriptions and performance appraisals
6. Delivery of care and documentation systems
7. Change process

These areas reflect the clinical nursing practice structures that must support and encourage the use of nursing diagnosis.

Examination and analysis of these areas will be influenced and directed by philosophical issues, and these have been discussed in the first step of the implementation process. The remaining six areas encompass a vast amount of information about the clinical nursing practice environment. A brief discussion will be provided here, and specific issues will be addressed in the remaining chapters in Part II.

Staff

An evaluation of the current status of the nursing staff must cover four important areas. These will include:

- the percentage of registered nurses and their educational preparation
- their knowledge and expertise in using nursing process
- their attitudes and beliefs about autonomy and accountability for nursing practice
- their knowledge and expertise in using nursing diagnosis[25]

TABLE 5–3. VALUES CLARIFICATION EXERCISE #1

What I Believe about Nursing Process and Nursing Diagnosis

1. What do I believe about nursing process?
   What do I do that demonstrates these beliefs?
2. What type of patient problems/conditions are commonly seen in the population that I work with?
   What problems do I spend most of my time working on?
3. What are the most important responsibilities of the registered nurse on the nursing unit for a given shift?
   What are the most time-consuming or frequently performed activities of registered nurses for a given shift on my unit(s)?
4. What do I believe about nursing diagnosis?
   What do I do that demonstrates these beliefs?
5. What do I believe about the role of nursing process in the present clinical nursing practice culture?
   What can I detect in the present clinical practice environment the supports or enables the professional nurse in using nursing process?
6. What do I believe about autonomy and accountability in nursing practice?
   What autonomy and accountability for nursing practice can be found in the present clinical nursing practice culture?

VALUES CLARIFICATION EXERCISE #2

Priorities of Action: Clinical Situations

Rank the statements in each cluster based on your priorities.

1. ____ Helping a patient understand the purposes of a diagnostic test
   ____ Assisting a blind patient to eat
   ____ Planning a patient care conference with the multidisciplinary team to set goals for a patient's treatment
2. ____ Teaching a patient to change an ostomy bag
   ____ Administering scheduled 6 P.M. medications
   ____ Transcribing a physician's orders to the Kardex
3. ____ Obtaining a sputum specimen from a patient with pneumonia
   ____ Performing a nursing history and physical assessment on a newly admitted patient
   ____ Contacting a social worker for a patient who will be discharged in a few days
4. ____ Notifying hospital security about visitors who will not leave after visiting hours
   ____ Identifying a nursing diagnosis and care plan for a patient who has just been told the biopsy result was malignant
   ____ Performing wound care for a patient with an infected decubitus
5. ____ Cleaning and providing skin care for an incontinent patient
   ____ Assisting a discharged patient out of the hospital to her car
   ____ Assessing a patient who has just returned from an angiogram
6. ____ Responding to a post-operative patient's request for pain medication
   ____ Contacting the dietician to talk with a patient who is dissatisfied with the food
   ____ Holding a patient while the physician obtains a blood sample
7. ____ Giving a tube feeding to an unconscious patient
   ____ Determining the most effective nursing interventions for the patient with Impaired Physical Mobility
   ____ Assembling equipment for a discharged patient to take home
8. ____ Offering a supportive presence as a nursing intervention for Anxiety related to hospitalization
   ____ Assisting a physician to obtain an autopsy consent
   ____ Preparing a room for a patient being transferred out of the ICU
9. ____ Restraining a confused, disoriented patient
   ____ Assessing the patient's response to chemotherapy to identify nursing diagnoses and a nursing care plan
   ____ Shampooing the hair of a patient who is unable to do so

TABLE 5—3.   (Continued)

Priorities of Action: Clinical Situations

10.   ____   Making a referral to the social worker for a patient who has an Alteration in Health
              Maintenence related to lack of resources
       ____   Consulting a dietician for a nutritional assessment of a patient receiving tube feedings
       ____   Requesting advice from the physical therapist about transfer techniques for a stroke patient

What type of situations did you choose as high-priority? Were they task-based or nursing diagnosis-based?
Are there consistencies in the types of activities that you chose as most important? What insights have
you gained about your priorities?

VALUES CLARIFICATION EXERCISE #3

Priorities of Action: Administrative Situations

Answer the following questions twice. The first time answer with a YES or NO based on what you think the
ideal situation would be. The second time answer with YES if you believe this statement is an accurate
description of the situation that you are currently working in. Answer with a NO if you believe that the
statement is not accurate. Answer all questions.

____/____   I believe that the most skilled staff members should be assigned to the sickest/most difficult
            patients.

____/____   There is a place on my unit for all levels of nursing staff (RNs, LPNs, nursing assistants).

____/____   Staff meetings should focus on administrative issues.

____/____   Monitoring the care that nursing staff provides is the job of quality assurance.

____/____   The supplies and equipment that are needed to provide nursing care to patients are always
            available on the unit.

____/____   Registered nurses must have the time to do nursing care plans and documentation of patient
            care.

____/____   Dividing the number of patients by the number of nursing staff is the best way to make assign-
            ments for a shift.

____/____   A medication nurse to administer all medications for the shift is the most efficient way to get
            this work done.

____/____   Nursing diagnosis is too complicated for most nurses to use.

____/____   Staffing issues take very little of my time.

____/____   The model of nursing practice on my unit(s) is effective in supporting the registered nurse in
            making nursing diagnoses and nursing care plans.

____/____   RNs, LPNs, and nursing assistants have clear roles and responsibilities on my unit(s).

____/____   Giving feedback and assistance to RNs about nursing diagnosis and nursing care planning is
            something that I enjoy doing.

____/____   How well RNs do nursing care planning is an important part of their performance evaluation.

____/____   Patient care conferences and educational programs occur regularly on my unit.

____/____   There is little distinction between RNs and other nursing personnel on my unit in terms of
            actual work done.

____/____   I monitor nursing care planning on my unit(s) regularly.

____/____   Staff meetings, patient care conferences, and team conferences are times for sharing clinical
            problems and group problem solving.

____/____   Nursing and medical staff are colleagues and work together on my unit(s).

____/____   Nursing diagnosis is a helpful framework for nurses on my unit to use in identifying patient
            problems for nursing care planning.

____/____   LPNs on my unit participate in nursing care planning by contributing data to the assessment,
            carrying out nursing interventions, and reporting patient progress.

(continued)

TABLE 5–3. (Continued)

Priorities of Action: Administrative Situations

____/____   *Nursing staff on my unit works well together.*

____/____   *Nursing care planning issues are regularly included in shift report.*

____/____   *Shift report is a time for reporting information, not problem solving or discussion of nursing care plans.*

____/____   *The documentation on my unit(s) consistently meets the quality assurance standards of the organization.*

____/____   *Nursing staff often stay after their shift is over to complete documentation responsibilities.*

____/____   *The documentation requirements and standards make sense to the nursing staff on my unit(s).*

____/____   *The nursing care plan is an important part of the documentation of the patient's care.*

____/____   *The written nursing care plan is used to provide nursing care.*

____/____   *Nurses respect the nursing care plans developed by their colleagues and carry out the plan as indicated.*

____/____   *Nursing diagnosis makes doing nursing care plans more difficult for many of my staff.*

____/____   *LPNs and nursing assistants understand the purpose of the nursing diagnoses and nursing care plans.*

____/____   *There are clinical role models and resources available to help with nursing diagnosis and nursing care planning.*

How well do your ideal and real situations match? The purpose of this exercise is to identify discrepancies between the things that you value as ideal administrative practices and real situations that you might want to make closer to your ideal.

The information derived from this evaluation will provide an important foundation for designing the implementation plan.

The assessment of the existing staff situation may be compared with the two conditions that must be present for organizational change: a sufficient number of registered nurses who are capable of diagnosis-based practice and a clinical practice environment that enables and supports the professional nurse in that practice. If the existing staff resources, mix of categories, knowledge, expertise, and attitudes are not consistent with the conditions for diagnosis-based practice, narrowing the gap provides the focus and direction for the implementation plan.

Consider a nursing unit consisting only of registered nurses and nursing assistants. RNs account for 85 percent of the staff and half of these are baccalaureate prepared. The quality assurance audits show that this unit develops and uses nursing care plans for the majority of their patients, and that their documentation is consistent with the standards of the organization. A strong sense of professional accountability is evident in their primary nursing model of practice.

In order for this unit to meet the two conditions for organizational change to diagnosis-based nursing practice, movement from existing state to desired state will be small. The major thrust of the implementation program will focus on the knowledge, skills, and attitudes necessary to work with nursing diagnosis. Many of the other supporting conditions are already present.

Consider another unit with different circumstances and a nursing staff composed of registered nurses, licensed practical nurses, and nursing assistants. The percentage of RN staff if 30 percent, only a few of which have baccalaureate degrees, while the LPN group comprises 55 percent and the remaining 15 percent are nursing assistants. The quality assurance audits indicate that nursing care plans are infrequently done, although the quality is good. Other documentation standards are inconsistently met.

An informal survey of the entire staff reveals a group of energetic, concerned individuals who are frustrated with their failure to meet documentation standards but proud of their ability to meet the physical needs of their patients. The RNs wish they had the opportunity to address more of their patients' needs than just physical care, but the LPNs and assistants are confused by the RNs desire to "do all that talking and paperwork." The model of nursing practice is a modified form of total patient care, wherein each staff member has a group of patients assigned for the shift with nominal supervision by the charge RN.

To meet the conditions for organizational change on this unit, a number of issues must be addressed to support diagnosis-based practice, and these need attention either before the introduction of nursing diagnosis or during the early part of the implementation process. In order to have a sufficient number of nurses who are capable of diagnosis-based practice, the number of RNs on this unit needs to be increased or the model of nursing practice must be adjusted so that the existing number of RNs can be used most effectively for diagnosing and planning nursing treatment. Changing the model of nursing practice to a team model, with clear accountability for nursing process for all patients on the team vested in the team leader, might be a way to work with the present staff numbers and mix.

A change in the model of nursing practice would also address the second condition, a clinical practice system that supports the registered nurse in diagnosis-based practice. By organizing the work activities of the unit so that the professional nurse has the clear accountability and the time to make nursing diagnostic and treatment decisions, the skills of the existing RN staff can be employed with maximum benefit. On the other hand, if responsibilities for nursing diagnosis and care planning are simply added to the nurse's current set of tasks and duties, the possibility of success is very slim, and frustration and resentment can be the result rather than improved nursing care planning.

An important area in the evaluation of the tasks and activities that occupy nursing time is the rites and rituals of the clinical practice culture. The standards of acceptable behavior and ways in which procedures are carried out are tangible indicators of the strength of the culture. Although these rituals may seem ineffective or trivial, they are often very powerful factors for maintaining the culture. Attempts to change these behaviors can meet with strong resistance.[26]

Many activities on the nursing unit can hold the force of ritual. Shift report is often endowed with certain ritualistic aspects; who sits where, whether questions are allowed, who attends report, or whether it is acceptable to smoke or drink coffee. Clinical procedures also may have an element of ritual. The use of draw sheets, certain pre-op routines, and the location of equipment at the patient's bedside are just a few of the rituals that can be seen in clinical nursing practice. In the absence of a clearly defined model of nursing practice, assignments may have an element of ritual, and there is grief for the new nurse who does not follow the accepted ways of doing things. An agreed-upon set of ground rules can have a tremendously liberating effect.[27] These rituals provide a sense of structure and security for the individuals in the culture. On a busy nursing unit very few things are predictable. These rituals of unit routine or clinical procedures are a way to achieve some semblance of structure and predictability.

The positive effects for the organizational culture may be overshadowed if the rituals are no longer accomplishing their purpose. Changing rituals that are ineffective, or obsolete can be very difficult because the force of culture is behind them. Recognizing the ritual value of certain activities on the nursing unit and analyzing the purposes that they serve is an important part of the evaluation of the nursing unit culture prior to implementing nursing diagnosis.

One question that always arises about the implementation of nursing diagnosis is: Where will the time come from for staff nurses to make nursing diagnoses and care plans? An analysis of the tasks and duties that consume nurses' time on the units is a critical part of the staff evaluation. The performance on non-nursing tasks can take up the time of the professional nurse to the exclusion of nursing care activities. One study of five Boston hospitals in the mid-

1970s showed that 77 percent of registered nurses spent 28 percent of their time on simple tasks such as locating and setting up equipment and transporting patients.[28] Think of what could be accomplished with that time if the nurses' activity was focused on diagnosing and treating patient problems.

If the professional nurse is to have the time necessary for diagnosis-based nursing practice, then non-nursing activities must be delegated to non-nurses. Toth states:

> We cannot afford to empty the trash on the 11 P.M. to 7 A.M. shift, wrap bedpans for central supply, clean stretchers for housekeeping, do medication inventories for pharmacy, serve trays for dietary, or transport patients for other ancillary departments unless indicated for nursing reasons. We must give up the traditional handmaiden tasks to free us to do nursing care only. Anyone who is not willing to fight to relinquish non-nursing tasks does not belong in nursing management today.[29]

Many times nurse managers wonder how they can ask their nursing staff to do one more thing. Furthermore, in the midst of a nursing shortage the hiring of more nurses is not likely, nor is it the solution to this issue of non-nursing tasks.

Perhaps nurses have not been able to rid themselves of non-nursing tasks because there has been no clearly defined nursing activity that justified this. Diagnosis-based nursing practice provides this justification. It is a way for nurses to spend their time nursing: assessing patients, diagnosing human responses, designing and implementing care plans, and evaluating their effectiveness. If non-nursing tasks are delegated to the appropriate non-nurses, then the time of the professional nurse becomes available for providing nursing care.

When the time is provided for diganosis-based nursing practice, nurse managers can set standards and expectations for nursing care with a sense of the possible rather than the sense that they are overloading their nursing staff with "paperwork." Providing the time, however, is not all; staff nurses must be guided in the diagnostic process, in working with the language of nursing diagnosis, and in identifying the most effective nursing interventions. Time and skill issues both must be addressed in the initial assessment and the implementation plan.

Standards of Nursing Practice

A standard is defined as "something set up as a rule for measuring or as a model to be followed."[30] Standards of nursing practice are designed as mechanisms for measuring the care that patients receive and the practice of nursing necessary to accomplish this care. Many professional nursing organizations have developed and published nursing practice standards, and these standards are often brought down to the organizational level by the development of policies, procedures, or other types of operational guidelines.

If there is inconsistency between the written standards of the nursing department and the present clinical practice activity, this can cause a number of problems, and it would be best if they were resolved prior to or as a part of the early phases of the implementation of nursing diagnosis. Making nursing practice more consistent with the written standards and clarifying the role of standards in directing the nursing care that patients receive can decrease confusion about the purpose of nursing diagnosis in the care of these patients. (See Chapter 2 for a discussion of the relationship between standards and nursing diagnosis.)

The existence of written standards, congruent with clinical practice, and an active quality assurance program provides fundamental mechanisms for measuring and determining the current quality of nursing care delivery. If these two clinical practice structures are deficient or absent, the development and implementation of programs to establish or improve written standards of care and a quality assurance program should take place before the implementation of nursing diagnosis. (See Chapter 8 for a discussion of Quality Assurance and Nursing Diagnosis.)

Resources

An assessment of the resources for the implementation of nursing diagnosis should examine a number of areas. Those resources of the administrative and clinical leadership groups are the first area. A strong philosophical commitment to professional nursing practice shared by the majority of this group is one of the most critical resources for the implementation of nursing diagnosis.

The administrative and clinical leadership is also an important source of talent in the form of clinical and administrative role models. The talents that should be tapped included skill in formulating nursing diagnoses, using nursing diagnoses in patient care conferences, incorporating nursing diagnoses and care plans into shift reports, designing assignment strategies to support the professional nurse in diagnosis-based nursing practice, and the ability to share and develop these skills in others. Representatives of the administrative and clinical leadership should be involved in any committees, task forces, or other problem-solving groups that are active in the implementation process.

The standing committees of the department of nursing are an invaluable resource in the implementation process, both for planning and implementation itself. The Care Planning Committee will do a tremendous amount of work in reviewing and revising nursing care plans for the organization that incorporates nursing diagnosis. The Policy Committee must develop policies for documentation, assignments, and other aspects of diagnosis-based practice. Specialized clinical groups, such as the critical care nurses or the pediatric nurses, may wish to explore issues that have implications for their patient populations. This type of committee activity can be a powerful mechanism for involving the grass-roots clinical staff in the planning and implementation of nursing diagnosis.

Another important resource area for the implementation process is the informal leadership on the nursing units. The informal leaders, whether RN, LPN, clerk, or an employee in another job category, can play an essential role in the cultural acceptance of the change process. The identification of these individuals and their active participation in the implementation process is critical.

Oftentimes, the resource area that is first targeted for the implementation of nursing diagnosis is the staff development department. While the implementation of nursing diagnosis does require that new information be provided, it is a myth that sending nurses to a workshop on nursing diagnosis will be adequate.[31] This does not mean that there is not an important role for staff development nurses in the implementation process; that role, however, should be based on the unique characteristics of the organization. One critical characteristic is the educational backgrounds, experience, and familiarity with nursing process and nursing care planning of the nursing staff. If the nursing staff consists of predominantly baccalaureate-prepared, recent graduates who learned about nursing diagnosis in school, then the focus of the staff development department can move beyond presentation of basic concepts into diagnostic thinking and differential diagnostic issues. On the other hand, a nursing staff that had little previous exposure to nursing diagnosis requires more comprehensive educational programs to support the implementation process.

The talents within the administrative and clinical leadership is another characteristic of the organization that influences the role of the staff development department. In the presence of strong clinical practitioners on the nursing unites, the staff development department can assume a coordinating, supportive role, providing educational materials, programs away from the nursing unit, and consultative assistance to the frontline people. If this frontline expertise is unavailable, then it is very important for the staff development instructors to be available on the nursing units to assist with nursing diagnositic questions as they arose.

Nursing faculty and students can also be a valuable resource for the implementation process. Those nursing units that provide clinical experiences for students can take advantage of student learning activities such as nursing care plans using nursing diagnosis and conferences where nursing diagnoses are discussed. In this situation, the students and the nursing staff can learn about nursing diagnosis together.

A number of resources may be found outside the department of nursing. If part of the implementation process involves changes in documentation and chart forms, the Medical Records Committee of the hospital can be very helpful in setting up special forms or flow sheets. The involvement of this committee in the planning process also facilitates the approval necessary to make the new forms part of the permanent record.

Those organizations that have computerized information systems can find many helpful resources in the Information Systems Department. In fact, this group is a critical resource and should be consulted and involved in any documentation system changes that will become part of the information system. Consulting this group early in the implementation planning can provide important advice and guidance, and help avoid time-consuming or costly errors. A discussion of nursing diagnosis and nursing information systems is presented in Chapter 9.

Another critical resource is financial support for a change in nursing practice. An important financial consideration for the implementation program described here is nursing salary hours for educational programs, unit conferences, and committee meetings. If a full-time change agent is designated for this project, there is a financial outlay, either in salary or in hiring someone to assume the previous duties of that individual. There also are expenditures for books, development or purchase of educational materials, travel expenses for national meetings of the North American Nursing Diagnosis Association (NANDA) or other groups, and external resources such as computer time or consultants from outside the organization.

Job Descriptions and Performance Appraisals. The job descriptions and performance appraisals of the registered nurse should be evaluated in order to determine their support for diagnosis-based nursing practice. One key area to examine are the tasks and duties of the registered nurse: Do these include nursing diagnosis and nursing process? Are the requirements for these activities clearly described?

To answer these questions, the job description for the registered nurse should include specific statements for each step of the nursing process. The phrase "Utilizes nursing process in clinical practice" is not sufficient as a job description criterion, nor does it serve as a useful appraisal standard. The following are examples of statements for an RN job description:

- Assesses all assigned patients using functional health patterns and body systems formats, documents assessment in accordance with documentation policy
- Makes nursing diagnoses of human responses that are amenable to nursing interventions, based on assessments, for assigned patients; nursing care plans are developed for these nursing diagnoses, and progress is monitored and evaluated; patient assignments for nursing diagnoses and care plans are made in accordance with unit model of nursing practice and documented in accordance with documentation policy

The inclusion of nursing diagnosis and nursing treatment in the job description and performance evaluations of the professional nurse are essential organizational supports for diagnosis-based nursing practice.

The job descriptions and performance appraisals for other nursing roles also should reflect the requirements of diagnosis-based nursing practice. For head nurses, job descriptions should include statements about monitoring nursing diagnoses and care plans and assisting nursing staff in the development of diagnostic skills as well as providing a model of nursing practice that supports staff nurses in making and acting on nursing diagnoses and nursing care plans.

Nurse managers at all levels should work from job descriptions and evaluation criteria that define their roles in maintaining and strengthening diagnosis-based nursing practice. The responsibility for nurse managers to advocate for the role of the professional nurse should be stated in operational terms. The inclusion of job description criteria that support diagnosis-based practice in all levels of nursing service is an important philosophical statement that nursing diagnosis and professional nursing practice is valued by nursing service.

Delivery of Care and Documentation System. The model of nursing practice is the mechanism by which nursing care is delivered on the nursing unit. The model of nursing practice is a key factor for the establishment of diagnosis-based nursing practice, and the determination of the distribution of work responsibilities that a model of nursing practice offers plays an important role in the documentation systems. If the documentation system requires the RN to assess patients and plan their nursing care, and the model of nursing practice does not support this, then it is unlikely that documentation standards will be met.

The model of nursing practice should be evaluated for its support of diagnosis-based nursing practice. The role of the professional nurse and the tasks that consume RN time are particularly important in this analysis. It is essential that nursing diagnosis and nursing care planning are incorporated into the clinical practice systems rather than simply added on to the workload of the RN. If the introduction of nursing diagnosis is perceived as an additional workload of indeterminate benefit, then it is doubtful that the change to using nursing diagnosis will become a part of the clinical practice culture.

The importance of the model of nursing practice to support diagnosis-based nursing practice cannot be overemphasized. Chapter 6 presents a comprehensive review of the recognized models: functional nursing, team nursing, total patient care, primary nursing, and case management. While functional nursing is not compatible with diagnosis-based nursing practice, the other four can be used successfully to provide professional nursing care. The choice of a model of nursing practice can be based on a number of factors, such as patient characteristics and staff mix, that permits the most effective and efficient use of nursing resources.

The documentation system also must be reviewed for its support of professional nursing practice. The nursing documentation requirements should be analyzed for a logical flow of information that reflects the nursing process. For example, the initial nursing history and physical assessment can be organized with a nursing focus that assists the nurse in identifying nursing diagnoses, or it can follow traditional medical model format. This latter situation does not support the nurse in diagnosis-based nursing practice.

The nursing documentation requirements, formats, and policies must include mechanisms for recording nursing assessment data, nursing diagnoses, nursing care plans and their implementation, and evaluation of the patients' progress. Unless there is a logical progression in the documentation framework, nurses will be confounded in attempts to record all of this information. The issues affecting nursing documentation are influenced by professional, organizational, and legal mandates. Incorporating nursing diagnosis into the existing system of an organization can be challenging and exciting. A discussion of specific issues, problems, and strategies for documentation systems using nursing diagnosis can be found in Chapter 7.

Change Process. An analysis of the past experiences that the nursing department has had with change projects can provide important information for planning the implementation of nursing diagnosis. Factors to be considered in this evaluation are:

What changes are going on currently in the nursing department and the organization?

What methods of change have been most successful or least effective in the past? Are the same methods available or appropriate now?

What factors will support or inhibit a change at this point in time and the change to using nursing diagnosis?

What types of reactions to nursing diagnosis can be anticipated from nurses, physicians, other disciplines, and non-professionals? What groundwork or politicking should be carried out to gain support from these groups?

What evaluation methodologies are required by the change to nursing diagnosis? What evaluation methodologies are available?[32]

Information gained from this evaluation of the nursing department and organization can be used in planning the change to diagnosis-based nursing practice. This planning must be based on a realistic and accurate appraisal of the situation at hand.

The second step of the implementation process consists of a careful and realistic analysis of the clinical practice systems, the personnel resources, and the change history of the organization. This information provides foundations for the planning aspect of the implementation of nursing diagnosis. Steps 3, 4, and 5 are concerned with planning and preparation for the implementation of nursing diagnosis.

Step 3. Develop an operational definition of nursing diagnosis to guide the implementation process

In Step 2, the current state of nursing practice is examined and serves as the baseline description of the clinical practice systems and culture. The next step is to develop an operational definition of nursing diagnosis that can direct the implementation process and provide a standard against which the success of the implementation program may be judged.

The operational definition of nursing diagnosis is the foundation of the implementation plan. In order to select the appropriate change strategies for implementation, there must be a clearly defined statement of what a nursing diagnosis is, why and when it will be used, and who will be responsible for making it. The choices that an organization makes in determining its operational definition of nursing diagnosis and subsequent implementation strategies will be guided by the goals and mission of the organization, the values of the clinical practice culture, the available personnel and material resources, and the vision of its nurse leaders.

The operational definition provides a vehicle for the organization or agency to bridge the gaps from the existing clinical practice systems, structures, and culture to the abstract, conceptual descriptions of nursing diagnosis. This definition should contain two components that deal with the current issues about nursing diagnosis and the organizational philosophy and mission: a conceptual statement about nursing diagnosis and a logistical description for the use of nursing diagnosis.

The first component, the conceptual statement, must define nursing diagnosis, the reasons for its use, and its place within the context of the nursing process. A key component of this part of the operational definition is the delineation of the role of nursing diagnosis and the scope of nursing practice. Of critical importance in this discussion is the differentiation of nursing and medical diagnoses. The direction of nursing care by policy, procedure, standards, or protocols must also be defined in relation to the direction provided by nursing diagnosis.

The second component must address the logistics of nursing diagnosis within the clinical practice systems of the organization. This refers to the practical realities of who makes nursing diagnoses, when these should or should not be made, where the nursing diagnoses and related nursing interventions are documented, and against which criteria they will be evaluated. This logistical statement must be clear and descriptive enough to guide the formulation of supporting policy, procedure, and protocol that direct how these logistical decisions are carried out.

In order to develop an operational definition for nursing diagnosis that will be useful in directing the implementation process, three areas should be considered. An important consideration for the conceptual component of the operational definition is the philosophical approach to professional nursing practice in the organization. The unique characteristics of the organization are important determinants of the logistical component of the operational definition. The characteristics of the clinical practice culture should also be used to direct the choices for the operational definition. A sample operational definition is presented in Chapter 2.

The operational definition of nursing diagnosis is the foundation of the implementation plan. Steps 3, 4, and 5 are concerned with the development of the implementation plan. This plan should consist of the operational definition, clearly identified outcomes for the implementation process, and the specific strategies for accomplishing this change. (See Table 5–4.)

Step 4. Identify outcomes, including broad goals and specific measurable objectives

In order to direct the change process and to evaluate its success, it is necessary to identify what the change is supposed to accomplish. The desired aims of the change should be clearly

---

TABLE 5–4. THE PLAN FOR IMPLEMENTING NURSING DIAGNOSIS

Part 1: The Operational Definition of Nursing Diagnosis *(Step 3, also see Chapter 2)*
Philosophical statement about the use of nursing diagnosis in the organization
Logistical statement about who will make nursing diagnoses, when they will be made, how they will be documented, and against which criteria they will be evaluated

Part 2: Goals, objectives, and outcomes of the implementation process (Step 4)
Outcomes are identified as the desired aims of the change project in clear, measurable terms
Broad goals for both task accomplishment and system maintenance are set
Objectives are developed that give direction for carrying out the activities necessary to accomplish the desired goals

Part 3: Specific strategies to be carried out to meet the objectives and accomplish the desired goals *(Step 5, also see chapters in Part 3)*
Strategies that should be implemented before the implementation of nursing diagnosis
Strategies to prepare for nursing diagnosis
Actual implementation strategies:
   clinical activities
   system activities
   administrative activities
   educational activities
Strategies to monitor, evaluate, and maintain the use of nursing diagnosis

and precisely described in observable, measurable terms. These outcomes of change can provide guidance in the selection of change strategies, in the utilization of resources, and in the development of methods for determining the effectiveness of the change program.

Goals represent a desired condition that may be value-laden; goals can serve as a focus for work. They are generally stated in broad or conceptual terms. Nurses often describe goals for a patient as: improve nutritional state or maintain optimal function. The goals that nurses might identify for their unit or organization can be stated as: provide high-quality care for our patients or offer patient education for all patients.

The goals of an organization can be divided into two categories: task-achievement goals and system-maintenance goals. For the implementation of nursing diagnosis, goals are required for both categories. Task-achievement goals for the nursing staff include achieving skill in making nursing diagnoses, designing a documentation system that supports nursing diagnosis, or revising the Quality Assurance Program to reflect the use of nursing diagnosis in the organization.

There also are system-maintenance goals in the implementation plan for nursing diagnosis. The recruitment and retention of clinically expert nurses, the establishment of committee for care plan development or speciality nursing issues, and the delivery of nursing care through a defined model of nursing practice are examples. Once the appropriate system-maintenance goals have been determined, the next step is to develop specific objectives.

Objectives should be clear and descriptive enough to direct the activities of the organization. Four components of objectives have been suggested:

1. The activity to be done or the change desired
2. The persons responsible for the activity
3. The time frame for the activity
4. An acceptable outcome, in measurable terms[33]

The linkage between objective and outcome is essential. The objective must be written so that it gives adequate direction for the persons in the organization who must carry out the specified activity. The clarity of the objective is important in determining a measurable outcome of the activity.

Consider a nursing unit that is dissatisfied with its documentation system and the time it requires. A goal is developed that states: improve overall the quality of documentation. For this goal to be accomplished, it must be restructured into tangible objectives that can direct work to attain the goal and that can define measurable outcomes. Specific direction for developing objectives are based on the unique characteristics of the unit as well as the personnel and material resources that are available.

Objectives for the goal of improving the quality of documentation might consist of designing a flow sheet for numerical and repetitive data, developing a format for progress notes that focuses on descriptive and evaluative information, and creating a set of charting guidelines for certain clinical conditions. These objectives address task issues for the documentation system. A set of objectives concerned with system maintenance would address the participation of the unit staff in the development of the objectives and planning for the documentation change as well as strategies for staff education about the new documentation system. (See Table 5–5.)

This example demonstrates the movement from broad goal statements to action-oriented objectives. The next step is to identify clear, measurable outcomes for the change project. This same movement can occur with the development of goals, objectives, and outcomes for the implementation of nursing diagnosis.

TABLE 5–5. GOAL AND OBJECTIVES FOR CHANGING OUR DOCUMENTATION SYSTEM

Goal #1
Improvement of the quality of overall nursing documentation

Objectives:
1. *Design a flow sheet for bedside recording of numerical and repetitive data (vital signs, I & O, unit tests, repeated procedures or nursing treatments, AM care)*
2. *Develop a progress note format that focuses on descriptive and evaluative information about the patient's condition*
3. *Create a set of charting guidelines for common patient situations (post-op assessment, admission of new patient, and specific surgical or diagnostic procedures)*
4. *Survey nursing staff for ideas and suggestions*
5. *Offer initial information about the documentation system changes in staff meetings and a one-hour instructional and practice session*
6. *Develop audit criteria for the new documentation system; conduct periodic audits and share the results in staff meetings*

Outcome Measures:
1. *A flow sheet in designed, formatted, and in use by —/—/—*
2. *A progress note format is designed and in use by —/—/—*
3. *Charting guidelines for post-op assessment, admission of new patients, and three surgical procedures (identified from staff survey) are developed by —/—/—*

The broad goals for the implementation of nursing diagnosis include the development of skill in making and using nursing diagnosis for all registered nurses in the organization, the revision or modification of models of nursing practice to support diagnosis-based nursing practice, and the implementation of rewards and structure to maintain the use of nursing diagnosis within the clinical practice culture. The goals for a particular health care organization should reflect its unique characteristics and resources. For example, if there is a computerized hospital information system, then one goal might focus on the incorporation of nursing diagnosis into that system.

Goals should be established that address both the task-accomplishment activities of implementing nursing diagnosis and the system-maintenance requirements as well. Some examples of goals for these areas are presented in Table 5–6.

An important consideration in establishing goals is the necessity to determine whether the goal has been met. In developing goals and associated objectives, two underlying questions should always be: How can this goal be measured? What methods are currently available and what methods would be needed to show accomplishment of this objective? If these questions are raised in the planning process, then the necessary evaluation methodology can be obtained or developed as a part of the implementation process.

The determination of specific objectives and measurable outcomes for these goals play an important role in the selection of strategies to accomplish the implementation of nursing diagnosis. Oftentimes, the objective and the strategy might look like the same thing. An example of this is:

Goal:	Increase knowledge about nursing diagnosis within the RN staff
Objective:	Present educational programs on nursing diagnosis for all RNs
Strategy:	Offer the educational programs that cover identified content areas about nursing diagnosis to all RNs on the shifts
Outcome:	Based on pretest, posttest evaluation method, obtain at least a 20 percent increase on posttest scores for at least 80 percent of the RN staff

TABLE 5–6. SOME EXAMPLES OF TASK AND MAINTENENCE GOALS FOR THE IMPLEMENTATION OF NURSING DIAGNOSIS

Task Accomplishment	System Maintenence
skill in using nursing diagnosis	recruit/retain expert nurses
implement a model of nursing practice that encouraged diagnosis-based nursing practice	establish committees to support nursing diagnosis
adapt documentation system to incorporate nursing diagnosis	set-up rewards/recognition for excellence in using nursing diagnosis in clinical practice and in documentation
revise Quality Assurance Program to reflect changes in nursing practice and nursing documentation	establish mechanism for Quality Assurance results to be reported to staff with clear relationships between nursing practice and results
	incorporate nursing diagnosis and nursing process into all patient care conferences, continuing education programs, unit inservices on clinical topics
	include nursing diagnosis and nursing care planning as job description requirements and performance criteria for all levels of registered nurse

Step 5: Select Specific Implementation Strategies

The specific strategies used in the implementation of nursing diagnosis are a critical part of the implementation plan, and the selection of these strategies is the fifth step of this process. This step is concerned with the selection of strategies to accomplish the desired goals, the sequence and timeframes for these strategies and the allocation of the appropriate resources that are required by the selected strategies.

It is helpful to examine the types of strategies that can be used in the implementation of nursing diagnosis in four categories: educational strategies, clinical strategies, systems strategies, and administrative strategies. While there may be considerable overlap at times, the distinctions among categories can offer some guidance in targeting certain groups for responsibility or in making choices about sequencing and the timeframes for implementation. The strategies that might be used in each category are presented first. Many of these strategies can be used as a part of all three phases of change: unfreezing, moving or changing, and refreezing. The sequencing of the selected strategies will be discussed in Step 6.

Educational Strategies

Educational strategies play an important role in the implementation of nursing diagnosis. These strategies are a primary means for accomplishing the first level of change, change in knowledge. The concept, language, and clinical use of nursing diagnosis will be new to many nurses.

The selection of specific educational strategies must be based on analysis of the existing knowledge and experience of the nursing staff about nursing diagnosis. In many organizations there will be a great deal of variability in the knowledge levels of different categories of nursing personnel. For example, staff nurses, particularly new graduates who worked with nursing diagnosis in their educational programs, may have more information than nurse managers who are several years away from their educational experiences. There also might be both more and less knowledgeable individuals in any of the nursing job categories.

This diversity of levels of experience or knowledge about nursing diagnosis means that a variety of educational strategies are needed. One approach is classroom instruction, particularly for those nurses who have had little or no exposure to nursing diagnosis. These programs should include information about the concept of nursing diagnosis, its historical development, the role of nursing diagnosis within the scope of nursing practice, and the language of nursing diagnosis.

The diagnostic process is another topic that is helpful to present, particularly to experienced clinicians who are novice diagnosticians. Nursing diagnosis must be presented as a useful tool in clinical nursing practice. Educational strategies such as case studies and decision trees can be effective in assisting nurses with the diagnostic process and using the language of nursing diagnosis.

The nursing diagnoses approved by NANDA should be presented. A useful educational strategy is to introduce these nursing diagnoses as a starting point rather than as an all-inclusive list. This approach focuses diagnositic thinking on recognized diagnositic labels; however, it avoids the frustration of trying to make patients "fit" into nursing diagnoses when the situation might be one for which an approved label does not yet exist.

The classroom setting is also useful for presenting information about the system changes that are a part of the implementation process. Classes or workshops about new documentation formats, quality assurance criteria, or particular clinical issues and their relationship to nursing diagnosis can be very effective. Nursing diagnosis should be included in the orientation of new staff.

In order for educational strategies to be effective, the instructor must be able to make nursing diagnoses and use them effectively in clinical practice. The goal of any educational strategy must be the clinical application of the information provided. If the information provided about nursing diagnosis is too abstract or theoretical to be applied to patients, then that information cannot be incorporated into behavior, the third level of change. For this reason, educational strategies must move out of the classroom.

The classroom setting has significant limitations in teaching experienced nurses how to diagnose. Educational strategies that go to the patient's bedside should be an important part of the implementation plan. Activities such as supervised patient assessment and practice in developing nursing diagnoses, pairing nurses to review and critique each other's diagnositic techniques, and group diagnosing in patient care conferences can be used very effectively. These strategies move nursing diagnosis from the abstact, theoretical classroom to clinical practice reality, and this is essential for successful implementation of nursing diagnosis.

Clinical Strategies

Clinical strategies for implementing nursing diagnosis are those activities that take place within the context of actual nursing practice; they occur on the nursing unit, at the patient's bedside. These strategies are essential because nursing diagnosis must be applied to patients within the context of nursing practice if the implementation process is to be successful. Clinical strategies are an important mechanism for accomplishing the first three levels of change: changes in knowledge, changes in attitudes, and changes in individual behavior. If these levels of change are not successful, organizational change cannot occur.

A key factor in the success of any clinical strategy is role modeling in the use of nursing diagnosis in nursing practice. In fact, the identification and development of nurses who can provide this role-modeling function is a critical strategy in all of the categories of implementation strategies. A variety of clinical strategies for specific clinical areas are presented in the chapters in Part III.

A useful starting strategy is to identify a few nursing diagnoses that occur frequently on a nursing unit and to encourage nursing staff to work with those specific nursing diagnoses. For example, a nursing unit with a large medical cardiology population might find it helpful to begin working with the following nursing diagnoses:

Activity Intolerance related to imbalance between oxygen supply and demand
Self Care Deficit related to fatigue
Fluid Volume Excess related to dietary indiscretion
Knowledge Deficit related to new diagnosis (specify) _____

Encouraging staff nurses to begin with a few nursing diagnoses permits them to get a feel for the language and to explore the use of nursing diagnosis in a manageable fashion. As individual nurses develop skill in diagnosing patients' problems, they come to recognize the specific applications of these particular nursing diagnoses and express interest in others.

An especially useful clinical strategy is to examine the nursing care requirements of the patient population on a particular nursing unit in order to determine which nursing activities can be organized and streamlined for best effectiveness. There are a number of situations where certain aspects of nursing care for groups of patients can be predicted and provided because the patients share common characteristics. Examples of such patient situations include routine hygiene or skin care, consistent pre-operative routines, tube feeding or bowel-training regimes, safety precautions for suicidal patients, and some patient education programs.

Consider a surgical unit where the patient population is admitted the day before surgery and stays anywhere from four to seven days. By defining the pre-op routine, including appropriate patient teaching, the nurses on this unit can meet the routine, predictable needs of these patients consistently and easily. Time is then available for identifying particular patients' individual responses and dealing with these through nursing diagnoses and nursing treatment. In the absence of a clearly defined pre-op routine, time might be less effectively used in offering the routine preparations, sometimes referred to as "re-inventing the wheel." For a more detailed discussion about the role of protocols or clinical guidelines, see Chapter 2.

The choice of clinical strategies depends upon the available resources at the unit level. Consider a nursing unit with several expert clinicians who have a strong interest in nursing diagnosis. These nurses carry out clinical strategies such as giving reports using nursing diagnoses, talking about nursing diagnoses during lunch or informal discussion, developing clinical protocols or guidelines, and consulting with other nurses on patient assessment, diagnoses, or treatment questions. These clinical strategies provide role modeling for the use of nursing diagnosis, and there is also a reeducative aspect in that new ways of working with patient problems could be learned.

In the absence of strong, unit-based resources, different clinical strategies could be employed. Emphasizing diagnostic thinking in patient care conferences, presenting patient problems for group discussion and diagnosing, or consulting resources such as clinical nurse specialists or nursing faculty might be helpful in developing the diagnostic skills of the nursing staff at the unit level. Strategies that focus on this development of diagnostic skill and the ability to use the language of nursing diagnosis are an essential part of the implementation plan. The individual behavior change to working with nursing diagnosis must occur before organizational change can be accomplished.

One of the most important clinical strategies is to get everyone on the nursing unit and, indeed, within the nursing department, to begin talking about and working with nursing diagnosis. At the unit level, this means discussing nursing diagnoses for patients in report, patient care conferences, informal conversations, and any other time that patient issues are discussed. At the nursing department level, nursing diagnosis should be included in Nursing

Grand Rounds, continuing education programs, and consultation provided by other nurses, such as Clinical Nurse Specialists. Administrative meetings should provide a forum of ideas about how to support nurses in working with nursing diagnosis, as well as ways that this aspect of nursing practice should be included in administrative supervision and feedback sessions and performance appraisals.

Clinical strategies must also include activities to incorporate nursing diagnostic and treatment activity into the existing clinical practice situation. Unless nursing diagnosis and nursing process are woven into the fabric of clinical activity in the health care organization, the benefits of diagnosis-based nursing practice can not be realized. Instead, nursing diagnosis is just another task added into the busy day of the staff nurse, and it will probably be last on the list in importance.

Systems Strategies

Incorporating nursing diagnosis into clincial practice systems shifts the implementation strategies into another category, the systems strategies. Systems strategies are a critical part of the implementation plan. Only if nursing diagnosis is incorporated into the clinical practice system and culture will organizational change be accomplished.

The systems strategies and the administrative strategies share a number of concerns, and their separate presentation is for purposes of discussion only. In reality, the strategies for each of these categories must proceed together as part of a total implementation plan. The need for this is apparent in the first of the systems strategies: revising or reinforcing the model of nursing practice.

The model of nursing practice is the most important system in the clinical practice environment for the implementation of nursing diagnosis. If the model of nursing practice supports and enables the registered nurse in diagnosis-based nursing practice, then the success of the implementation process is much more likely; however, where the model of nursing practice does not distinguish between the levels of nursing personnel, or the time of the registered nurse is occupied with non-nursing tasks, then the success of the implementation process is much less likely.

The systems strategies should be selected in order to move the existing model of nursing practice toward a model that supports diagnosis-based nursing practice. This choice depends upon the characteristics of the patient population, the available personnel resources, and the philosophy of the organization. A detailed discussion of model assessment and selection is presented in Chapter 6.

The model of nursing practice is a critical factor in the delivery of nursing care. Other factors that play a role in nursing care delivery are material resources and support services. If nurses are spending their time locating equipment, reordering medications, or completing tasks for other disciplines, then there is little time or energy for diagnosis-based nursing practice. In the presence of problems in this area, systems strategies must be used to address the availability of adequate resources on the nursing unit and the delegation of non-nursing tasks such as reordering unit supplies, cleaning equipment, or emptying trash cans.

Another important system strategy is the adaption of the nursing documentation system to include nursing diagnosis. The requirements for nursing documentation is diagnosis-based nursing practice must reflect the nursing process. Assessment of the patient, organized in a nursing framework, is the first part of such a system. The identification of nursing diagnoses, based on this assessment, and the associated nursing treatments composes a major portion of the documentation system. It is also necessary to document appropriate evaluative information, again based on the nursing diagnoses, so that there can be measurement of nursing care against the standards of the organization.

Nursing documentation in a system based on the steps of the nursing process and focused on nursing diagnosis appears very different from the traditional notations seen in nurses' notes. "Appears sleeping," "Good day," "No complaints," or "Resting quietly" are general statements of opinion about the patient that have little, if any, relationship to individualized patient assessment, diagnosis, and treatment by professional nurses. Making changes in the documentation system to include the use of nursing diagnosis can be a powerful and effective systems strategy in the implementation process. Chapter 7 presents a discussion of the issues of incorporating nursing diagnosis into documentation systems, and Chapter 9 discusses the use of nursing diagnosis in nursing information systems.

Any changes in the documentation system must be supported by concomitant changes in the Quality Assurance Program. If the documentation system is based on nursing diagnoses, but the Quality Assurance Program focuses only on tasks or isolated indicators, a number of problems can result. Low scores on Quality Assurance audits, lack of feedback or reinforcement for the nursing diagnosis-based documentation system, and discouragement or frustration with the discrepancies between documentation requirements and Quality Assurance criteria are a few of the results of this situation. The role of nursing diagnosis and Quality Assurance Programs is discussed in Chapter 8.

These suggested systems strategies—a model of nursing practice revisions, documentation changes, and Quality Assurance modifications—must be supported by strategies that address personnel and job performance issues. The inclusion of nursing diagnosis as an expectation in the performance appraisal criteria for the registered nurse is a critical strategy for the implementation of nursing diagnosis. Identifying nursing diagnosis as a specific skill in the job description of professional nurses is a powerful statement about the value and importance of professional nursing practice. This also establishes the basis for a number of administrative strategies for the implementation of nursing diagnosis.

Administrative Strategies

Administative and systems strategies are closely related, and the implementation of the systems strategies will fall to nurse managers in most cases. While systems strategies are concerned with adapting, modifying, or supporting clinical practice systems that encourage diagnosis-based nursing practice, administrative strategies focus on the personnel supervision aspects of the nurse manager's role. The guidance and support that nurse managers provide as the implementation process takes place is a critical factor.

One of the most important administrative strategies is a positive attitude toward nursing diagnosis and nursing process. If nurses sense that their administrative leaders are skeptical, unsure, or negative about the implementation of nursing diagnosis, it has an effect on the implementation process. These attitudes may make other nurses hesitate to become involved in the change process.

Administrative strategies must include educational and skill development activities for the nursing leaders; activities should promote both positive attitudes about the implementation of nursing diagnosis and the necessary abilities to demonstrate its use. While nurse managers have many other demands to meet, the ability to use nursing diagnosis is essential in order to direct the administrative and systems strategies. Furthermore, these skills are essential in personnel supervision activities. Only if the nurse manager is able to use nursing diagnosis in clinical practice is it possible to provide the feedback, guidance, and supervision to nursing staff in diagnosis-based nursing practice.

In addition to setting the tone for the change to diagnosis-based nursing practice and role modeling, there are a number of other administrative strategies. An important one is the support and follow-through at the nursing unit level for the systems strategies that are a part of the implementation plan. Without this, successful implementation is highly unlikely.

Another important administrative strategy is the individual guidance, feedback, and supervision that the nurse manager provides to individual nurses. Nurses who are beginning to work with nursing diagnosis, or who are trying to improve their skills using nursing process, need encouragement and direction. This can range from verbal recognition to written statements in performance appraisals. This administrative reward for using nursing diagnosis, particularly if it is new to the nurse and involves some risk-taking, is a critical part of the implementation plan.

There are a number of ways that this administrative reward can be accomplished. Including nursing diagnosis and nursing process activities in performance appraisals is certainly a powerful and effective mechanism, but only if it is done in a positive manner. There should be emphasis on the quality and clinical accuracy of the nursing diagnoses and care plans. If the focus for performance appraisals is *only* on the number of care plans written by the nurse, with little or no attention to quality, then this approach reflects task-based nursing practice and might be perceived as punitive by nursing staff.

Administrative reward can also be provided within the context of unit systems. When the nurse manager selects a nurse who is expert in using nursing diagnosis to assist in orienting new staff, that is rewarding expert nursing practice. When the nurse manager supports a staff nurse's diagnostic or treatment expertise in a situation where a conflict arises, that is an administrative reward. Compliments and positive feedback about nursing diagnoses used in a particular patient's care plan or patient care conference can be rewarding, too.

This administrative reward strategy should not be reserved for staff nurses. Staff development instructors who incorporate nursing diagnosis into continuing education activities should be recognized. Clinical nurse specialists who base their consultation about patients on nursing diagnosis should receive acknowledgement of the benefits of this, both for the patient's care and the role modeling for nursing staff. Head nurses and supervisors who promote the use of nursing diagnosis in their areas, who design effective assignment methods to enable the professional nurse to accomplish care planning, and who are able to develop their staff members into skilled diagnosticians deserve a tremendous amount of recognition for their efforts. Nurse managers at all levels must recognize and reward the efforts of nurses at all levels to work with nursing diagnosis and to support diagnosis-based nursing practice.

Administrative reward must be combined with administrative strategies that assist and encourage nurse managers to incorporate nursing diagnosis into the clinical practice systems of their individual units or departments. Nursing directors must promote open communication among clinical and administrative leaders so that effective strategies can be shared. The problems that arise in the implementation process should be shared as well. They can provide a focus for exploring new ideas and creative problem solving.

This openness and willingness to share both problems and solutions is a critical administrative strategy. Whenever a change of this magnitude is undertaken, there are invariably problems that arise, and anxieties about these problems also surface. If these problems and anxieties are not dealt with, it may be difficult, if not impossible, to move forward with the change process.

For example, if there is a fear by several head nurses that the physicians will object to the use of nursing diagnosis, this could have a number of effects on the implementation process. If this fear is not shared or discussed, this group of head nurses might attempt to delay or halt the implementation process. This might occur by failing to schedule their staff for educational programs or consistently raising vague objections in planning meetings. These tactics can not only slow down the organizational implementation process, they can also be very distressing to those nurses who are strongly committed to nursing diagnosis and charged with carrying out the implementation plan.

If the fear about physician response to nursing diagnosis is discussed by the head nurse group, then steps can be taken to deal with it. The physicians can be surveyed for their opinions about the proposed change. In the event that the physician response is negative, then plans can be made to present information about nursing diagnosis to the physician group or to lobby more receptive physicians for support. It can also be that the physicians are in favor of the nurses using nursing diagnosis! In either case, by dealing with the fears about implementing nursing diagnosis, it is possible to move forward rather than getting stalled along the way.

The administrative strategies for implementing nursing diagnosis include a positive attitude about nursing diagnosis and nursing process, developing the diagnostic skills of nursing managers, role modeling of those skills, and providing administrative reward for diagnosis-based nursing practice. The implementation of the systems strategies falls to the nurse managers in most cases, and the follow-through for these system changes is an important administrative strategy in the implementation process. An important foundation for these strategies is open communication and willingness to share both problems and solutions that arise in the implementation process.

One strategy for the implementation of nursing diagnosis that crosses all of these categories is the use of a change agent. The activities of a formally designated change agent can be very effective. For that reason it is discussed separately.

The Role of the Change Agent in the Implementation of Nursing Diagnosis

The change agent is an individual who assists in the change process. In the change to diagnosis-based nursing practice, the strategy of selecting a change agent to guide, direct, and monitor the change process can be very effective. The types of changes included in the implementation of nursing diagnosis may cross many clinical and administrative areas, making coordination of the project a critical and challenging aspect of the change. A brief review of the role of the change agent and some specific aspects of the change agent in the implementation of diagnosis-based nursing practice are presented here.

The focus of the change agent's activity is the target population, the group that is being assisted with the change. Seven functions have been identifed for this role.[34] (See Table 5–7.) The nurse change agent is responsible for influencing a target population of other nurses to accomplish change. For the implementation of nursing diagnosis, the role of the change agent might be assumed by a number of different individuals within the nursing department. Many nurses may assume the role of change agent at different times in their practice. They generally engage in change activities as a part of their work responsibilities rather than as a full-time job.

TABLE 5–7. FUNCTIONS OF THE CHANGE AGENT

1. *Developing a need for change*
2. *Establishing a change relationship with the target population*
3. *Diagnosing the problem that the change will correct*
4. *Identifying alternative courses of action for the target population*
5. *Translating the desire to change into action so that the target population actually does change*
6. *Stabilizing the change in order to prevent discontinuance of the new behavior*
7. *Terminating the change relationship with the target population.*

(Rogers, E. M. Change Agents, Clients, and Change. In G. Zaltman, P. Kotter, & I. Kaufman (Eds.), Creating Social Change. New York: Rhinehart and Winston, 1972)

The change agent also may be formally appointed to that role. In the implementation of nursing diagnosis, it may be helpful to designate a project coordinator who can facilitate, direct, and monitor the change to nursing diagnosis. For implementation on a large scale such as an entire organization, this role can be invaluable. When the scope of the change is smaller, such as a single nursing unit, then the change agent functions can be carried out effectively by someone within the system, such as the head nurse or an experienced clinician.

In planned change, this role of formally appointed change agent has been described as the implementor-nurse change agent. In this situation the change agent does not spontaneously come forth to lead a change program but is appointed or designated by one group to develop and implement a change for another group. The implementor-nurse change agent may lack passion and dedication; however, this person has the administrative support to effect change.[35]

If it is decided to use an implementor-nurse change agent, the selection of this individual should be guided by a number of factors. First and foremost, the implementor-nurse change agent must be able to use nursing diagnosis in clinical practice, and this ability must be recognized by other members of the nursing staff. When the implementor-nurse change agent is perceived as too theoretical, or worse, unskilled in the nursing care of patients, it is very difficult for that individual to effect change in clinical nursing practice. The possession of expert power and the ability to use it effectively, are important factors to consider in selecting an implementor-nurse change agent.

A second factor to be considered is the ability of the implementor-nurse change agent to work with nurse managers effectively and collaboratively. The implementation of nursing diagnosis in any organization requires some systems strategies, and the implementor-nurse change agent must be able to assist the nurse managers with the necessary analysis of existing systems, the identification and execution of appropriate strategies to change or strengthen these systems, and the evaluation of these systems. Knowledge of the clinical and administrative systems as well as the priorities of the organization is important; however, the interpersonal skills to work closely with others on sensitive issues is also required.

Another factor in selecting an implementor-nurse change agent is the unique characteristics of the organization, especially the state of the nursing department. For example, if the implementation of nursing diagnosis involves changes in the hospital's computerized information system, then some facility in working with that system should be a factor in the choice. On the other hand, if the major focus of the implementation process is on nursing practice models and staffing issues, the implementor-nurse change agent should be knowledgeable and skilled in those areas.

The knowledge and skill necessary to direct the change to diagnosis-based practice provide a foundation of expert power for the implementor-nurse change agent. There can also be referent power, based on identification with the change agent, or legitimate power, based on internalized values relating to a standard or code of behavior.[36] Supplementing these forms of power with authority enhances the effectiveness of the implementor-nurse change agent.

Authority is the right to get others to do something by virtue of formal position in the organizational hierarchy.[37] For some implementor-nurse change agents, the authority to carry out the implementation program may be found in the line authority of their position in the organization. If the Director of Nursing or the Quality Assurance Coordinator acts as the implementor-change agent, the authority for change is located in those positions.

For many implementor-change agents, the formal authority to carry out the implementation process is found in the change agent's relationship with the nursing director or nurse managers. The position of the change agent within the administrative hierarchy must be identified clearly. If the implementor-nurse change agent is seen as external to the line of authority and as having no influence within that line, then the change agent role lacks the essential authority to accomplish change.

Consider this scenario. A clinically expert, highly-skilled instructor from the staff development department is appointed to the position of implementor-nurse change agent for the implementation of nursing diagnosis. The individual reports to the Director of Staff Development; however, this appointment was made by the Director of Nursing. This situation has the potential for a great deal of authority or very little.

The ability of the instructor to act as an effective implementor-nurse change agent depends upon several factors. One of the most important is the relationship between the Directors of Nursing and Staff Development. If these individuals are in agreement about the goals and strategies of the implementation project, including the appointment of the implementor-nurse change agent, this can offer a great deal of administrative support for the instructor. If there is disagreement or conflict at the director level, it has an inhibiting effect on the activities of the change agent.

Another important factor is the access that the instructor has to both directors. Without access, it is impossible for the implementor-nurse change agent to utilize the authority of these individuals in the change process. This access must also be accompanied by tangible activities on the part of the directors in support of the implementation process. For example, if the Director of Nursing only pays lip service to the issue of nursing practice models, the change agent will have very little success in assisting nursing units to establish defined models of nursing practice. On the other hand, were the Director of Nursing to include discussions of models of nursing practice and how to incorporate nursing diagnosis into these in all administrative meetings, that is a powerful message of support for the implementation process and the implementor-nurse change agent.

The selection of an implementor-nurse change agent should be done as early as possible. This permits the change agent to participate actively in the planning process and to begin unfreezing strategies as soon as the decision to implement nursing diagnosis has been made. During the early planning stages, the implementor-nurse change agent can capitalize on any existing frustration or dissatisfaction that can be channeled into the implementation process. This is also an excellent time to identify individuals who can act as supporter-nurse change agents.

Another change agent role in planned change is that of supporter-nurse change agent. This nurse assists the implementor-nurse change agent in the actual execution of the change program. The role of the supporter must be clearly defined and directed, and these nurses can play a key role in the implementation process.[38] For the implementation of nursing diagnosis, supporter-nurse change agents are essential to assist with the day-to-day, unit-level questions and problems that arise. Clinical nurse specialists, nurse educators, and other expert clinicians should be enlisted early in the planning process.

During the implementation process, the availability of a unit-based resource person who can answer questions, assist with diagnostic and treatment decision making, and monitor the responses of the nursing staff can make the difference between success and failure. The supporter-nurse change agents also provide a maintenance mechanism to prevent discontinuance of new practice. Channeling the energy and enthusiasm of spontaneous change agents into the role of supporter-nurse change agent can be a very effective stragegy.

The responsibilities of supporter-nurse change agents differ depending upon the clinical area and the usual role of the individual; however, there are several activities that can be very helpful. The first responsibility of supporter-nurse change agents should be as role models for the use of nursing diagnosis. This demonstration of the use of nursing diagnosis accomplishes two purposes: helping staff nurses learn to use nursing diagnosis dissipating its unfamiliarity.

The actual use of nursing diagnosis by the supporter-nurse change agents is a critical strategy for successful implementation, and the more nurses who are doing this, the greater the chance of success.

Another responsibility of the supporter-nurse change agent is to assist nurses in working within any new systems that are put in place as a part of the implementation process. Working with a new documentation system or a revised model of nursing practice can be challenging in and of itself; adding nursing diagnosis to that can be overwhelming. The supporter-nurse change agent can help in the day-to-day reeducation that must occur for these system changes to be incorporated into the clinical practice culture.

Other responsibilities of supporter-nurse change agents can be assigned based on particular characteristics of individuals and their jobs. The supporter-nurse change agent responsibilities of the staff development department will be determined by specific educational needs and programs. Nurses with special skills, such as computers or clinical protocol development, can also play important supporter roles. The available resources and the unique characteristics of the organization should be carefully analyzed for specific areas and individuals who can be utilized in the most effective and creative manner.

The selection of individuals to act as change agents is an important strategy for the implementation of nursing diagnosis. It is only one of many strategies, however. Strategies are simply part of the plan.

Step 6: Carry Out Implementation Strategies.

The implementation plan consists of the operational definition of nursing diagnosis developed for the organization, a set of broad goals with specific objectives and measurable outcomes, and a number of specific strategies. One of the most important aspects of putting the plan into effect is the timing and sequencing of the particular strategies.

For the implementation of nursing diagnosis, the timing of implementation can be approached in four stages. These four stages are:

1. Things to do *before* implementing nursing diagnosis
2. Things to do to *prepare* for nursing diagnosis
3. Things to do for the actual *implementation* of nursing diagnosis
4. Things to do to *maintain* the use of nursing diagnosis

These four stages reflect the phases of change: unfreezing, moving or changing, and refreezing. These stages are simply a more concrete delineation of those phases, specifically for the change to diagnosis-based nursing practice.

Before Implementing Nursing Diagnosis. The first stage consists of those things that should occur before the implementation of nursing diagnosis. This stage includes Steps 1 through 5, which encompasses the decision to implement nursing diagnosis, the philosophical consensus that ideally accompanies a decision of this magnitude, and the planning needed to support that decision. While much of the activity that is attendant to this process has an unfreezing effect on the clinical practice environment and culture, the unfreezing phase of change is a critical one, and it deserves particular attention.

To Prepare for Nursing Diagnosis. The second stage, things to do to prepare for nursing diagnosis, is similar to the unfreezing phase, and it is specifically concerned with getting everyone and everything in the clinical practice setting ready for change. The choice of strategies for this stage should be guided by the examination of the clinical practice culture and setting, conducted in step 2. Educational strategies might focus on presenting introductory information about nursing diagnosis within the context of existing programs. Clinical strategies that build on the current strengths and weaknesses rather than introducing new systems can lay groundwork for implementation strategies in the future.

In situations where nursing diagnosis is new for most of the nursing department, educational strategies can be useful unfreezing strategies. The programs should present information about nursing diagnosis to the learner group within a context that is meaningful rather than as a separate, discrete topic. At this point the information about nursing diagnosis would take the form of sensitizing doses as opposed to formal presentations about it.

For example, a management workshop for newly promoted nurse managers can include some information about nursing diagnosis within the evaluation process for registered nurses. Or a critical care course might discuss specific nursing diagnoses and nursing interventions for the multiple-trauma patient. A program on improving nursing documentation might introduce nursing diagnosis as an important professional trend.

Certain clinical strategies can be effective in unfreezing the clinical practice environment and culture. Revising models of nursing practice and assignment patterns can have an unfreezing effect. The examination of nursing practice necessary for the development of clinical protocols or guidelines can result in some unfreezing of the unit systems. Developing unit audit systems can provide information to analyze unit or organizational nursing practice. The congruence, or the lack of congruence, between actual and perceived nursing practice can have a powerful unfreezing effect.

Unfreezing strategies should be directed toward the individual nursing units and toward the administrative and clinical leadership. Consider approaches at the unit level first. For one nursing unit, the RN staff includes a high complement of recent graduates who were exposed to nursing diagnosis in their educational programs. One unfreezing strategy is to encourage these nurses to discuss their experiences with nursing diagnosis with other nurses on the unit who are unfamiliar with it. Conducting regular discussions in staff meetings about ways to improve nursing care planning is another way to begin the unfreezing of this unit. Encouraging the informal use of nursing diagnosis in patient care conferences and nursing care plans by *interested* nurses, and providing assistance, feedback, and recognition is another unfreezing strategy that can be used. Care should be taken with this approach, however, to avoid any elitist attitude about nursing diagnosis or nusing care planning as this can inhibit other nurses from attempting to use nursing diagnosis.

On another nursing unit, different unfreezing strategies would be used. The nursing unit whose nurses are always "too busy" to start report on time or have patient care conferences, much less do nursing care plans, needs a decidedly different approach to unfreezing. In fact, it may be that a number of systems strategies should be carried out before implementing nursing diagnosis is considered. Unfreezing strategies might consist of revising the model of practice and assignment patterns so that nursing care delivery is better organized. This unit might also benefit from developing several clinical protocols to streamline nursing care for their patient populations. The implementation of these systems strategies provides a framework for diagnosis-based nursing practice, and nursing diagnosis and improved nursing care planning can then be implemented within that context.

The unfreezing activities for the administrative and clinical leadership groups are critically important for the successful implementation of nursing diagnosis. Only if these leadership groups are genuinely in support of the diagnosis-based nursing practice is it possible to accomplish this change. Unfreezing experienced administrators and clinicians can be an extremely challenging task. These individuals may have developed their skills and expertise prior to the advent of nursing diagnosis, and the incorporation of nursing diagnosis into their thinking and working habits can be perceived as frustrating, unnecessary, challenging, or all of these.

One useful approach to unfreezing these groups is values clarification, which was discussed earlier in this chapter. Brainstorming, think-tanks, and other creative thinking activities can present opportunities to explore the issues and problems of professional nursing practice. It is essential that these sessions precede the decision to implement nursing diagnosis. The change to diagnosis-based nursing practice and the clinical thinking that accompany it must be firmly grounded in personal values. For the administrative and clinical leadership, coercive change may be necessary to start the unfreezing process, but it is much less effective in accomplishing the desired changes.

Unfreezing can be an uncomfortable time. There is a sense of loss, of giving up known, familiar activities or thinking patterns. Furthermore, the proposed replacements for these familiar habits can seem vague, risky, ineffective, or impossible to accomplish. Some examples of comments that might be heard during the unfreezing period are:

- *I think nursing diagnosis is a good idea for some patients, but not ours.*
- *Why rename what we do everyday?*
- *I already have a plan in my head.*
- *It's just a new name for the same old thing.* [39]

In selecting unfreezing strategies, there should be an effort made to address these feelings whenever possible.

Appointing a highly-respected and trusted individual as implementor-nurse change agent gives nurses a sense of confidence in the change process. Continuing certain established patterns of behavior such as walking report or clinical routines can reassure staff that everything is not being taken away from them. Soliciting suggestions and ideas from all levels of nursing is an invaluable strategy to make nurses feel involved in the change process. A thorough examination of the clinical practice environment, as discussed in step 2, will provide accurate and realistic information as well as demonstrating interest in what is really happening on the nursing units. Finally, one of the most important strategies to minimize the unsettled feelings that are a part of the unfreezing phase is maintaining open lines of communication, with frequent bulletins about the implementation process.

Unfreezing is also a time of experimentation and initial skill development with nursing diagnosis. An important strategy to minimize the frustration and anxiety of unfreezing is a clear recognition that making nursing diagnoses is different from intuition or simple problem naming; the allocation of time and energy for nurturing the development of diagnostic skills is an effective strategy. [40] This strategy can begin in the unfreezing phase, but it must continue through the actual implementation and refreezing phases.

Implementation. This stage is similar to the moving or changing phase described by Lewin. [41] At this point, the various educational, clinical, systems, and administrative strategies that were selected in step 5 are put into operation. While the specific strategies vary, there are several issues that arise in most organizations.

One issue of concern during the implementation stage is that the use of nursing diagnosis is a skill that takes time and energy for its development. A second related concern is the necessity of achieving the necessary levels of change for the use of nursing diagnosis to occur. There must be changes in knowledge about nursing diagnosis and its use, changes in attitudes toward nursing diagnosis and nursing care planning in general, and these changes must manifest themselves in changes in individual behavior, the use of nursing diagnosis in each nurse's clinical practice. For these reasons the implementation phase occupies a lengthy period of time.

These issues of skill development and levels of change necessary for individual nurses to become proficient in using nursing diagnosis are important driving forces in the implementation stage. The first implication of these issues for the implementation stage is that educational strategies are a critical first step; however, for the information about nursing diagnosis to influence clinical practice behavior, the educational strategies must focus on the application of nursing diagnoses to patient situations. Educational strategies must also be supported with clinical and systems strategies so that learning about nursing diagnosis is not lost in a practice system that continues to be task-based.

The skill-development aspect of nursing diagnosis has important implications for the implementation stage. While some nurses may welcome the clinical and intellectual challenge of identifying nursing diagnoses and appropriate nursing care plans, the more common situation is that writing a nursing diagnosis on a care plan or in a progress note feels very risky. This sense of exposing one's professional knowledge and judgment can inhibit capable nurses in their use of nursing diagnosis.

Several strategies can ease the apprehension associated with the skill-development phase of the implementation process. One strategy is to approach the implementation stage as a long-term project, the idea being that there is a discrete starting point, but no particular end. Nursing diagnosis is what is done from here on. In this approach refreezing strategies are carried out to maintain nursing diagnosis as an ongoing activity. This strategy reflects a commitment to nursing diagnosis, and it removes any anxiety about becoming an expert diagnostician in a few weeks from the implementation date.

Having an adequate number of resources and role models is another means of decreasing the apprehension of the skill-development portion of implementation. This is an important role for the supporter-nurse change agents, and there should be at least one of these resources for each nursing unit. It is easier and more comfortable for nurses to begin their work with nursing diagnosis when diagnostic questions can be answered promptly and effectively within their clinical context. This also minimizes the frustration of trying to do something new. Another benefit of this strategy is that misinterpretation of the implementation process can be avoided.

An important strategy to assist with the skill-development aspect of the implementation stage is the operational definition of nursing diagnosis. This definition can be used as a guide for questions that arise in the implementation process. Questions about the correct format for nursing diagnoses, where and how they should be documented, and the place of nursing diagnosis in the overall scheme of nursing practice can be referred to the operational definition. In the absence of an operational defintion for nursing diagnosis, it is very difficult, if not impossible, to obtain any degree of consistency in the nursing diagnoses used in the organization.

The administrative strategy of reward and recognition for nurses who use nursing diagnoses is particularly important at this stage. It is also somewhat more complex at this stage as well. As nurses are making initial attempts at nursing diagnosis, some highly creative diagnostic labels may result. The challenge is to encourage and reward the effort while tactfully correcting the language, the format, or even the clinical judgment involved.

Nurses who are beginning skill development in nursing diagnosis must be guided and directed in this process. To be most effective, this should occur on the nursing unit within the context of nursing practice activities. This guidance must be provided in a way that directs diagnostic and treatment thinking toward nursing diagnoses that are clinically accurate and consistent with the organization's operational definition. Comments, criticism, and feedback must also be offered tactfully, recognizing that the initial attempts at nursing diagnosis are risky and threatening to one's professional self-esteem.

The issue of developing skill in nursing diagnosis so that changes in individual behavior can take place is a critical one at this stage of the implementation process. Another pertinent issue is incorporation of the nursing diagnosis into clinical practice systems of the organization. Unless this is successfully accomplished, any changes in individual behavior will not be sustained or become a part of the organizational culture.

Resistance to change may occur at any point in the change process; however, during the implementation of specific strategies, resistance may take on significant proportions. Resistance to change must be analyzed and understood in order to intervene effectively. Often, change is anticipated only in terms of negative consequences for an individual or group. Other sources of resistance to change include threatened self-interest, inaccurate perceptions, objective disagreement, psychological reactance, and low tolerance for change.[42] Many of these sources of resistance can be minimized through effective planning and open communication about the planned change process.

Resistance to nursing diagnosis seems to have its basis in several related areas. The first of these is the familiarity and experience that most nurses have in using the medical model. Strongly supporting this are the rewards in the clinical practice culture for this type of thinking. Nurses who are skilled at identifying critical symptoms and assisting with medical treatments are recognized for these abilities by physicians and nurses, while expertise in nursing care planning has traditionally received little acknowledgement.

Closely related to the comfort with the medical model is the anxiety of trying something new, in this case nursing diagnosis. Furthermore, the nursing diagnosis must be written in the patient's record where it can be scrutinized by anyone. Minimizing this performance anxiety for nurses who are learning to use nursing diagnosis is essential to the success of implementation.

Another issue that may provide a stimulus for resistance to nursing diagnosis is the entry into practice debate. If nursing diagnosis is presented to nurses or perceived by them as something that only baccalaureate prepared nurses should do, then the implementation of nursing diagnosis will be highly threatening to nurses with associate degrees or diplomas of nursing. A motion was approved at the 1986 NANDA General Assembly which states:

> *Motion 23:* Moved that NANDA go on record as supporting the concept that only registered, professional nurses be responsible and accountable for identifying the nursing diagnoses for their patient population.[43]

This motion clearly places the responsibility for nursing diagnosis with the registered nurse; it does not, however, distinguish between types of educational preparation. Presenting this information *early* in the implementation discussions is a strategy to avoid some of the resistance that might be based on educational concerns.

There is a third source of resistance to nursing diagnosis that has no relationship to medical-model thinking or performance anxiety. That source is money. This resistance is based in the fear that implementing nursing diagnosis requires significant financial outlay in terms of more RN positions, educational programs, or other costly supports for diagnosis-based nursing practice. While a certain amount of financial support is necessary for the implementation of nursing diagnosis, the actual expenses depend upon the current state of the nursing department, the specific implementation strategies, and the scope of the implementation plan.

The clinical, systems, and administrative strategies needed to incorporate nursing diagnosis into clinical practice systems are highly specific for particular nursing units or patient groups. The strategies used in the critical care unit will differ considerable from those used in community health; however, whatever strategies are selected, there must be a mechanism for maintaining the systems and behaviors resulting from these strategies.

Maintaining Nursing Diagnosis. The methods for maintaining the use of nursing diagnosis must be built into the implementation plan. One of the most effective methods of maintaining a change in clinical practice is to structure the new behaviors into the systems and culture of the organization; this approach should direct many of the implementation strategies. Another important method is to establish a regular evaluation process. The information obtained through this process can be a powerful mechanism to reward practice, to detect problems or deviations from the planned change, and to reinforce the desired clinical practice behaviors.

In order to maintain the clinical practice behaviors, a mechanism is required for monitoring the use of nursing diagnosis and the systems that support its use. This mechanism should be included in the setting of goals and the identification of objectives and measurable outcomes. Most of the objectives will require regular and repeated evaluation. The maintenance stage, with its focus on evaluation and feedback, moves implementation into the next step of the process.

Step 7: Evaluate the clinical practice structure against the previously determined goals, objectives, and outcomes at appropriate time intervals

Evaluation of the implementation of nursing diagnosis is essential for three reasons. The first is that the change project must be evaluated for its success, or lack thereof, in achieving the goals of the project. This information gives direction for additional change activities, for modifying or revising existing strategies, and for identifying which strategies and activities were most or least effective.

The second reason for evaluating the implementation of nursing diagnosis is to determine the effects, benefits, or problems that are a result of the use of nursing diagnosis in clinical nursing practice for the organization. The outcomes established for the evaluation process should examine clinical outcomes for patient groups, whenever possible. Administrative outcomes such as changes in length of stay for patients or RN turnover rates should also be factored into the evaluation mechanism.

The third reason for the evaluation step is to use the information obtained in the evaluation process to reinforce and refreeze new behaviors. The first two reasons for evaluating the implementation process have to do with obtaining accurate data about its effects. This third reason is concerned with using that information to provide feedback to individual nurses and to nursing units. This information can be employed as administrative reward, as a stimulus for clinical or educational strategies, and as an indicator of the responses of clinical practice systems to the change process.

While the specific evaluation criteria must be based on the goals and objectives of the organization, these three reasons offer some general guidance for evaluating the implementation of nursing diagnosis. It is helpful at this point to review the purposes of evaluation and the activities involved in it. From this perspective, the particular issues of evaluating the implementation of nursing diagnosis can be examined.

The evaluation process consists of four activities. These are:

1. establishing the criteria for evaluation
2. evaluating goal achievement
3. assessing the variables that affect goal achievement
4. modifying the activity/structure under evaluation[44]

The first activity, establishing the criteria for evaluation, should be included in the planning for the implementation of nursing diagnosis; this was discussed in step 2. This offers a clear direction for the selection of specific strategies to use in the implementation process. It also is helpful in keeping the implementation process on target.

Evaluation Criteria. The evaluation of the implementation of nursing diagnosis must include evaluations of changes in knowledge, attitudes, individual behavior, and organizational behavior. The monitoring and data collection activities for this evaluation must occur at both the unit level and the nursing department level. Information obtained from this process should be used to reinforce and reward individual and unit practice as well as to adjust or modify implementation strategies, as indicated.

Evaluation approaches generally tend to fall into three categories: structure, process, and outcome. In the evaluation of the implementation of nursing diagnosis all three of these approaches will be needed. Structure and process criteria will be associated with certain systems strategies such as putting a defined model of nursing practice into place. There are also process criteria associated with the diagnostic skill-development part of the implementation process. Outcome criteria fall into two categories, outcomes of nurse behavior that indicate the use of nursing diagnosis and patient outcomes associated with certain nursing diagnoses or nursing interventions. This discussion focuses on the outcomes of nurse behavior as well as the structure and process criteria that indicate successful implementation of nursing diagnosis.

There are two essential areas of evaluation of the implementation of nursing diagnoses: the actual use of nursing diagnosis in clinical nursing practice and the effectiveness of clinical practice systems to support diagnosis-based nursing practice. While specific criteria vary in different organizations, these two areas serve as major themes for the evaluation process. Furthermore, the close relationship between the use of nursing diagnosis and the clinical practice systems of the organization makes the examination of both areas critical. (See Table 5–8.)

The use of nursing diagnosis by nurses in their daily practice requires changes in knowledge, attitudes, and individual behavior as well as the support of clinical practice systems. This provides an outcome measure of nurse behavior that can then be evaluated aginst specified criteria. Actual use of nursing diagnosis can be measured in a number of ways.

The nursing care plans, progress note documentation, and verbal communication in report, patient care conferences, or informal discussions are all sources of evaluation data. Formal mechanisms such as chart audits and informal strategies such as identifying themes in patient care conferences or report can be used to obtain this type of evaluative information.

The number and clinical accuracy of nursing diagnoses written in the patient record provides a great deal of useful information. One highly significant piece of information for nurse managers during the implementation process is which nurses are using nursing diagnosis and which are not. Another important finding is the clinical accuracy and relevance of the nursing diagnoses used. Are all patients receiving the same nursing diagnosis? Are new or "creative" nursing diagnoses appearing on care plans? This information can be utilized effectively in making decisions about clinical and educational strategies at both the unit level and for the nursing department.

TABLE 5—8. EVALUATION OF NURSING DIAGNOSIS IMPLEMENTATION

Use of Nursing Diagnosis in Clinical Practice	Systems to Support Diagnosis-Based Nursing Practice
Audit Patient Records for:	*Analysis of Systems:*
assessment of patient and recording of defining characteristics for appropriate nursing diagnoses	*Model of Nursing Practice*
	assignment patterns
nursing diagnoses on care plans, in progress notes	*clear definition of roles of RNs, LPNs, and other job categories*
interventions for identified nursing diagnoses	*Documentation system*
descriptive and evaluative information about the patient's responses to nursing intervention	*supports nursing diagnosis and avoids double documentation*
Unit Observation for:	*Quality Assurance Program*
use of nursing diagnosis in report, patient care conferences, inservices	*evaluates against diagnosis-based criteria rather than tasks or isolated patient indicators*
informal discussion about patients included nursing diagnoses	*RN Job Performance Criteria*
Survey/Test for:	*identifies nursing diagnosis as a job requirement*
knowledge of staff about nursing diagnosis	
attitudes about nursing diagnosis, change process, and strategies used	

It is also necessary to review the nursing diagnoses written in the patient record for their compliance with the structure criteria in the operational definition. The process criteria of the documentation guidelines also provide an evaluation mechanism. Another factor to be considered in the evaluation process is the timeliness of the documentation of nursing diagnoses. An example of this is the criterion that every patient have a nursing care plan developed within 24 hours of admission. Whether this criterion has been met can be easily determined through an audit procedure.

Another way to determine actual use of nursing diagnoses would be to tape record shift report. An analysis of task-based information and nursing diagnosis-based information can be used to identify clinical strategies to help nurses incorporate nursing diagnosis into their clinical thinking and practice. Information from tapes of shift report or patient care conferences might also provide some indication of whether unfreezing has occurred, what level of change is present, or why nursing diagnosis is or is not being used.

Monitoring and evaluation must be done within the context of the clinical practice systems and the culture of both the nursing unit and the organization. Consider a nursing unit where shift report consists almost entirely of tasks that have been done or that remain to be done. This is a busy medical unit that also has a large population of long-term, physically dependent patients. Many of these patients require tube feedings or must be fed by the nurses, and there are always several patients with tracheostomies, wounds, or isolation procedures.

The nursing staff on this unit works hard. Patients are turned and gotten out of bed; skin breakdown is a rare occurrence. Family members are often complimentary of the nurses' care and attention; however, only a few patients have nursing care plans, and the nursing documentation consistently falls below the Quality Assurance standard.

It is not surprising that shift report focuses on task-accomplishment, which is probably not a bad thing in view of the needs of this patient population. The monitoring and evaluation of nursing diagnosis on this unit must be done within the context of the clinical realities. For instance, clinical strategies to streamline routine nursing care activities for the patients on this unit should be one of the first implementation approaches, and its effectivenss then can be one of the first evaluation activities. If these strategies are not effective, the clinical practice environment will offer little, if any, support for the use of nursing diagnosis.

This example demonstrates the close relationship between the evaluation of the use of nursing diagnosis and the systems that support its use. Monitoring those systems during their implementation is a critical strategy if those systems are to be incorporated into the clinical practice culture. This is a critical responsibility for nurse managers.

The monitoring and evaluation of individual knowledge, attitudes, and behavior is an important strategy for front line nurse managers. In order to offer direction and guidance to the nurses under their supervision, nurse managers must have accurate, objective data about how nursing staff are actually using nursing diagnosis. The establishment of mechanisms for collecting this information and then using it to assist nurses in developing their diagnostic skills is a critical administrative strategy; it is one that plays a very important role in implementation and refreezing.

The establishment of monitoring mechanisms at the unit level should be guided by a number of factors. The first of these is the operational definition of nursing diagnosis. This definition sets the criteria for the format and use of nursing diagnosis. Other factors that have a significant effect on these monitoring mechanisms are the documentation guidelines for the nursing department, particularly if this is one of the systems strategies for implementation, and the Quality Assurance Program for the organization.

These individual and unit evaluations can be compiled into an evaluation of the nursing department. For this to be effective, however, there must be enough consistency in the unit-based evaluation, so that trends, results, or problems with implementation can be determined for the nursing department as a whole. A balance must be struck between obtaining the information that is pertinent to a departmental analysis of the use of nursing diagnosis, and the unit's needs to collect specific data that is unique to their patient populations. For example, all nursing units should evaluate the timeliness of nursing care planning and the clinical relevance of nursing diagnoses and nursing interventions. Specific data about the insertion of invasive lines or equipment used in the care of the patient have a higher priority for evaluation in the critical care or emergency area than in the medical/surgical areas.

Goal Achievement. The evaluation of goal achievement for the implementation of nursing diagnosis is a long-range evaluation, of necessity. Evaluation activities for the implementation of nursing diagnosis fall into two groups: monitoring activities and goal achievement evaluation. The determination of goal achievement in many cases may not be possible for months or years, depending upon the scope of the changes involved in the implementation process. During that time monitoring of progress toward goal achievement is essential.

Setting the criteria for goal achievement must be included in the initial planning for implementation. A critical component of this is the identification of timeframes and specific criteria to be monitored on a regular basis. Beginning the monitoring process fairly soon in the implementation of nursing diagnosis can provide very useful information about the effectiveness of change strategies, the responses of the nurses to the change, the resistance to the change that is present, and any problems that may be developing.

By starting to monitor fairly early in the change process, two things can be accomplished. The first is the availability of information, which can be used to modify or adapt the change strategies and to provide feedback for individuals and nursing units. Early monitoring also helps identify the use of interim behaviors that indicate progress toward the goals and outcomes of the program. This recognition of interim behaviors is important because refreezing of these interim behaviors should be avoided as this could result in significantly different outcomes than those specified in the implementation plan.

The levels of change may be used as a guide for the monitoring aspect of the evaluation process. Accomplishing organizational change means time must be allocated for the first three levels of change: changes in knowledge, changes in attitudes, and changes in individual behavior. Before the evaluation of the organizational change can be done, it is necessary to evaluate these other levels. Monitoring changes in knowledge, attitudes, and individual behavior can be used as a strategy both to provide reinforcement of new behaviors and as the components of a larger evaluation mechanism.

Examine this process for one nursing unit. This unit has completed its unfreezing stage, and several implementation strategies have been initiated in the last six months. An introductory educational program has been presented to all nursing staff, and many of the staff nurses are curious about nursing diagnosis and interested in trying to use it. There has been discussion in the last two staff meetings about changes in the model of nursing practice that would support the RNs in using nursing diagnosis. Another system strategy has been put into place in conjunction with the pharmacy department to decrease the amount of time that the RNs spend reordering medications.

Evaluation activities at this point should begin with monitoring changes in knowledge and attitudes. The educational strategies can use a pretest, posttest methodology, and the posttest can be repeated at regular time intervals. The changes in attitudes can be monitored through the topics, tone, or quality of discussion about nursing diagnosis in staff meetings. The willingness, or lack of it, to explore changing clinical practice systems might be another helpful indicator of attitudes. A staff survey of attitudes or the use of values clarification exercises in staff meetings are other strategies that can be used to monitor and evaluate attitudes during the change process.

As sytems strategies are put into place on this unit, the evaluation of individual behavior becomes more important. If a systems strategy is to modify the model of nursing practice on the unit, one evaluation strategy would be to monitor nurse-patient assignments to determine whether these were consistent with the model of practice. If individual nurses are not making nurse-patient assignments that meet the guidelines for the model, then individual change has not occurred. Organizational change takes place when most, if not all, of the nurses are using the assignment guidelines; this is dependent upon individual behavioral change in the majority of the nurses.

Changes in individual behavior could also be detected on this unit through audits of the patient records. This is particularly true if the implementation strategies include documentation changes. If a few venturesome RNs are making attempts toward using nursing diagnoses in their documentation, this would be a positive indicator that individual behavior change was beginning. At this point role modeling, administrative reward, and clinical guidance would take on critical significance as implementation strategies. Assisting these nurses in their efforts and encouraging other nurses to begin using nursing diagnosis then will provide more nursing diagnoses in the patient records for review and evaluation.

This example illustrates again that the evaluation of the use of nursing diagnoses and the clinical systems for nursing practice must proceed together. This example also gives an indication of the amount of time involved for reaching goal attainment. On a unit where a model of nursing practice revision and major documentation modifications are required, the successful implementation of nursing diagnosis can occupy the better part of two years or more.

Setting time frames for goal achievement should be done generously, and frequent, regular monitoring of progress toward those goals is essential.

The levels of change that are necessary for organizational change to take place can provide a framework for this monitoring process. In this way, the conditions present on nursing units and in the organization can be compared to the requirements for diagnosis-based nursing practice. (See Table 5–1.) The implementation plan and strategies can then be modified, adapted, or changed in order to maintain progress toward goal achievement.

Variables that Affect Goal Achievement. One variable that affects achieving the goal of diagnosis-based nursing practice is the state of the clinical practice systems. This is a critical variable, and its role and strategies to address it have already been discussed; however, there are a number of other variables that can be included in the evaluation activities. The decisions of which ones should be a part of the evaluation depends upon the unique characteristics and needs of the organization.

A variable that comes first to mind for many nurses when considering the implementation of nursing diagnosis is staffing. The numbers of available staff and the mix in job categories of nursing staff is an important variable. A number of studies have examined the use of specific models of nursing practice; however, there is very little information available about the effects of staff mix and the implementation of nursing diagnosis.

One reported study does examine the costs of nursing care on one unit with a predominantly RN staff (72 percent) and one unit with a more traditional staff mix of 40 percent RNs, 40 percent nursing aides, and 20 percent LPNs.[45] On both units RNs were asked to identify nursing diagnoses for their patients. An established engineering technique measured direct nursing time. The salary cost of delivering direct nursing care averaged over $25 per day *less* on the RN staffed unit. Halloran suggests that more staff may not be the answer, but a shift to more qualified staff that can deal with total patient needs can be a cost-effective strategy.[46]

More research in this area is necessary, and the evaluation of the implementation of nursing diagnosis can provide important descriptive information. Staffing variables that should be factored into the evaluation process are staff mix, educational preparation, experience levels of RN staff both in nursing practice and in using nursing diagnosis, and attitudes of nursing staff. Attitudes toward nursing diagnosis can be an important variable in the implementation process. One factor that influences attitudes toward nursing diagnosis is the evolving state of nursing diagnosis. Those nurses who are uncomfortable with ambiguity, flexibility, or change may have less positive attitudes toward nursing diagnosis. This can be a critical variable in planning strategies for those nurses and also in interpreting the evaluation data on units where such attitudes may be prevalent.

The attitude variable should not be limited to attitudes toward nursing diagnosis. Professionalism, autonomy, and job satisfaction are other attitudes that can provide important information in planning, monitoring, and directing the implementation process. Two other areas where evaluation of attitudes may offer useful insight are attitudes toward patient populations and attitudes toward management styles used on the nursing unit. These areas require different approaches for their evaluation, but they can yield useful information for modifying the implementation process or for reasons why the process is encountering difficulties.

A variable that is related to nurse staffing is the availability and quality of the services that support the nursing unit. Pharmacy, linen, housekeeping, food and nutrition services, or central supply all can have a tremendous impact on the nursing care delivery on nursing units. If linen and supplies are unavailable, if the medication carts are stocked inadequately or incorrectly, and if the arrival of meal trays is unpredictable, nurses find themselves tied up dealing with these situations. The time spent dealing with these issues is time that is lost from professional nursing practice.

The support services variable varies in different organizations. In many situations it should be included in the pre-implementation assessment, planning, and subsequent evaluation of the implementation process. When the implementation plan calls for systems strategies to address problems with support systems, the evaluation of these strategies provide very useful information. This variable also should be examined for nursing units where implementation activities are not progressing as well as they could be. It may be that the time nurses spend on obtaining the necessary supplies or services for patient care may be interfering with professional nursing practice.

Another important variable that influences the implementation of nursing diagnosis is the patient population. A critical factor is the evolving state of nursing diagnosis. Certain clinical specialty areas have a relatively large body of research and literature describing the application of nursing diagnosis. Journal articles and textbooks present nursing care, using nursing diagnosis, for medical/surgical nursing[47,48] critical care,[49] and neuroscience nursing.[50] Other areas such as pediatrics and maternal-child have fewer resources to guide the clinical application of nursing diagnoses for these patient populations.

The acuity of the patient population also can have an effect on the implementation of nursing diagnosis. This reflects both physiologic instability and the rapid turnover seen in some patient groups. In both situations the nurse's time with the patient is occupied with a great deal of medical management activity, and this time crunch is further exacerbated by the short time period that the nurse has available for assessing the patient and indentifying nursing diagnoses.

The presence of any of these variables should be identified in the implementation plan, and evaluation criteria established at that point. Consideration of variables that affect the implementation process can occur through the identification of specific strategies to address these. For example, for a nursing unit with an average length of stay of 3 days, implementation strategies can include a very specific, concise initial nursing assessment tool that assists in identifying nursing diagnoses. This tool also could serve as both initial assessment and care plan. The nursing diagnoses and other clinical information recorded on this tool, the timeliness of its completion, and the ease of use for the nursing staff would be the major areas for evaluation of this strategy.

Modifying the Evaluation Criteria. Certain variables might indicate that the timeframes for implementation should be modified. For a nursing unit with a number of unfilled RN positions, evaluation of the implementation process may need to be adjusted to reflect the staffing situation. Monitoring changes in knowledge, attitudes, and individual behavior should still occur; however, the criteria that deal with aspects of organizational change must be interpreted within the context of the clinical practice reality. Evaluating this unit against a criterion such as 90 percent of patients will have a nursing care plan initiated within 24 hours can and probably should still be done. When only half of the budgeted RN positions are filled, a finding that only 35 percent of patients met this criteria will be very disheartening for that staff unless there is a description of the staffing shortage along with the score on the evaluation.

A number of variables can influence the implementation process, and they must be taken into account in the evaluation process if the evaluation is to be meaningful. Some of these factors are numbers of available staff, staff mix, educational preparation, attitudes, level of experience, the availability of support services, and the characteristics of the patient population, including acuity and length of stay. The purpose of evaluating the effects of these variables is to identify their role and influence on the implementation of nursing diagnosis. This information then can be used to interpret the evaluation data, modify the implementation strategies, or in identify new or different strategies.

CONCLUSION

The implementation of nursing diagnosis is the first step in establishing diagnosis-based nursing practice. Moving nursing practice from the use of the medical model for clinical thinking, from a focus on tasks and chores, is a major exercise in cultural transformation. The process of change is seldom easy, and the change to using nursing diagnosis, as the foundation of clinical nursing practice, involves changes in knowledge, attitudes, individual behavior, and organizational behavior for all nurses and many others in the health care organization.

One of the most helpful hints for implementing nursing diagnosis is to recognize the magnitude of the change that is involved. It can be extremely comforting to the change agents, to supporters of this change, and to the nurses at all levels who are trying to change to realize that planned change can take years to accomplish. While it is essential to set goals for the implementation of nursing diagnosis, and these goals may be very ambitious, it is absolutely essential to allow enough time for goal achievement. Unrealistic timeframes can be fatal to the change project, as well as to the hopes and dreams of those nurses who are committed to the implementation of nursing diagnosis.

Another helpful hint concerns the response to resistance. It is effective to approach resistance as a positive, active response to the change activities. While the response may be more active and less positive than is desirable, resistance indicates that people are listening, thinking about, and responding to the issues of nursing diagnosis and professional practice. This is better than having these issues ignored or treated in a blasé fashion. In fact, for the change agent with a stout heart and hardy spirit, stirring up resistance can be a highly effective strategy to bring hidden anxieties and fears about nursing diagnosis out into the open. These anxieties and fears may be tremendous blocks to the implementation process as long as they are hidden. By airing these concerns and identifying strategies to address them, the implementation process can continue to move forward.

It is also helpful to recognize that change rarely occurs in a homogeneous manner. Some individuals make the changes to diagnosis-based nursing practice very quickly and easily, some accomplish this only with great difficulty, and some nurses may never be at ease with nursing diagnosis. The same is true for nursing units. A nursing unit predicted to make the change to diagnosis-based nursing practice easily and smoothly may encounter unanticipated problems. Another unit that seems to lack many important resources and supports may do very well.

Implementing nursing diagnosis may be new for many nurses, nursing units, and organizations. The unpredictability of planned change projects in general, and the implementation of nursing diagnosis in particular, makes the monitoring and evaluation component of the implementation process essential. Only if there is a mechanism to obtain measurable, objective data about the implementation process, can the necessary modifications and adaptations be made.

Living through a major change process can make people react in a highly subjective fashion. Changing thinking and working habits can be perceived as risky or threatening, and the resulting anxiety can cloud judgment. While subjective evaluation and certain assumptions can be very useful in many situations, it is essential that there are clear and precise goals, objectives, and outcome criteria for the change process. Without the guidance provided by these tools, the change process can get bogged down in details, personal reactions, and vague apprehensions.

It is important to realize that in a change of this magnitude there are going to be times when the individuals directing the change may disagree. Differences of opinion can be very distressing, especially when there may be only a small core of individuals acting as change agents, and the environment is still significantly unfrozen and unreceptive to the idea of implementing nursing diagnosis. If it is possible to use these differences of opinion constructively, by all means do so. There may also be points where it may be best to leave the issue alone for awhile. Remember, it is going to take years to accomplish this change; there is plenty of time.

In keeping with the same theme of working together to implement nursing diagnosis, the establishment of supportive peer groups or work groups can be a very effective strategy. Formal groups, such as the Care Planning Committee or the clinical nurse specialists, can provide a great deal of professional and personal support for individuals during the change process. Informal groups can and should be encouraged, as well. The "diagnosis for lunch bunch," where interested nurses can meet and discuss diagnostic problems and challenging patients, can be productive and fun. Journal clubs, casual discussions in the nurses' lounge, staff meetings, and nursing rounds on the unit are just a few ways to deal with both the clinical issues of nursing diagnosis and the support that nurses need in attempting this change.

One last helpful hint is this: Have fun with nursing diagnosis! Nursing diagnosis offers a challenge to all nurses, to examine nursing practice and the ways in which nurses go about it. An approach that sees the humor as well as the serious issues can go a long way toward diminishing some of the anxiety associated with change. There is enough stress and pressure in the practice of nursing; efforts must be made during the implementation of nursing diagnosis to avoid adding to it if at all possible. Humor, peer support, and an optimistic attitude can be highly effective implementation strategies.

The implementation of nursing diagnosis must be approached as an organizational change, affecting knowledge, attitudes, individual behavior, and the clinical practice culture. In order to accomplish this, careful and deliberate planning is essential; this change is too large and unwieldy to be undertaken lightly. Including monitoring and evaluation methodologies from the beginning of the process provides valuable information on which to base decisions about modifications of the plan and goal achievement.

Meeting the requirements for diagnosis-based nursing practice is the driving force for the implementation process. The establishment of a philosophical base for the use of nursing diagnosis at all levels of the nursing department is an essential requirement. An adequate number of nurses who can use nursing diagnoses effectively in clinical practice is the foundation of diagnosis-based nursing practice; however, the use of nursing diagnosis in clinical practice must be supported by the clinical practice systems of the nursing unit. The following chapters in this section will present a more detailed discussion of the assessment, planning, and implementation strategies for the clinical systems that are needed to support diagnosis-based nursing practice.

REFERENCES

1. Jacox, A. Role restructuring in hospital nursing. In L.H. Aiken & S.R. Gortner (Eds.), *Nursing in the 1980s: Crises, opportunities, challenges.* Philadelphia: J.B. Lippincott, 1982
2. Palisin, H.E. Nursing care plans are a snare and a delusion. *American Journal of Nursing,* 1971, *71,* 1, 63
3. Benner, P. *From novice to expert: Excellence and power in clinical nursing practice.* Menlo Park, CA: Addison-Wesley, 1984
4. *Ibid.*
5. Massie, L., & Douglas, J. *Managing—A contemporary introduction.* Englewood Cliffs, NJ: Prentice-Hall, 1973

6. Hersey, P., & Blanchard, K. *Management of organizational behavior: Utilizing human resources* (3rd ed.). Englewood Cliffs, NJ: Prentice-Hall, 1977
7. Massie & Douglas
8. *The Merriam-Webster Dictionary.* New York: Pocket Books, 1974
9. Mauksch, I.G., & Miller, M.H. *Implementing change in nursing.* St. Louis: C.V. Mosby 1981
10. Hersey & Blanchard
11. Mauksch & Miller
12. *Ibid.*
13. *Ibid.*
14. *Ibid.*
15. Zaltman, G., & Duncan, R. *Strategies for planned change.* New York: John Wiley & Sons, Inc., 1977
16. Lewin, K. Frontiers in groups dynamics: Concept, method, and reality in social sciences; social equilibrium and social change. *Human Relations,* 1947, *1,* 1, 5
17. Lancour, J. Implementation of nursing diagnosis: acute and long-term care settings. In M.E. Hurley (Ed.), *Classification of nursing diagnoses: Proceedings of the sixth conference.* St. Louis: C.V. Mosby, 1986
18. Steele, S.M. Values and values clarification. In S.M. Steele & V.M. Harmon, *Values clarification in nursing* (2nd ed.). Norwalk, CT: Appleton-Century-Crofts, 1983
19. Deal, T.E., & Kennedy, A.A. *Corporate culture: The rites and rituals of corporate life.* Reading, MA: Addison-Wesley, 1982
20. *Ibid.*
21. Steele
22. *Ibid.*
23. Steele
24. Lancour
25. *Ibid.*
26. Deal
27. *Ibid.*
28. Goldstein, H. & Horowitz, M.A. *Utilization of health personnel: A five hospital study.* Germantown, MD: Aspen Systems Corp., 1978
29. Toth, R.M. Reimbursement mechanism based on nursing diagnosis. In M.J. Kim, G.K. McFarland, & A.M. McLane, *Classification of nursing diagnoses: Proceedings of the fifth national conference,* St. Louis: C.V. Mosby, 1984
30. *The Merriam-Webster Dictionary.* New York: Pocket Books, 1974
31. Lancour
32. *Ibid.*
33. McFarland, G.K., Leonard, H.S., & Morris, M.M. *Nursing leadership and management: Contemporary strategies.* New York: John Wiley & Sons, 1984
34. Rogers, E.M. Change agents, clients, and change. In G. Zaltman, P. Kotter, and I. Kaufman (Eds.), *Creating social change.* New York: Holt, Rhinehart, and Winston, 1972
35. Mauksch, & Miller
36. McFarland, Leonard, & Morris
37. *Ibid.*
38. Mauksch & Miller
39. Young, M.S., & Lucas, C.M. Nursing diagnosis: Common problems in implementation. *Topics in clinical nursing,* 1984, *5,* 4, p. 70
40. Lancour
41. Lewin
42. McFarland, Leonard, & Morris
43. Approved motions from NANDA general assembly, seventh national conference, 1986. In A.M. McLane (Ed.), *Classification of nursing diagnoses: Proceedings of the seventh conference.* St. Louis: C. V. Mosby, 1987
44. Alfaro, R. *Application of nursing process: A step-by-step guide.* Philadelphia: J. B. Lippincott, 1986
45. Halloran, E.J. RN staffing: More care—less cost. *Nursing management,* 1983, 14, 9, 18
46. *Ibid.*
47. Thompson, J.M. et al. *Clinical nursing.* St. Louis: C.V. Mosby, 1986
48. Carpenito, L.J. *Nursing diagnosis: Application to clinical practice.* Philadelphia: J.B. Lippincott, 1983
49. Roberts, S.L. *Physiological concepts and the critically ill patient.* Englewood Cliffs, NJ: Prentice-Hall, 1985
50. Snyder, M., Ed. *A guide to neurological and neurosurgical nursing.* New York: John Wiley & Sons, 1983

CHAPTER 6

Models of Nursing Practice: The Basis of Diagnosis-based Nursing Practice

Judith Rocchiccioli and Brenda B. Colley

The model of nursing practice is the most important organizational structure in the implementation of nursing diagnosis. A defined model of nursing practice must support the professional nurse in practicing in a manner that is diagnosis-based, rather than task-based. While issues about nursing practice models are not new, there are a number of factors in the current health care climate that make the establishment of a model of nursing practice based on nursing diagnosis more important and more complex.

There are four recognized models of nursing practice: functional nursing, total patient care, team nursing, and primary nursing. These models of nursing practice, also referred to as nursing care delivery systems, have developed as part of the historical evolution of nursing itself. Each model has specific attributes and characteristics in a defined combination; however, in the clinical practice environment, many nursing units may incorporate characteristics from more than one model into their individual nursing care delivery system, although one model may be predominant. This chapter will describe the characteristics and attributes of each model. An examination of these characteristics for their support of diagnosis-based nursing practice will be followed by specific strategies for incorporating nursing diagnosis, within the context of nursing process, into each model.

The Benefits of a Defined Model of Nursing Practice

The benefits of changing to an effective model of nursing practice on a unit are significant. It has been suggested that an effective, professional nursing practice model could insure increased job satisfaction among nurses, thus lowering turnover and increasing productivity. In a study of five nursing units in three hospitals, the implementation of a professional nursing model that incorporated nursing diagnosis resulted in signficant increases in job satisfaction, nurses' attitudes toward organizational effectiveness, and patient satisfaction.[1] Kron states that job satisfaction in nursing comes from being able to provide quality work and knowing that the quality is recognized and appreciated.[2]

When the expectations for nursing care delivery are clearly defined in a professional model, feedback about job performance is clear, accurate, and linked with day-to-day activities. Feedback needs to be genuinely positive when positive feedback is indicated. Critical feedback needs to be given fairly and tactfully. An appropriate model of nursing practice provides the opportunities and the structure for the registered nurse to obtain these types of feedback, an essential part of job satisfaction.

Another component of job satisfaction that results from a defined practice model is the support it provides for multidisciplinary team work. Collaborative relationships between the interdisciplinary team members are improved with well-defined role responsibilities. Change strategies that support the continued work of the multidisciplinary team should be included in the planning process.

Health Care Trends

Offering quality patient care in the face of an extreme nursing shortage will be the challenge of nursing in the 1990s and throughout the first quarter of the 21st century. The nursing shortage is real, already present, and intense. It poses a serious threat to the quality of health care services. The shortage of qualified nurses is nationwide, and particularly acute in the Middle Atlantic, Pacific, and East North Central regions of the country.[3] Nationally the vacancy rates for registered nurses in hospitals more than doubled between 1985 and 1986, up from 6.3 percent to 13.6 percent according to a recent survey conducted by the American Hospital Association.[4] It also was found that 83 percent of hospitals reported RN vacancies in 1986, compared with 65 percent in 1985.[5]

Of further concern to nursing leaders is the decreasing number of qualified applicants applying for basic nursing education programs. Data reported in 1987 by the National League for Nursing showed enrollments down 4 percent in Baccalaureate programs, down 8 percent in Associate Degree programs, and down 18 percent in Diploma programs as compared to similar data collected in 1984.[6] While the number of graduates has increased in all levels of basic education except Diploma programs, this number of nursing graduates is insufficient to cover the present demand for qualified nurses today.

The anticipated demand for nurses in the future is significantly greater than the current need. Additionally, the U.S. Department of Health and Human Services predicts an imbalance in the educational preparation of registered nurses. By 1990 the nation will face a shortage of 390,000 nurses with bachelor's degrees and a surplus of 368,000 of nurses with associate degrees and diplomas.[7] A number of trends are directly related to the present nursing shortage, and these make it more important than ever to determine the best nursing model for the institution.

Changes in health care reimbursement have resulted in a decreased length of stay for the hospitalized patient, with a simultaneous increase in acuity. The patient population is older and sicker, has multiple system involvement, and has more chronic problems than ever before. Furthermore the technology is increasingly complex and rapidly changing. In a review of its patient acuity and nursing productivity, one hospital found that in 1969, 42.3 percent of their patients were ambulatory and that nursing salaries accounted for 17.8 percent of the hospital budget. In 1985 only 18 percent of the patients were ambulatory; however, the percentage of the hospital budget spent on nursing salaries decreased to 14.7 percent despite a major increase in the hiring of more costly RNs over LPNs and aides.[8]

Another trend of significant importance in health care today is increasing consumer awareness and perceptions of quality care. Kalisch[9] predicts that by the year 2010 the health care market will be influenced heavily by some type of "Buyers Guide" for consumers. Developed for the consumer public, it will include drug information data, present charge rates and fees; it also will report overcharging by health care providers, data concerning length of stay, surgical morbidity rates for physicians, infection rates, and malpractice suits against hospital and professionals.

All of these factors affecting the health care environment—a nursing shortage, increasing patient acuity, consumerism, and prospective payment—exert tremendous pressures on nurses and nursing. Nursing must not lose the ground it has gained in the last 25 years as it has moved toward professionalism. It is absolutely essential the best method be determined for offering high-quality, professionally directed nursing care. The selection of the most appropriate model of nursing care for the unit and institution determines how care is delivered. The use of nursing process and nursing diagnosis within the framework of diagnosis-based nursing practice will facilitate organization of nursing care and assure the quality of its delivery.

THE NURSE AND THE MODEL OF NURSING PRACTICE

While nursing process describes how one nurse plans and carries out nursing care for a particular patient, a nursing practice model describes how a group of nurses, such as the nursing staff assigned to a particular nursing unit, provides care for an entire group of patients. A carefully selected nursing practice model, incorporating the use of nursing diagnosis, will support diagnosis-based nursing practice—the key to the future in planning and organizing nursing care.

A review of nursing literature describes three distinct models of nursing practice: functional nursing, team nursing, and primary nursing. A fourth model, which is frequently found in clinical practice but not well-defined in the nursing literature, is total patient care. In addition to these, a new model called case management is making an appearance in a variety of nursing care settings. Modular nursing is another term sometimes used, describing a nursing practice model that is actually a geographic patient assignment format in which an RN and one or two other nursing personnel provide nursing care for patients located in a particular area or module.

The following definitions of these major models of nursing practice will be used throughout this chapter.

Functional Nursing:	An assembly-line method assigns each nurse to perform a specific task or set of tasks for every patient.
Team Nursing:	A group of nursing personnel, including LPNs and nursing aides, are led by an RN team leader in providing care for a group of patients.
Primary Nursing:	A single RN is responsible and accountable for providing comprehensive nursing care to a group of patients during their entire hospital stay; delegation of tasks to non-RN personnel is reduced but not eliminated.
Total Patient Care:	A single RN is responsible for providing the nursing care to a group of patients for one shift. Nurse accountability does not extend beyond that shift.
Case Management:	An extension of primary nursing whereby an RN provides care prior to, during, and after hospitalization, including telephone consultation and home care visits.
Modular Nursing:	An RN accompanied by one or two other nursing personnel provide care for a group of patients located in a particular geographic area.

The development of functional and team nursing occurred prior to the introduction of the nursing process, the recognized model of thinking for the nursing profession. Over the years, new models of nursing practice emerged, and a number of adaptations were made in these older models. One of the most important modifications in these recognized models of nursing practice is the incorporation of nursing process.

Nursing process is basic to nursing practice regardless of the model. Gordon describes nursing process as a problem identification and problem-solving approach to client care that is the basis for building a helping relationship characterized by knowledge, reason, and caring.[10] Through nursing process, the professional nurse directs patient care by using nursing diagnosis to name patient problems and to guide treatment of these. This is diagnosis-based nursing practice.

The role of the professional nurse in any model of nursing practice includes:

1. Assessing patients needs
2. Diagnosing real and potential patient conditions
3. Determining observable, measurable patient outcomes
4. Planning specific patient interventions
5. Evaluating outcomes and reassessing patient needs

In order to provide an efficient system of safe patient care, the nursing practice model must support the professional role of the nurse in diagnosis-based care planning and in nursing care delivery. In order to accomplish this, there must be congruency in the philosophy of nursing service and the selection of a nursing care delivery modality.

To survive in the competitive, cost-constrained health care environment of today, nursing service departments must develop efficient systems for delivery of safe patient care. The most efficient care delivery system is dependent upon staff numbers, mix, and experience, as well as the characteristics of the patient population, particularly patient acuity. The purpose of this chapter is to review the current accepted models of care delivery, and to present specific strategies and examples that incorporate nursing diagnosis into these models. Particular emphasis will be placed on analysis and assessment of the nursing unit, as well as systems planning to incorporate the use of nursing diagnosis.

MANAGEMENT CONSIDERATIONS

One of the first and most critical responsibilities of the unit management team is an analysis of the model of nursing practice that is currently in use. This assessment should include the philosophy and values of the management team and unit staff as well as the logistical and staffing issues. In the event that a model change is indicated as a part of the implementation of nursing diagnosis, there are a number of issues that must be considered.

Clues that a change is needed may be very specific, such as low quality assurance scores in documentation of nursing process. Indications for a change may also be very subtle, such as dissatisfaction of nursing staff about assignments, tasks, and interactions among staff. Such dissatisfaction may be seen in high turnover rates for staff and lack of participation in patient care conferences and staff meetings. Failure to complete special projects and intershift conflict are further evidence that a change is needed. Additional clues may include incomplete work assignments, decreased patient satisfaction with nursing care as evidenced by complaints, deterioration of nurse/physician relationships, JCAHO standards that are not attained, and increased absenteeism.

Two distinct stages of change are essential for managers to consider and accomplish if change is to be effective: diagnosis and implementation.[11] In diagnosing a need for change and determining what change may be appropriate, nurse managers should attempt to describe what is happening now, what will happen if no change occurs, what ideally needs to happen, and what are the constraints in moving toward the ideal.

Specific areas of assessment should include demographic data, quality assurance, scores, nurse satisfaction/nurse turnover, patient length of stay, patient acuity, and allocations of nursing staff. Other assessment data include patient satisfaction in relation to nurse's technical skills, educational/teaching abilities, and counseling and communication skills. Staff meetings, assignment methods, change of shift report, patient care conferences, staff orientation, paper flow, and patient education systems also should be examined as critical aspects of the nursing care on the unit.[12] No matter what the result of the assessment, the reality of the unit situation must be considered.

A strategy to assist nurse managers in this assessment is the development of a consultative service within the department of nursing. This approach has been used at the Medical College of Virginia Hospitals to help nursing units identify and implement appropriate models of nursing practice.[13] Here, nursing units were assisted with both the diagnostic and implementation stages of accomplishing a change in the model of nursing practice. A critical aspect of this consultative process was the selection of the model with the best fit for the patient care requirements, staff numbers and skill mix, and the philosophy of nursing of the nursing unit staff and management. Specific criteria for model selection will be presented in each individual model discussion later in the chapter.

Selection of a nursing practice model that best fits the nursing unit is followed by the implementation stage. An extremely important part of implementing the chosen model is careful planning and structuring of the model change. This planning is best done at the unit management level.

The unit management team is the cornerstone to the success of any model of nursing care delivery. The team consists of the head nurse and the assistant head nurses. Other leadership positions on the unit, such as clinicians, practitioners, teachers, or permanent shift charge nurses should also be considered as a part of the team. The unit management team, collectively and individually, are accountable for planning, decision making, and problem solving around the anticipated model change. Responsibilities of team members are found in Table 6–1.

TABLE 6–1. MANAGEMENT TEAM RESPONSIBILITIES IN MODEL IMPLEMENTATION

1. *Acting as role models and teachers*
2. *Monitoring the quality of nursing care as evidenced by depth and completeness of nursing history and physical assessment, nursing diagnosis, nursing plan of care, documentation of care, patient education, discharge planning, and patient care conferences based on the nursing diagnosis format*
3. *Evaluating staff individually and assisting them to formulate objectives for development and enhancement of clinical skills, communication skills, nursing process skills, and the ongoing development of appropriate, accurate nursing diagnoses*
4. *Problem-solving around obstacles and difficulties that may arise or do arise that impede the practice of the designated model of nursing care*
5. *Determining goals and timetables for implementation of the planned model change*
6. *Supporting, complementing and challenging the professional growth of the nursing staff*
7. *Planning developmental programs to meet individual staff members' learning needs*
8. *Designing orientation of new staff to incorporate the principles of the model of care delivery*
9. *Maintaining all systems (including clerical, educational and unit) to provide a nursing process/nursing diagnosis-based model of care delivery system*
10. *Incorporating nursing process and nursing diagnosis into overall employee performance evaluations*

In order to ensure the success of a model, the management team must subscribe to the philosophy of the model. As a team, they must identify the strengths of the unit as well as obstacles to both changing the model of practice and working with nursing diagnosis. While considering strengths and weaknesses, the team must define short- and long-term goals to support the change to the selected model of nursing and diagnosis-based nursing practice.

The management team must be able to communicate these goals clearly to their unit staff and to hospital and nursing administration. The goals of this planned model change must fit and must be congruent with nursing administration and institutional goals. For instance, implementation of primary nursing on a unit reflects a philosophical commitment to independent, autonomous nursing practice. However, if the personnel resources allocated to that unit are predominantly new graduates who have not yet developed the necessary skills for autonomous nursing practice, there is a lack of fit between the expressed philosophy and the decisions regarding resource distribution. Any nursing care delivery change is doomed to failure unless common philosophies and goals are shared by the unit and the health care organization.

Planning for Change

Preparing for a change in a model of practice requires deliberate and strategic planning. A classic theory of the change process developed by Lewin has three main phases: unfreezing, moving, and refreezing.[14] Nursing management must determine the necessary strategies for these phases based on their assessment of the existing practice model and their goals for the change project.

It is imperative to have clearly articulated goals as a foundation for developing a comprehensive change plan. While the interest and discussions about a new model of practice or working with nursing diagnosis will provide preliminary unfreezing of the environment, the unfreezing step is critical, and the change plan should include specific steps for it. Although a comprehensive plan is needed at the outset of change, adaptations will need to occur throughout the process as assessment data indicates.

Implementation of change is simply the translation of assessment data into goals and plans, strategies, and procedures.[15] Change strategies should be identified for each stage of Lewin's three phases: unfreezing, changing, and refreezing. Specific strategies for each phase are discussed in the next section.

Unfreezing. A strategy frequently used for unfreezing is the empirical rational strategy that is based on the assumption that people are rational and will adopt change if there is reason to justify the change and if they will experience some gain from the change.[16] For example, simply sharing unsatisfactory nursing process scores with staff, or sharing assessment findings that include a summary of staff preference for a model of nursing may be all that is necessary for unfreezing a unit.

Educating the staff to a different method of delivering nursing care, one that provides more benefits than the presently used model of care is an essential strategy. This is a normative-reeducative strategy.[17] This strategy educates so that attitudes and values are altered to allow a commitment to a new method of care delivery.

The power-coercive strategy,[18] in which the more powerful direct the less powerful, is a third unfreezing strategy. Such a strategy may include a nursing administrative decision that all nursing units will practice one particular model of nursing, based on an assessment by nursing administration of elements in the environment. This may be the most appropriate strategy when nurses are reluctant or unwilling to change. Use of this strategy may be necessary after other strategies have failed to result in planned change. It is important to recognize that change that occurs as a result of this strategy is often short-lived, as the desire to change is a response to an administrative threat and does not alter an individual's value system.

Moving. Once a nursing unit is unfrozen, the nurses are ready for change. After a unit assessment has been completed and an appropriate model of nursing has been selected, deliberate and strategic planning needs to occur prior to implementation of the model. Beyers suggests the use of planning techniques when designing and implementing change that involves many people and various departments.[19] Use of a planning format also serves as an information tool about the change, allows people to prepare for change adequately, and conveys that the expectation for the change is serious business and not just "talk."[20]

In order to ensure successful change, it is important that staff nurses feel and be an important part of the change process. This can be accomplished by having staff nurses serve on committees where they can have input in the decision-making process and the change plans. Improved motivation and satisfaction result from being involved, which can be factors in recruitment and retention of qualified nurses.[21]

The moving phase of the change process is dependent upon the quality and specificity of the change plan. Indeed, with a well-defined plan for change, with clearly articulated goals, objectives, and strategies, the moving phase simply consists of carrying out the plan. While the reality of making change is not quite so simple, this aspect of change can be greatly facilitated through the existence of a clear plan for the change. Further discussion of the change process is presented in Chapter 5.

Refreezing. Refreezing is the process in which the changes that have been made are internalized and incorporated into daily practice. When implementation of the model has occurred, refreezing strategies are initiated so the change will be maintained. Implementation of a model of nursing practice is perhaps the easy part. Maintaining that change may be quite difficult, and this requires the use of specifically planned refreezing strategies.

One specific strategy to accompany refreezing is to incorporate the desired behaviors into orientation of new personnel. This allows the new staff to practice the chosen model, thus supporting the present staff in their practice change.

Another refreezing strategy is the generous use of positive feedback. This can come from administration when looking at reduced turnover, improved nursing process scores, or improved morale of nursing staff. Patients may also be a source of positive feedback by speaking directly to the nursing staff or in filling out patient satisfaction surveys. The key element is that the nurses must hear the good news so they will feel the change has been worth the effort and must be maintained.

Recognition is another useful refreezing strategy. Once an effective model has been made, it is worthwhile to allow personnel from the unit to share their practice changes through nursing grand rounds or nursing newsletters. These strategies will vary depending on the organization, and this can be an opportunity for a great deal of creativity.

A critical refreezing strategy is accurate and effective evaluation. Evaluation of a model of nursing practice is essential to its success and to the quality of patient care. The evaluation process, which must occur at regular and frequent intervals, also provides another opportunity for feedback, enhancing the satisfaction levels of the nursing staff. An essential role of the nurse manager is to monitor the quality, accuracy, and appropriateness of the nursing care plan. The use of nursing diagnosis as the framework for nursing process allows for a smooth flow between the elements of nursing process; therefore, evaluation of the clinical relevance of nursing diagnosis is an important part of the evaluation process.

The actual evaluation of the model of care should encompass four areas: task completion, patient satisfaction, nurse satisfaction, and institutional satisfaction. Specific strategies for monitoring task completion are presented in Table 6-2. These questions can be used to develop assessment tools for an individual unit.

Evaluation of patient satisfaction may be monitored through surveys and interviews with patients. Informal feedback to the nursing staff as well as the physician should be considered in this evaluation, too. Evaluation strategies to monitor patient satisfaction must be deliberate.

Nurse satisfaction may be evaluated through assessment of turnover rates, absenteeism, and ongoing feedback. Formal tools have been developed and can be developed to survey nurse satisfaction with the model. For instance, a Level of Concerns tool developed by Hall can quickly identify problems prevalent in the care delivery system.[22,23]

Evaluation of institutional satisfaction should take into account perceptions of nursing care by physicians, hospital administrations, fiscal analysts, and allied health professionals.

Young and Lucas identify major problems in the refreezing phase.[24] One of these is lack of reinforcement. For refreezing to occur, reinforcement must be continuous. When the desired behaviors are demonstrated by role models, nurses learn the desired skills quickly and easily. Immediate, consistent positive feedback for the desired actions can then serve to promote and sustain the desired nursing model. Intermittent reinforcement may be utilized after the initial change has occurred.

Another problem is the lack of goals, outcome criteria, and evaluation. It is difficult to sustain or maintain a model of nursing practice if there is ambiguity in what is to be done, or the standards against which the nurse will be evaluated are unclear. (See Chapter 5 for a discussion of goal setting and evaluation of the implementation of nursing diagnosis.)

Still another problem is refreezing the wrong thing. Particularly when a change project is large and complex, there may be interim behaviors which indicate progress toward goals. If these interim behaviors are refrozen, rather than continuing in the change process until goals are accomplished, the results of the change project may be very different than anticipated.

Refreezing strategies are mandatory for the continued success of a model change. Strategies should be directed toward continuous and intermittent reinforcement as well as clearly defined goals, outcome criteria, and evaluation standards of both patient care and staff performance.

MODELS OF NURSING PRACTICE

The selection of a model of nursing practice must be based upon a number of factors: hospital and nursing philosophy, patient acuity and case mix, patient length of stay, numbers and mix of professional and nonprofessional staff, and development and skill of professional nurses. The variability of these factors at the nursing unit level means that there may be a number of

---

TABLE 6–2. MONITORING TASK COMPLETION

1. *Are assignments completed?*
2. *Are assignments made in a manner consistent with the model of nursing practice and appropriate to the level of staff?*
3. *Are all personnel practicing at their highest level?*
4. *Are some levels of staff consistently working overtime while others always leave on time?*
5. *Are ongoing assessment and care planning occurring?*
6. *Are unit systems efficient and effective?*

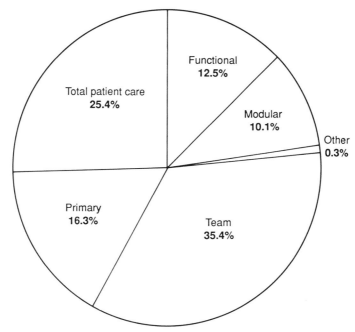

Figure 6–1. Use of nursing practice models. *(From AHA's New Data Shed Light on Hospital Staffing,* American Journal of Nursing, *1984, 84, 6, 809).*

different practice models in one institution. For instance, a hospital may practice functional, team, and primary nursing on different nursing units. Should this be the case, then institutional philosophy should ascribe to the use of different models, and it must allow for the flexibility and autonomy necessary to maintain a varying model practice structure. (See Fig. 6–1.)

Historical Development. It is interesting to note that the oldest model of nursing practice began in the late 1800s, when one nurse had total nursing responsibility for the patient. The private duty nurse often lived in the patient's home and provided nursing care that was highly individualized, including grooming, providing comfort, and cleaning house. The nurse worked under the auspices of a physician and performed very few skilled activities. The hospital boom between 1900 and 1910 moved nurses into the hospital,[25] but nurses continued to be directed by the physician to complete tasks.

After World War I patients were more often treated in hospitals than in their homes, and there was usually only one registered nurse or practical nurse to a ward. Of necessity, the focus shifted from individualized patient care to a task-oriented checklist approach. Functional nursing became prevalent after World War II when large numbers of less skilled health care workers were available for minimal pay and industrial engineering techniques were popular. Organizing patient care was done in the most functional manner with the nurse working directly under the umbrella of the physician. LPNs, nursing aides, and orderlies became the main source of hospital labor, while RNs were removed from the bedside to perform managerial functions.

The effects of having too few registered nurses to provide adequate supervision of task-trained personnel led to the development of team nursing. The team leader was responsible for assigning tasks to the team members and for supervising the delivery of nursing care. Initially, the tasks were divided functionally with the aide completing baths, the LPN performing treatments, and the RN administering medications. The work of the team was defined by tasks that needed to be completed in a given shift rather than providing responsive care over an extended period of time. This description may seem very familiar to nurses practicing in today's health care organizations.

Total patient care evolved as a way to allow a nurse to accept total responsibility for a patient for one shift of care. Unlike the team nursing and primary nursing models which resulted from specific, planned development, total patient care does not have widespread recognition.[26]

Physician-controlled and directed nursing practice continued for the first half of the twentieth century, until nursing education moved to the academic centers and away from hospital nursing programs. With the advent of college-educated nurses, the profession began to search seriously for ways to provide holistic nursing practice—a result of the science and liberal arts backgrounds experienced by college- and university-educated nurses. A growing need for professional accountability for meeting patient needs using a theoretical basis for nursing practice perhaps led to the development of primary nursing.[27]

Each of the models being discussed has evolved as a result of changing resources in personnel or needs of the health care organization. While each model has its own design characteristics, they also share commonalities with other models. Each of these models, with the exception of functional nursing, can be used to accomplish professional nursing practice using nursing diagnosis. The requirements, guidelines for selection, and strategies to implement each model are discussed in the next section.

Functional Nursing

Functional nursing is the method of organizing nursing tasks to maximize the technical skills of nursing service personnel. In this modality, one professional nurse supervises the care of a large number of patients. Thus nursing care is provided by many levels of nursing personnel, each completing tasks they are trained to do.[28] Tasks, not patients, are assigned to personnel so that the tasks requiring the least skill are assigned to the least skilled staff member. A typical assignment sheet for a unit employing functional nursing will outline task responsibilities, such as charge nurse, medication nurse, treatment nurse, and bedside care nurse.

Although functional nursing is still utilized in many health care settings, the basic drawback remains that the patient's needs are often lost in the process of completing tasks. In addition, job satisfaction for nurses and patient satisfaction with nursing care are minimal. Functional nursing does not allow for holistic patient care, assessment of patient needs, nursing autonomy, clinical judgment or decision making, or diagnosis-based nursing practice.

Even though functional nursing is the least desirable modality of nursing from both holistic and professional viewpoints, economic and staffing constraints may foster its use. The realities of clinical practice might dictate that a functional model may have to be used for short periods of time when professional nursing staff is inadequate. For example, as a result of sick calls, the staffing mix on a very busy medical-surgical nursing unit might consist of one RN, one LPN, and two nursing assistants. Although the usual model of nursing might be team, in this situation staffing is inadequate to practice in that model. Consequently, short-term use of a functional modality might be appropriate.

It must be emphasized, however, that functional nursing is not conducive to professional nursing practice. If the usual modality of practice is functional, consideration should be given to moving toward a model that encourages professional practice and focuses on holistic patient care.

Team Nursing

Team nursing is a method of organizing nursing care in which nursing personnel of all levels are assigned to a team, and the team is responsible for a specific group of patients.[29] A nursing team is composed of the RN team leader and team members who may be RNs, LPNs, aides, and clerical staff. Professional leadership of smaller teams allows closer supervision of auxiliary staff.

Team nursing is founded on the belief that nursing is patient centered and that care is best delivered through the functioning of a team. Quality of care is linked directly to the abilities of the charge nurse and team leader in supervising and evaluating task completion and in executing collaborative functioning of team members.[30]

The team leader is responsible for assessing, diagnosing, and planning for each patient's care. This responsibility may also be delegated to another professional nurse on the team. The nursing care plan is then carried out by various team members. The team must think of themselves as a cohesive group with the skills of individual members valued and utilized. This calls for sensitivity and responsiveness to each other, as well as to patients, and communication among team members is essential. In essence, a professional nurse coordinates the activities of the team and is accountable for the nursing care delivery on that shift. The staff use all their skills in completing their assignments. For example, LPNs might administer medications to patients as well as complete treatments and give bedside care.

Integrating nursing process and nursing diagnosis into the team model is absolutely essential for the maintenance of quality care. In the absence of an individualized patient care plan, nursing care may become generic to all patients of similar medical diagnoses, inconsistent from shift to shift, responsive to physical but not psychosocial needs, depersonalized, or disorganized. The common language of nursing diagnosis and comprehensive care planning incorporated into a team nursing approach can promote holistic care for the patient.

Team nursing is the most widely used model in hospitals today. (See Fig. 6–1.) Brown suggests that team nursing is the dominant model of nursing today because of the economic benefits.[31] These economic benefits include the substitution of lower-paid employees with less skill for higher-paid professional nurses and a reduction in the time and expense of training nursing personnel.

Roles.   There are three roles in team nursing: charge nurse, team leader, and team member. To ensure professional practice, the charge nurse and team leader must be registered nurses. In addition, a registered nurse may function as a team member. Regardless of which role the RN assumes, the identification of nursing diagnoses and a nursing care plan will be an important aspect of that role.

The charge nurse is the designated RN who has overall accountability for all patients on the nursing unit for the assigned shift. The charge nurse is responsible for maintaining overall shift functioning and decision making. She functions as primary communicator with allied health professionals and hospital departments concerning unit functioning. The charge nurse also serves as resource and collaborator for her staff. Table 6–3 lists the charge nurse's responsibilities.

The team leader is the RN designated to provide for the health care needs of a group of patients through assessing, diagnosing, planning, implementing, and evaluating nursing care. The team leader directs and supervises team members and is accountable for all patients assigned to the team. (See Table 6–4). Identifying nursing diagnoses based on nursing assessment and formulating a plan of care to meet the patient's needs is a major responsibility of the team leader. Delegation of work load among the team leader and team members must

TABLE 6–3. CHARGE NURSE ROLE IN TEAM NURSING

1. *Making team assignments and reviewing individual patient care assignments with the team leader*
2. *Maintaining significant working knowledge of each patient's status and dynamic changes throughout the shift*
3. *Making rounds of all or specific patients every shift and prn, observing patient condition and the environment*
4. *Assigning unit operational tasks to be completed*
5. *Serving as resource for team leaders concerning patient care issues, conflict management, or problem solving*
6. *Assuming a minimal patient care assignment and/or serving as team leader*
7. *Assessing and arranging staffing for the oncoming shift*

be done so that the team leader has the time and opportunity to fulfill this function. An essential function for team leaders is the direction of team members to implement the care plan and to provide feedback for updating the plan.

The team member is the individual designed to provide for the nursing needs of assigned patients. Team members are accountable for the nursing care delivery that is congruent with their skill levels, job descriptions, and state practice acts. Table 6–5 describes the team member's responsibilities.

Team nursing lends itself to development of new graduates by allowing them to "pair" with an experienced nurse to progress from initial skill development toward comprehensive patient care and indepth diagnosing and care planning. Precepting provides an ideal method to accomplish role transition. Developing the team member or team leader requires a concentrated effort by all staff and unit management. Table 6–6 lists the criteria by which to assess the readiness of a team leader candidate.

Of critical importance to the successful practice of team nursing is the internalization of the concepts of cooperation and collaboration. The "spirit" of team nursing must be fostered in orientation, in clinical practice, in problem solving, and in care planning. Cooperation and collaboration are evidenced in unit pride and in quality care. Lack of these essential concepts may lead to unit dysfunction, fragmented practice, nurse dissatisfaction, and increased nursing turnover.

TABLE 6–4. TEAM LEADER ROLE IN TEAM NURSING

1. *Maintaining a thorough working knowledge of each patient's status throughout the shift*
2. *Making patient assignments for the team, matching team member's skills with patient needs. Assignment-making includes providing coverage for breaks and meals, educational activities, and meetings*
3. *Assuming or delegating to RN team members responsibility for formulating nursing diagnoses and care plans*
4. *Delegating responsibility for special assignments to individual team members*
5. *Serving as the central team communicator within the team, between teams, with the charge nurse, and with other disciplines*
6. *Making patient rounds on the team prior to and following report and prn*
7. *Checking periodically with team members for task completion/workload and providing assistance as needed*
8. *Processing new orders on team patients and delegating to team members as appropriate*
9. *Reviewing lab data and test results and communicating information to appropriate personnel*
10. *Delivering and documenting patient care to a minimal number of patients as determined by unit need and team leader responsibilities*
11. *Monitoring documentation of team members*
12. *Planning/conducting patient care conferences*

Criteria for the Selection of Team Nursing. The appropriateness of implementing team nursing on a specific nursing unit is dependent upon a careful analysis of criteria for conversion to team nursing. An important criterion is philosophical agreement between hospital and nursing management, between nursing management and unit management, and between unit management and unit nursing staff. Lack of congruency in philosophy of care will result in failure to successfully implement the model, potentiate nurse turnover, and generate dissatisfaction.

A second criterion is staffing. Numbers, mix, and experience of staff must be analyzed. There must be one RN for each team for each shift. The proportion of RNs to ancillary staff is less than required for primary nursing, but more than needed for functional nursing. The number of nurses who can administer medications must be sufficient to handle the work load without converting to functional nursing.

Nursing turnover in team nursing does not appear to have as detrimental an effect as may be seen in other nursing practice models. For successful team nursing it is important to have a core group of experienced, clinically skilled, registered nurses to maintain safe, quality practice. With an experienced, capable team leader, new nurses, float nurses, or other nursing personnel who are not familiar with the unit can be incorporated into the team with relative ease because their activities are guided and directed by the team leader; however, chronically overloading the team leader with new or unfamiliar team members can have a detrimental effect, and this should be avoided.

One modification of team nursing that may enhance professional nursing satisfaction and patient satisfaction is to superimpose a primary documentation responsibility onto the team nursing model. While the daily assignment of patient care may best fit the team model, the assessing, diagnosing, care planning, and evaluating of nursing care for a given number of patients may be assumed by one RN. This primary documentation nurse is responsible for directing the patient's care from the time of admission to the time of discharge. The primary documentation nurse makes appropriate referrals, plans for discharge, facilitates patient care conferences, and provides patient teaching. In this adaptation of team nursing, the primary documentation nurse must interact with the patient frequently, but may not necessarily deliver the nursing care every day. This modification may be ideal for units that desire to provide continuity of professional nursing care for their patients but lack the staff numbers or skill mix required in other nursing practice models.

Total Patient Care

Total patient care is a method of organizing nursing care in which the professional nurse is accountable for the assessing, diagnosing, planning, implementing, and evaluating of nursing care to an assigned group of patients for one shift of duty. Total patient care differs from

---

TABLE 6–5. TEAM MEMBER ROLE IN TEAM NURSING

1. *Maintaining thorough working knowledge of assigned patients*
2. *Making rounds with the team leader and prn*
3. *Delivering and documenting patient care to an assigned number of patients using all skills and requesting assistance as needed*
4. *Communicating to the team leader patient status and environmental concerns ongoing throughout the shift*
5. *Participating in patient care conferences and team conferences, contributing information for nursing diagnoses and care plan formulation*
6. *Assisting other team members with tasks as needed*

TABLE 6–6. ASSESSING READINESS TO BECOME A TEAM LEADER

1. *Determine the applicant's knowledge of team nursing*
2. *Assess knowledge of and past experience with the nursing process*
3. *Assess present knowledge of and use of nursing diagnosis*
4. *Determine ways that the applicant feels orientation to team nursing and nursing diagnosis might best be facilitated*
5. *Assess knowledge of nurse applicant's technical skills; after assessment, a comprehensive orientation to the team model must be systematically planned; the plan should be goal directed, evaluative, and include the individual goals of the future team leader and the institution; implementation of this plan needs to be initiated early in unit orientation*

primary nursing in that the nurse is accountable for patient care only for the assigned shift rather than throughout a patient's specific unit stay or overall hospital admission. Thus, overall patient care may be fragmented due to the number of possible care givers during the course of his hospital stay.

Total or comprehensive patient care are bywords that became popular in the 1950s.[32] Brown suggests that total patient care falls on a continuum between team and primary nursing in relation to job design characteristics.[33] There is, however, little in the literature that describes total patient care as a modality of nursing care, but rather as one of the components of either team nursing or primary nursing. Essential elements of total patient care include autonomy, accountability, and responsibility delegated on a shift-to-shift basis. Autonomous practice requires staff with developed clinical, theoretical, communication, and documentation skills.

While total patient care is appropriate for short-term settings, it is not as supportive of diagnosis-based nursing practice in longer-stay areas. Due to the professional requirements of assessing, diagnosing, and care planning for the patients, total patient care as a modality of care requires an all-RN staff. Assignments are made that utilize each staff member's talents and abilities.

Roles. There are two roles in total patient care: charge nurse and total patient care provider. The charge nurse is the designated RN with overall accountability for all patients on the unit, responsibility for maintaining unit work flow and decision making, and who functions as collaborator and resource for other nursing staff. (See Table 6–7).

The total patient care provider is a RN designated to provide for the health needs of a group of patients through diagnosing, planning, implementing, and evaluating patient care, and is accountable for the assigned patients for the shift of duty. This RN is the central communicator between the interdisciplinary team and the assigned patients, and is available to other care

TABLE 6–7. CHARGE NURSE ROLE IN TOTAL PATIENT CARE

1. *Maintaining significant working knowledge on each patient's status and dynamic changes throughout shift*
2. *Making rounds on all or specific patients, observing patient status and environment*
3. *Making assignments matching patient needs and staff skills*
4. *Delegating unit operation tasks as appropriate*
5. *Serving as resource to total patient care providers concerning patient care issues, conflict management, or problem solving*
6. *Providing and documenting patient care to assigned patients*
7. *Assessing and arranging staffing for the oncoming shift*

TABLE 6–8. PATIENT CARE PROVIDER IN TOTAL PATIENT CARE

1. *Maintaining a thorough working knowledge of each assigned patient's status*
2. *Making rounds on assigned patients*
3. *Providing and documenting comprehensive patient care to assigned patients*
4. *Assuming responsibility for formulating nursing diagnoses and care plans*
5. *Processing orders for assigned patients*
6. *Reviewing lab data and test results, and communicating information to appropriate personnel*
7. *Communicating changes in patient's condition to the charge nurse and physicians*

givers as a resource and a collaborator. Table 6–8 describes the responsibilities of the total patient care provider.

Criteria for Selection of Total Patient Care. Total patient care is best selected as a system of nursing care delivery in situations when nurse-patient interaction is time-limited, such as in the recovery room, ambulatory surgery, ambulatory care setting, or the emergency room. Ideally the length of stay should be less than 24 hours. Total patient care should not be the model of choice when patients have special emotional or physical needs that require a long-term, trusting relationship. At times, total patient care may be appropriate when the RN staff is unwilling or unready to accept responsibility for meeting the patients' needs on a continuing basis.

As in team nursing, continuity of care from shift to shift is possible only when the professional nurse communicates patient care needs through an individualized plan written in a common language—that of nursing diagnosis. For instance, a patient admitted to ambulatory surgery for a therapeutic abortion might be diagnosed to have Anxiety related to situational crisis: abortion. Effective nursing interventions identified by the admitting nurse can best be communicated to nurses on following shifts through the written plan of care. Indeed, in the absence of a consistent care giver, the written plan assumes critical importance.

Primary Nursing

Primary nursing is a system of nursing care delivery in which the registered nurse is account-able for assessing, diagnosing, planning, implementing, and evaluating patient care for a specific patient from the time of admission to the time of discharge. Primary nursing is both a philosophy and a modality of professional nursing care delivery that focuses the nurse's attention upon patient outcomes rather than tasks.[34] Primary nursing is concerned with keeping the nurse at the bedside, actively involved in "hands on" patient care while planning comprehensive, goal-directed, individualized nursing care.

The primary nurse is responsible for the initial assessment of the patient and for formulat-ing the initial nursing diagnoses. As patient situations and conditions change, other nurses may assume these responsibilities while caring for a primary nurse's patients. Of great importance in primary nursing is the concept that there can be no rigid rules or guidelines because the patient and each nurse is unique.

A review of the literature[35–37] indicates considerable confusion about many of the opera-tional elements of primary nursing. The confusion seems to be both in clearly understanding what these attributes are as well as how to locate, hire, or develop these attributes in potential primary nurses. The most critical of these elements are accountability, authority, assertiveness, commitment, and communication. Without possessing these elements it is impossible to guarantee success in the practice of primary nursing.

Brown suggests that the key word in primary nursing is accountability.[38] Zander states,

"Primary nursing makes the distinction between task responsibility and case-outcome accountability."[39] Responsibility is the means to an end, while accountability is answering for the results or outcomes of responsible actions.[40] For example, an outcome for a patient with the nursing diagnosis Ineffective Airway Clearance related to thick secretions might be breath sounds will be clear, bilaterally by (specified date). The nurses on each shift are responsible for carrying out the prescribed interventions in the nursing care plan and monitoring the status of the patient's breath sounds and any response to the interventions. The primary nurse is accountable for establishing and evaluating the effectiveness of the plan. This is accomplished by comparing the state of the patient and the outcomes. If the outcomes are met or there is movement toward these outcomes, then the primary nurse and the plan have been successful.

Many nurses have exhibited considerable fear and anxiety regarding the primary model. Some of these fears have been that they would constantly be plagued on their off days or that there would be a greater legal liability in primary nursing; however, liability for patient care is not altered in any model of practice. Zander states that "the product of nursing service is not nursing care, but rather the individualized set of outcomes of care for each patient."[41] The impact of this statement cannot be underestimated. Outcomes are observable and measurable in terms of physical and emotional status, activity levels, and knowledge. Primary nurses are evaluated on the outcomes of patient care, and not the tasks and responsibilities performed by staff nurses on a day-to-day basis. In essence, accountability speaks to the overall evaluation of patient outcomes and not the evaluation of the implementation of patient care.

If the primary nurse is to be held accountable for patient outcomes, then the authority must be given to practice autonomously and make independent nursing decisions. It is essential for administration not only to grant this authority, but to support autonomous practice. Both clinical and administrative policies and systems must support this type of nursing practice.

The use of nursing diagnosis in the primary nursing model offers an important contribution to independent, autonomous nursing practice. By clearly identifying the patient conditions for which the primary nurse has assumed treatment responsibility, nursing diagnosis serves as an important communication mechanism and as a way to evaluate the nursing care provided by the primary nurse. The clarity and direction for assessment, nursing care planning, and outcome evaluation provided by nursing diagnosis make the use of nursing diagnosis a key element in a primary nursing model of practice.

Roles. There are four roles in primary nursing: primary nurse, associate nurse, charge nurse, and assistant nurse. The role of the primary nurse is central to the successful implementation of the primary nursing model. The primary nurse is a registered nurse who has accountability, authority, and autonomy for the delivery of quality nursing care for an assigned group of patients from admission to discharge from a unit. Table 6–9 lists the primary nurse's responsibilities. The primary nurse must have demonstrated clinical competency in the delivery of nursing care and must have a thorough knowledge of nursing assessment and nursing diagnosis or must be in the process of being actively developed as a primary nurse.

The associate nurse is responsible for assisting in patient care planning in the absence of the primary nurse and for performing those nursing functions delegated by the primary nurse. The associate nurse is accountable for setting short-term goals and implementing interventions on that shift. The associate nurse is not responsible for long-range planning. It should be clearly noted that associate nurses may also function as primary nurses for their own designated groups of patients. (See Table 6–10.)

In essence, associate nurses "step" into the primary nurses' role of providing direct care in accordance with the nursing diagnosis care plan in the absence of the primary nurse. It is

TABLE 6–9. PRIMARY NURSE ROLE IN PRIMARY NURSING

1. Assessing and identifying patient problems at admission and throughout hospitalization on a nursing history and physical assessment form
2. Developing accurate, appropriate nursing diagnoses based on patient assessment at admission and throughout hospitalization
3. Initiating, evaluating, and updating the patient care plan for the nurse's primary patients
4. Delivering direct comprehensive safe patient care to primary and other assigned patients
5. Maintaining a thorough working knowledge of each assigned patient's status
6. Accepting responsibility for special assignments as delegated by the charge nurse
7. Planning and conducting patient care conferences based on the nursing diagnosis format for the nurse's primary patients for purposes of staff development and communication
8. Delegating specific tasks to deliver effective patient care when necessary
9. Formulating patient education and discharge plans using appropriate methods provided by the institution
10. Maintaining clinical and professional competence through educational programs

not unlikely that associate nurse may care for another nurse's patient for a lengthy period of time based on the realities of nursing practice; however, the associate nurse still must work collaboratively, collectively, and cooperatively with the primary nurse.

The charge nurse is the designated registered nurse accountable for overall unit functioning on a given shift. Facilitating unit work flow as well as collaborating with nursing staff for clinical decision making and problem solving are principle responsibilities of the charge nurse. The charge nurse on a primary nursing unit should have extensive expertise in nursing diagnosis in order to be a resource for other staff members as they gather assessment data and determine appropriate nursing diagnoses based on documented patient needs. Table 6–11 describes the charge nurse's responsibilities.

The assistant nurse is responsible for providing nursing care to selected patients in accordance with the nursing care plan. (See Table 6–12.) The assistant nurse may be an RN, LPN, aide, or nursing student. Responsibility for care planning does not belong to the assistant nurse. Changes in patient status requiring an immediate updated plan of care are the responsibility of the charge nurse. Registered nurses who are developing their skills as primary nurses may function initially as assistant nurses. In situations where primary or associate nurses are not available, such as absenteeism, vacations, reassignments to other units, an assistant nurse may be assigned to care for select patients.

TABLE 6–10. ASSOCIATE NURSE ROLE IN PRIMARY NURSING

1. Assisting with identifying patient problems, formulating nursing diagnoses, and updating the care plan throughout hospitalization in the absence of the primary nurse
2. Delivering direct, comprehensive, safe nursing care to assigned patients
3. Maintaining a thorough working knowledge of each assigned patient's status
4. Communicating and collaborating with charge nurse and other disciplines in the absence of, or as delegated by, the primary nurse
5. Accepting responsibility for special assignments as delegated by the charge nurse
6. Assisting in patient care conferences based on a nursing diagnosis format as directed by the primary nurse
7. Implementing patient education and discharge plans under the direction of the primary nurse in congruence with institutional procedure and policy
8. Seeking appropriate consultation for knowledge and skill development
9. Maintaining clinical and professional competency through planned inservices and self-development education programs

TABLE 6–11. CHARGE NURSE ROLE IN PRIMARY NURSING

1. *Maintaining a significant working knowledge on each patient's status and dynamic changes throughout the shift*
2. *Serving as a resource to other staff members when determining pertinent and correct nursing diagnoses based on assessed and/or perceived patient need*
3. *Reviewing staffing for oncoming shifts based on patient acuity and census*
4. *Checking with all care givers for task completion and workload*
5. *Delegating unit operation tasks such as narcotic count and emergency equipment checks*
6. *Supporting attendance at patient care conferences and staff inservices; these conferences should be designed to utilize a nursing diagnosis format*
7. *Documenting patient information according to a nursing diagnosis format and according to hospital and nursing policy*
8. *Assigning responsibility for setting short-term goals in the care plan when assistants are registered nurses*

Criteria for the Selection of Primary Nursing. As with the other models of nursing practice, there must be several criteria present in order to convert to primary nursing. The most important criterion is the presence of a group of experienced, professional registered nurses who are capable of autonomous nursing practice. Assertiveness and communication skills are essential requirements for nurses practicing primary nursing. Efforts to implement primary nursing in the absence of this criterion, or lack of adequate steps to achieve this criterion, will most probably result in frustration at best or failure at worst.

Another very important element essential to successful implementation is congruency in philosophies of the health care organization, the nursing administration, and the nursing unit. This philosophy must subscribe to the belief that holistic care is important, that primary responsibility produces nurse satisfaction and patient satisfaction, and that professional nursing is highly desirable.

A third essential element is staffing. A primary nurse must be an autonomous practitioner who is clinically skilled. This requires clinical experience, as well as decision-making and problem-solving skills. The ratio of registered nurses to nonprofessional nursing staff should be greater than 50 percent. If the proportion of experienced professional nurses is low, then the ratio of professional to nonprofessional staff must be even greater.

The ratio of primary nurses to number of patients must be maintained in order to ensure quality care. The clinical setting has an effect on the number of patients a primary nurse can care for. For example, a primary nurse in an ambulatory care setting can assume primary responsibility for many more patients than a primary nurse in a critical care setting.

Since the practice of primary nursing suggests a need for experienced nurses, it is important that an organized approach for developing primary nurses be implemented. The development of the primary nurse includes two areas: knowledge of the primary nursing model and development of a sound clinical knowledge base. This development must be systematically planned and initiated as early as unit orientation. At this time the nurse should

TABLE 6–12. ASSISTANT NURSE ROLE IN PRIMARY NURSING

1. *Delivering direct, comprehensive, safe nursing care to assigned patients*
2. *Maintaining a thorough working knowledge of each assigned patient's status*
3. *Keeping the charge nurse informed of changes in patient status and environmental concerns*
4. *Accepting responsibility for special assignments as directed by the charge nurse*
5. *Seeking appropriate consultation for knowledge and skill development*

practice as an assistant or associate nurse and plan primary nursing care with the help of a resource primary nurse. This pairing will allow the applicant to better conceptualize and learn the role of primary.

Another consideration in deciding to convert to primary nursing is the patient length of stay. The long-term patient with complex needs is most in need of a primary relationship and, therefore, strongly supports a primary nursing model. A very brief length of stay makes it difficult to establish a relationship, and other models may be more appropriate. In general, the minimum amount of time to establish a primary nurse/patient relationship is three days. Primary nursing is an appropriate model for use in the outpatient, public health, and clinic settings since interactions with these patients, although episodic, are generally long-term. It has been suggested, however, that primary nursing is appropriate for those patients with shorter lengths of stay as well.

In the primary nursing model, the primary nurse must have authority as well as autonomy, and responsibility as well as accountability. Primary nursing cannot succeed in a traditional hierarchical structure. The need and the desire to change to a primary nursing model must be thoroughly assessed and the environment must be adequately prepared prior to implementation of this model change.

Case Management

A model of nursing practice that is being discussed by many nurses and nursing organizations today is case management. This model has resulted from both changes in hospital reimbursement and the issues of nurse staffing and job satisfaction. The case management model expands the primary nursing concept to include pre-admission outpatient care, inpatient care, and post-discharge home care. The case manager is accountable for patient outcomes and possesses authority that extends across nursing unit boundaries for an episode of illness.[42]

The continuity and accountability found in the case management model offers many exciting possibilities for nursing, for patients, and for health care organizations. Potential effects of using this model include reduced length of stay, improved patient satisfaction, enhanced nurse-physician collaboration, and increased job satisfaction for nursing. This new model of nursing practice demonstrates the responsiveness and creativity of nurses and nursing to changes in the health care environment. What the future holds for case management remains to be seen, but the possibilities are challenging, stimulating, and consistent with the values and goals of professional nursing practice.

CONCLUSION

Never before has the delivery of nursing care been more important to health care organizations. Present and future trends indicate that nurse manpower will be at a premium for the rest of this century and the first quarter of the twenty-first century. Consequently, nursing services must effectively and efficiently use their resources. This demands the selection of an appropriate model of nursing care delivery that incorporates the use of nursing diagnosis.

Nursing diagnosis is the framework upon which nursing practice should be structured, communicated, and evaluated. This framework is already being used in nursing education. Future predictions indicate that nursing diagnosis will be the basis for costing out nursing services and that reimbursement for nursing time and services will be determined by diagnosis related groups in conjunction with nursing diagnosis.

It is essential to recognize that the imminent nursing shortage makes it imperative that efficiency prevail in nursing process as well as in operationalizing safe nursing practice.

Consequently, it is essential that the nursing profession adopt nursing diagnosis as the common language for effective communication in the profession. Additionally, nurses must engage in research to explore the best, most cost-effective model of care that preserves and promotes nursing autonomy and professionalism.

REFERENCES

1. Anderson, M. A., Duke, L., Haslan, W. B. A study of the professional use of nursing diagnosis related to registered nurse job satisfaction, perceived organizational effectiveness and patient satisfaction. Paper presented at the Meeting of the North American Nursing Diagnosis Association, St. Louis, 1988.
2. Kron, T., *The management of patient care: Putting leadership skills to work* (4th ed.). Philadelphia: W. B. Saunders, 1976.
3. RN shortage threatens quality of care. *The American Nurse*, 1987, *1*, 11, 14.
4. U.S. hospitals facing severe shortage of nurses. News release of American Hospital Association, Chicago, January 28, 1987
5. RN shortage, 14
6. National study shows sharp drop in the number of college freshmen planning nursing careers. *American Journal of Nursing*, 1987, *87*, 4, 530.
7. U.S. hospitals facing severe shortage, American Hospital Association.
8. Donovan, M.I. & Lewis, G. Increasing productivity and decreasing costs: The value of RNs. *Journal of Nursing Administration*, 1987, *17*, 9, 16
9. Kalish, B. Nursing and nursing diagnosis in the year 2010. Paper presented at the Nursing Diagnosis: Impact in Professional Practice workshop sponsored by the Mid-Atlantic Nursing Diagnosis Association and the George Washington University Medical Center Department of Nursing, Washington, D.C., March 12–13, 1987
10. Gordon, M. *Nursing diagnosis: Process and application.* New York: McGraw-Hill, 1982
11. Hersey, P. & Blanchard, K. *Management of organizational behavior: Utilizing human resources* (4th ed.). Englewood Cliffs, N.J.: Prentice Hall, 1982
12. Murray, K. V., et al. Professional practice consultative service: Guide for consultative services. Unpublished paper, Medical College of Virginia Hospital, Richmond, VA, 1983
13. *Ibid.*
14. Lewin, K. Frontiers in groups dynamics: Concept, method, and reality in social sciences, social equilibrium, and social change. *Human Relations,* 1947, *1,* 1, 5
15. Hersey & Blanchard
16. Haffer, A. Facilitating change: Choosing the appropriate strategy. *Journal of Nursing Administration,* 1986, *16,* 4, 18
17. *Ibid.*
18. *Ibid.*
19. Beyers, M. Getting on top of organizational change: Part 1, process and development. *Journal of Nursing Administration,* 1984, 32
20. *Ibid.*
21. *Ibid.*
22. Hall, G.E. The concerns-based approach to facilitating change: The research and development center for teacher education. *Education Horizons,* 1979, *57,* 4, 202
23. Hall, G.E. The concerns-based perspective on personnel preparation, program development, and dissemination. *Teacher Education and Special Education,* 1981, *4,* 2, 51
24. Young, M., & Lucas, C. M. Nursing diagnosis: Common problems in implementation. *Topics in Clinical Nursing,* 1984, *5,* 4, 68
25. Zander, K.S. *Primary nursing: Development and management.* Germantown, MD: Aspen Systems Corporation, 1980
26. Brown, B.J. *Perspectives in primary nursing: Professional practice environments.* Rockville, MD: Aspen Systems Corporation, 1982
27. Zander. *Primary nursing*
28. Marram, G., Barrett, M.W., & Bevis, E.O. *Primary nursing: A model for individualized care* (2nd ed.). St. Louis: C.V. Mosby, 1979
29. McClure, M.L. & Nelson, J.M. Trends in hospital nursing, in L.H. Aiken (Ed.)., *Nursing in the 1980s: Crises, opportunities, challenges.* Philadelphia: J.B. Lippincott, 1982, p. 67
30. *Ibid.,* p.4
31. Brown
32. McClure & Nelson, p.66
33. Brown
34. McAdam, E. Primary nursing *demands change. Nursing Management,* 1982, *13,* 5, 50
35. Zander, K. Second generation primary nursing: A new agenda. *Journal of Nursing Administration,* 1985, *15,* 3, 18
36. Weeks, L.C., Barrett, M., & Snead, C. Primary nursing: Teamwork is the answer. *Journal of Nursing Administration,* 1985, *15,* 9, 21
37. McAdam
38. Brown
39. Zander. Second generation primary nursing, p. 19
40. *Ibid.*
41. *Ibid.,* p. 18
42. Zander, K. Nursing case management: Strategic managements of cost and quality outcomes. *Journal of Nursing Administration,* 1988, *18,* 5, 23

CHAPTER 7

Documentation of Diagnosis-based Nursing Practice

Emmy Miller

The documentation of nursing care serves a number of important purposes. These purposes include communicating patient information to the health care team, providing patient data for planning care, and for comparison of data over time, as well as maintaining a permanent record of the patient's care. This permanent record may then be used to evaluate the quality of care, to provide data for clinical research, and to serve as an account of the patient's care for legal purposes. (See Table 7–1.)

If the purposes of documentation are to be accomplished, then the information that is recorded in the patient's record must be accurate, pertinent, and presented in a meaningful fashion. Such a documentation system for nursing practice demands hard choices. Critical choices must be made about the types and amounts of patient data the nurse must record, the framework for recording professional nursing judgments, and the fact that many health care professionals use the same patient data in documenting their individual contributions to the care of the patient.

The choices that must be made about these documentation issues are not always easy ones. Our sophisticated health care technology makes it possible to obtain tremendous amounts of important data about patients. How can decisions about which data are essential for the patient record be made? Documenting pertinent patient data and the professional judgments of nursing practice, while avoiding repetitious recording of information, is the goal of a nursing documentation system. In order to develop such a system, it is helpful to examine the types of patient data that nurses deal with and how that data is processed into meaningful information for and about nursing practice.

A starting point for this discussion is the relationship between data and information. The distinction between data and information has been described as:

> *Data* is derived from the Latin verb *do, dare,* meaning "to give," and refers to unstructured raw facts . . . The term *information* is derived from the Latin verb *informo, informare,* meaning "to give form to." Information is data that have been given form or structure and are organized.[1]

TABLE 7–1. PURPOSES OF DOCUMENTATION

1. *Communicate patient information to the health care team*
2. *Provide patient data for planning care and for comparison of data over time (patient progress)*
3. *Evaluate care delivery*
4. *Serve as a source for research*
5. *Provide a permanent legal record of the care received by the patient*

Data from the patient are given form through the clinical thinking processes of the nurse. The diagnostic reasoning process is one way that data are converted into information. Critical pieces of data are identified, and clusters or patterns of data are recognized and named.

The identification of essential data from the patient, which are then formed into pertinent information for nursing practice, offers a useful approach to the practice of nursing. Such an approach can also serve as a guideline for documenting nursing practice that is grounded in the clinical practice of nursing. Unfortunately, many factors influence the requirements for documenting the care that patients receive, and it sometimes seems that legal concerns or regulatory requirements for documentation supercede the issues of professional nursing practice.

The purposes of documenting nursing care must not be confused with the purposes of nursing care. Confusion may result if there is a discrepancy between what the nurse does and what the nurse is required to write. While the nursing process is the recognized thinking model of the nursing profession, a review of nursing documentation reveals a very different perspective. Nursing documentation frequently consists of recording technical procedures.[2]

Task-based nursing documentation is often a response to numerous and conflicting pressures from today's health care environment, such as increasing patient acuity, technological sophistication, quality-of-care issues, and the requirements of the prospective payment system. Task-based documentation may also be the result of task-based nursing practice. In that case, moving from task-based nursing practice to diagnosis-based nursing practice is a way to make the values of nursing and the practice of nursing more congruent. In diagnosis-based nursing practice, clinical thinking shifts from tasks to those human responses that nurses can diagnose and treat. The documentation requirements for nursing care must then shift as well.

Accurate recording of nursing care activities requires time, thought, and synthesis of information, as well as some risk taking.[3] In this era of high patient acuity and shortage of nurses, nurses' time must be used for best advantage. The time constraints that busy nurses often experience can also contribute to task-based documentation of nursing care. Indeed, issues of time have been identified as major factors which hinder documentation of nursing diagnoses, particularly not enough time, short staffing, and the feeling that providing nursing care takes precedence over documenting that care.[4]

Issues Affecting Nursing Documentation

A number of forces influence the documentation requirements of nursing care, and these factors have contributed to conflict and confusion about exactly what nurses should document. Professional practice standards play a significant role in the documentation of nursing care; indeed, the use of nursing diagnosis for documentation purposes is a reflection of this. The development of nursing diagnoses has provided a useful framework for clinical nursing practice and the documentation of this. Other professional forces affecting the documentation requirements for nursing care include higher patient acuity, specialization, and technological advances.

Another critical influence on nursing documentation issues is the role of legal considerations and concerns. Patient records often serve as evidence in court cases involving malpractice, personal injury, disability, or mental competence issues. Furthermore, the patient record is also the single most important document available to a hospital when a lawsuit occurs. Anxiety about the legality of nursing documentation is often used as a rationale for documentation requirements, as well as for resistance by nurses to expressing certain types of judgments in the patient record. (See Chapter 11 for a discussion of the legal issues related to nursing diagnosis.)

The issue of the quality of nursing care has an important place in any discussion of documentation. Rising health care costs have resulted in close scrutiny of health care delivery by those who must pay the bills. This concern about the costs of health care has been accompanied by concerns that health care dollars are spent on effective, efficient, and appropriate services. The quality of health care services is generally evaluated retrospectively, based upon the documentation of those services. The Joint Commission on Accreditation of Health Organizations (JCAHO) has developed standards for nursing documentation in order to ensure the quality of nursing care. Compliance with the JCAHO standards is often cited as a rationale for documentation requirements.

The economic ramifications of cost and quality considerations are also a significant issue for nursing documentation. Lynnhoke states:

> Documentation has always been important but the prospective payment system of diagnosis related groups (DRGs) has made it critical. What is charted can bring in or lose reimbursement dollars.[5]

The necessity to document patient information that will meet the criteria for prospective payment adds another set of documentation requirements for health care providers in general and nurses in particular.

Professional standards, legal considerations, quality of care concerns, and prospective payment are important and powerful forces in the practice of nursing and in how that practice must be documented. Unfortunately, these forces result in confusing and sometimes conflicting demands for documentation of nursing care. As a result, documentation requirements may be designed to accomplish the recording of tasks and raw data rather than describing information about the condition of the patient and the efforts of the nurse to deal with this.

Using nursing diagnoses, within the context of the nursing process, is a way to meet many of the documentation requirements for nursing care that are imposed by today's health care environment. The nursing diagnosis is a sound method of operationally summarizing patient problems in terms that are meaningful to nurses.[6] Shifting the focus of documentation requirements from tasks, technical procedures, and repetitive data to the problems of patients provides a structure for documentation which reflects the professional thinking and values of nursing. This approach to documentation does not mean that tasks, technical procedures, and repetitive data do not have a place in a system for recording nursing care; rather, these are placed within the context of the conditions of the patient and the clinical judgment of the nurse.

What Information Is Important for Nursing Documentation?

It is helpful to examine the information that nurses need to document in the patient record and the pertinent raw data from which this information is derived. When the critical types of information necessary for nursing practice are known, this knowledge can be used to determine what data nurses should collect and document, and it can also guide decisions about the framework for recording the data and related information. Three categories of information are essential for the professional practice of nursing: information about human responses, disease-related information, and additional information. (See Figure 7–1)

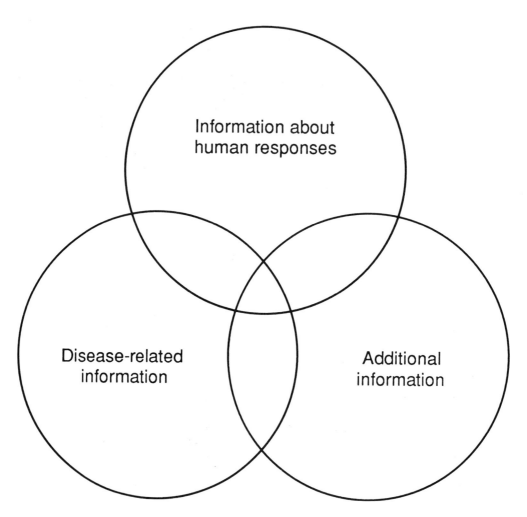

Figure 7–1. Categories of information needed for the professional practice of nursing.

The first category, information about human responses, is comprised of pertinent assessment data and nursing diagnoses, as well as implementation and evaluation of the nursing care plan. The nursing diagnosis is the foundation of this category of information for nursing documentation because nursing diagnoses describe those human responses to actual or potential health problems nurses treat. Independent nursing practice and much of interdependent nursing practice will be recorded in this category, therefore, the nursing process is a useful and effective framework for documenting this information.

Nursing diagnoses describe those human responses that are the focus of nursing practice. Using nursing diagnosis as a focal point for documentation will deal with many issues in nursing documentation, particularly the professional component of nursing practice, but it does not address those nursing responsibilities associated with the disease or medical condition of the patient. The practice of nursing includes both of these areas, and so must any approach to nursing documentation.

The second category of information for nursing documentation, describing disease-related information, includes the documentation of signs and symptoms of diseases and medical conditions, the effects of medical therapeutics, and the execution of medical orders. Information in this category should be described using medical terminology and does not usually fit into the nursing process framework.

Clinical findings, however, can be used as data to formulate both nursing and medical diagnoses. For example, the presence of agitation, restlessness, and disorientation are data that could be indicative of a nursing diagnosis or a disease-related situation. If this cluster of data was observed in an elderly patient only during the night shift, it might best be described with the nursing diagnosis. Potential for Injury related to confusion at night. If this cluster of data was observed in a recently admitted patient with a myocardial infarction, then this cluster represents a highly significant observation that must be reported to the physician and treated with medical therapeutics. Determining whether certain data should be included in information about human responses or in the disease-related category is complex and must be based in the realities of the clinical situation.

Additional information includes those data that are not directly linked to either the patient's disease condition or human responses to this. Oftentimes, this category reflects information necessary to meet legal, regulatory, or organizational requirements. An example of this type of requirement, found in many hospitals, would be that all patients have a notation in their record that the side rails are elevated and the bed is in low position. While this information is important, the impetus for recording it on all patients, irrespective of disease condition or human responses, is found in risk-management and legal concerns rather than clinical considerations.

Requirements for nursing documentation must be derived from the necessities to record and communicate information in clinical nursing practice; furthermore, these requirements must be organized in a way that encourages the documentation of meaningful information while providing mechanisms to handle large volumes of raw data. A documentation system designed to meet these requirements must include strategies for documenting all three categories of information that are used in nursing practice: information about human responses, disease-related information, and additional information. Although the distinctions between these categories may be blurred at times, documentation requirements based on these categories can be very useful in organizing data and information from nursing practice.

A BRIEF REVIEW OF GUIDELINES AND FORMATS FOR NURSING DOCUMENTATION

A system for nursing documentation must clearly identify the types of data and information that should be recorded as well as a framework for organizing this in a meaningful fashion. Many guidelines and formats have been proposed for the documentation of nursing care, and it is helpful to review these briefly before discussing ways in which nursing diagnosis can be incorporated into nursing documentation.

Guidelines for Nursing Documentation

The nursing process has been recognized as a guide for the documentation of professional nursing practice; however, use of the nursing process does not solve all of the problems associated with the documentation of nursing care. While providing an effective framework for documenting information about human responses, it does not include mechanisms for the disease-related information and additional information categories. These categories often consist of large amounts of repetitive or numerical data that the nursing process framework was never intended to cover. A system for documenting nursing care that does not address the need to record a variety of data and information will be frustrating and time consuming to use.

Legal concerns are often cited as a guide for nursing documentation requirements. Such guidelines tend to focus on the responsibility of the nurse to record disease-related information or directives for charting that minimize the possibility of misinterpretation of the written documentation. Legal guidelines for nursing documentation tend to emphasize avoiding those charting practices that have been cited in malpractice cases, and this is certainly valuable and important knowledge. Legal concerns however, generally provide little direction for developing a system for documenting nursing care that reflects the issues and contributions of professional nursing practice.

There are other sets of guidelines that do focus on the issues related to the quality of nursing care, and these are the guidelines set by regulatory groups, the best known being JCAHO. (See Table 7–2). These standards for nursing documentation focus on the identification of the patient's problems, nursing interventions for these, and discharge planning. Inherent in these standards is the concept of individualized nursing care for patients, reflecting a philosophy that "Standardized care plans will be okay when we have standardized patients" In section NR.5.6.5, the necesssity of organizing large volumes of repetitive data found in nursing practice is addressed, and strategies for accomplishing this will be discussed later in this chapter.

Professional, legal, and quality guidelines for nursing documentation identify broad content areas for a nursing documentation system. Another concern in developing a system for documenting nursing care is the format or structure for organizing the data and information which should be recorded. Two basic formats will be discussed here: the narrative, descriptive approach and the problem-oriented record.

Formats for Nursing Documentation

The narrative format for documentation is one in which observations and nursing care activities are recorded in paragraph form. Notations are made in chronological sequence. This traditional format is often used in source-oriented records where the patient record is divided

TABLE 7–2. JCAHO STANDARDS FOR NURSING DOCUMENTATION

NR.5.6 *Documentation of nursing care is pertinent and concise and reflects patient status.*

NR.5.6.1 *Nursing documentation addresses the patient's needs, problems, capabilities, and limitations.*

NR.5.6.2 *Nursing intervention and patient response are noted.*

NR.5.6.3 *When a patient is transferred within or discharged from the hospital, a nurse notes the patient's status in the medical record.*

NR.5.6.4 *As appropriate, patients who are discharged from the hospital requiring nursing care receive instructions and individualized counseling prior to discharge.*

NR.5.6.4.1 *Evidence of the instructions and the patient's or family's understanding of these instructions is noted in the patient's medical record.*

NR.5.6.4.2 *Such instructions and counseling are consistent with the responsible medical practitioner's instructions.*

NR.5.6.5 *The nursing department/service is encouraged to standardize documentation of routine elements of care and repeated monitoring of, for example, personal hygiene, administration of medication, and physiological parameters.*

Joint Commission on Accreditation of Health Organizations (JCAHO), Accreditation Manual for Hospitals. (Chicago: JCAHO, 1988), p. 146

into sections according to the source of data. In the source-oriented record, there are separate sections for nurses' notes, physician progress notes, and social service notes.[7]

In the narrative format, observations and events are recorded as they happen although some versions of this format permit the nurse to record a summary of events, in paragraph form, at the end of the shift. While this format may be useful in encouraging the documentation of descriptive information and timely documentation of events, the narrative format offers no mechanism for handling numerical, repetitive data nor does it establish any organized flow of information, other than chronological. Narrative, source-oriented recording does permit easy access to the documentation of various health care providers. Disadvantages of this documentation format include a lack of clear problem definition, difficulty identifying multidisciplinary approaches to problems, lack of integrated documentation of the patient's responses to intervention, and difficulty in auditing the record for quality of care.[8]

To deal with some of the documentation difficulties in the traditional approaches to documentation, the problem-oriented record (POR) was developed. This is a format that structures data into categories consisting of baseline data, problem list, plan of care, flow sheets, progress notes, and discharge summary.[9] The problem-oriented record provides mechanisms to clearly identify the patient's problems and to track the progress of these. Another advantage is the use of flow sheets, making the recording of large volumes of numerical or repetitive data easier and more meaningful.

A unique feature of the problem-oriented record is the format for the progress notes. This format is generally identified by the acronym SOAP, which stands for Subjective data, Objective data, Assessment, and Plan. Sometimes this SOAP framework may be extended to SOAPIER, where I is for the Implementation of the plan, E represents the Evaluation of the plan's effectiveness, and R indicates the Resolution of the problem. It may not be necessary to include each component of the SOAPIER format in every progress note: for an unconscious patient the S will not be included, an initial note for a newly identified problem would only consist of SOAP until the plan could be carried out, and the R for resolution would only be indicated for problems that were satisfactorily resolved.

The problem-oriented record offers a number of benefits for the documentation of nursing care such as a logical progress note format, flow sheets for repetitive data, and a clear flow of information. One disadvantage to this format is the tendency to identify only medical diagnoses on the problem list. Another disadvantage is that:

> the patient may get lost between the lines . . . On reading the progression of a patient problem record one can find out how a wound is healing or how a disease is progressing but not how the patient is doing. The problem-oriented system can be very dehumanizing—a terrible thing for such a humanistic profession [such as nursing] to promote.[10]

This is indeed a concern for nurses who want to provide pertinent, meaningful documentation of the condition of the patient and the nursing care associated with that condition.

A variation of the problem-oriented record, which has been designed to highlight the patient and also to organize the data that nurses record, is Focus Charting.[11] In this documentation format, the term "focus" is used rather than "problem" to avoid a negative approach to the patient. A focus may be a nursing diagnosis, a current patient concern or behavior, a significant change in patient status, or a significant event. A focus is *not* a medical diagnosis.

The Focus Charting system uses three columns to organize information in the progress note section of the patient record: date and time, focus, and notes. The notes are organized according to the following categories:

Data: Information which supports the stated focus or describes pertinent obser-
                         vations of the patient
Action: Immediate or future nursing actions to address the focus and evaluation
                         of the present care plan, along with any changes required
Response: Description of patient responses to any part of the medical or nursing
                         care

These categories also correspond to the steps of the nursing process with the data category representing the assessment step, action corresponding to the planning and implementation steps, and the response category fulfilling the evaluation step of the nursing process.[12]

Another documentation model that is similar to the problem-oriented record is Outcome Charting, which uses six components to guide the recording of objective, specific data and information about the patient's progress in achieving expected outcomes.[13] The six components are baseline data, problem identification, expected outcome, checkpoints and deadlines, nursing orders, and transfer/discharge summary. These components are used as horizontal headings for a document that serves as the basic care plan.

Charting by exception[14] is an alternative documentation method in which only abnormal or unusual findings are recorded. This method has been designed to use nursing time effectively and to address issues of costs, quality of care, legal standards, and nursing care planning. Here the emphasis is on documenting important findings and changes in the patient's condition rather than repeating normal assessments over and over again. Guidelines for charting, care planning, evaluation of nurse time spent in documentation, specialty applications, and shift report are included in the charting-by-exception framework.

PRINCIPLES OF DOCUMENTATION IN DIAGNOSIS-BASED NURSING PRACTICE

A system for documenting diagnosis-based nursing practice must include mechanisms for recording data and information for the three categories of information about human responses, disease-related information, and additional information. Different documentation strategies will be required for varying types of data and information. While documentation issues will vary in different clinical settings, there are certain principles which can be used to guide the documentation of diagnosis-based nursing practice. (See Table 7–3).

Analyzing the types of information that nurses must record, the data necessary to support this information, and some approaches to organizing this information is an essential foundation to a discussion of the role of nursing diagnosis in a documentation system. In

TABLE 7–3. PRINCIPLES FOR DOCUMENTATION OF DIAGNOSIS-BASED NURSING PRACTICE

Principle # 1	*Information documented in the patient record must be supported by data, and data should be linked to information*
Principle #2	*Use flow sheets or special forms to record repetitive numerical data and categorical information whenever possible*
Principle #3	*Descriptive data and information require an expository documentation format*
Principle #4	*Determining which documentation format to use will depend upon which category of information is to be documented: information about human responses, disease-related information, or additional information*
Principle #5	*Information about human responses can be effectively documented using the nursing process*

diagnosis-based nursing practice, nursing diagnosis is the driving force; the same is true for a documentation system for that practice. In order to examine the place of nursing diagnosis in a documentation system for diagnosis-based nursing practice, the place of other types of data and information that nurses deal with must be defined as well.

The distinction between data and information plays an important role in this approach to nursing documentation. Information is simply data that have been given form or structure; however, the accuracy and validity of information can only be judged if the supporting data are available. From the perspective of documenting nursing practice, both data and information are essential.

Consider a patient with a fractured femur in skeletal traction. A nursing diagnosis of Ineffective Coping related to physical dependency has been recorded on the nursing care plan. Observation of the patient reveals a pleasant, animated young man who is reading a magazine. In the patient's record there are no descriptions of behaviors that have been identified as defining characteristics for this nursing diagnosis, such as verbalizing feelings of inability to cope, inability to problem solve, or inappropriate use of defense mechanisms.[15] The absence of supporting data in the patient record makes the accuracy and validity of this nursing diagnosis open to question.

A similar example of the importance of recording both data and information also can be seen in the area of disease-related information. When the nurse records the amount of a medication given to treat the patient's pain and the time of the dose, those facts are data. If the patient's response to the medication or any patterns or trends in the patient's descriptions of the pain are also documented, then information about the patient's pain experience and treatment is available. The availability of this information enables the physician and nurse to evaluate the effectiveness of the pain medication and the patient's responses to the particular medication and dosage schedule, making modifications as indicated. If only data about the times and amounts of medication were recorded, it would be difficult, if not impossible, to determine the effectiveness of the medication or the patient's pain experience.

Principle #1: Information documented in the patient record must be supported by data, and data should be linked to information.

Much of the information recorded in the patient record is comprised of the professional judgments of health care providers. For example, a diagnosis reflects the clinical judgment of the health care professional, nursing or medical. That diagnosis must be supported by data, in the form of signs and symptoms or defining characteristics, in order for the diagnosis to be considered valid and accurate. Information about the treatment of the identified diagnosis must also be supported by the appropriate data. A clear and logical linkage between data and information is essential for a useful and meaningful documentation system for nursing practice.

Principle #1 raises another issue that concerns the choices made about the types and amounts of data recorded in the patient record. The amount of data that could be collected from an individual patient is tremendous. It is necessary to make choices about types and frequency of data collection in order to avoid becoming overwhelmed by the magnitude of available data.

Choices about data collection and recording must be guided by information needs. Information about human responses is the foundation of nursing practice; therefore, the choices about the types and amounts of data that nurses collect should be based on those data necessary for the diagnosis and treatment of human responses. An example of such a choice is the decision to use a nursing assessment framework, such as the Functional Health Patterns,[16] to guide and focus the data that nurses collect toward identification of nursing diagnoses and treatment plans for these.

The concept of a linkage between data and information also applies to the disease-related information category. The essential data that nurses must collect in this category are concerned with signs and symptoms of diseases and medical conditions, the effects of medical therapeutics, and the execution of medical orders. The nurse converts these data into information such as changes in the disease or medical condition, detection of highly significant signs or symptoms, identification of critical events, and responses to medical therapeutics. Nurses are continually called upon to make judgments about disease-related information that include reporting the observations to the physician, carrying out or withholding existing medical orders for the problem, executing palliative treatment based on nursing judgment, or some combination of these.[17]

Information about human responses and disease-related information can often share the same supporting data, and both contain a diagnostic/assessment component and a treatment component. By examining information about human responses and disease-related information in terms of diagnosis and treatment, it becomes easier to identify the necessary data for each of these information categories. This analysis is presented in Table 7–4.

Information about human responses, reflecting professional nursing practice, should be documented within the context of the nursing process. Disease-related information often lends itself to a different approach. Finally, data in either of these categories must be handled in a way that is efficient, meaningful, and avoids repetition. These issues lead to our second principle for documentation of diagnosis-based nursing practice.

TABLE 7–4. DOCUMENTATION OF DIAGNOSIS-BASED NURSING PRACTICE

	Data		Information	
	Type	*Format*	*Type*	*Format*
Information about Human Responses	*Assessment: behaviors statements physiologic measurements*	*special forms* *flow sheets* *flow sheets*	*nursing diagnosis*	*problem-oriented record, Focus Charting, Outcome Charting, nursing care plan*
	Treatment: *Nursing interventions, what and when*		*change in status of the nursing diagnosis*	*descriptive or narrative formats*
Disease-Related Information	*Observations: statements behaviors physiologic measurements*	*special forms* *flow sheets* *special forms*	*critical event signs & symptoms response to medical therapeutics*	*descriptive, narrative*
	Treatment: *execution of medical orders*		*Responses to medications, procedures*	*descriptive, narrative*
Additional Information	*demographic data*	*special forms*	*(May be clustered with data from other categories)*	
	socioeconomic data	*special forms*		
	miscellaneous	*special forms*		

Principle #2: Use flow sheets or special forms to record repetitive numerical data and categorical information whenever possible.

Data refer to facts. Clinical data about patients include such facts as vital sign measurements, intake and output measurements, testing of body fluids, routine nursing care activities, and observations of patient behavior. These clinical data contribute to both the diagnostic aspect and the treatment aspect of information about human resources and disease-related information. For example, certain trends in physiologic measurements play a crucial role in the diagnosis of patients with a variety of conditions. In the treatment area, routine monitoring or nursing care activities are important data that must be recorded.

Flow sheets are a very functional documentation tool. They can increase the efficient use of nurses' time spent in documentation, while legibility and accuracy of the data may also be enhanced. Recording serial data collections on a flow sheet also permits comparison of data and easier detection of significant trends. Nursing and medical treatment activities, including turning, range of motion exercises, mouth care, wound care, and tube feedings, can also be recorded effectively on flow charts.

Designing and using documentation flow sheets can accomplish a number of positive results. A flow sheet can jog one's memory, organize observations and judgments, schedule activities, establish communications, assure continuity, and provide a record of what has been done; furthermore, well-designed forms can "take the punishment out of the [documentation] process."[18] Some general guidelines for developing flow sheets are presented in Table 7–5.

Flow sheets present a concise overview of numerical data over time. Another useful documentation strategy is the development of special forms for certain types of categorical information. One example of this approach is a body systems assessment form on which the pertinent data category may be checked off rather than written out. In the intensive care unit, the respiratory assessment might include indicators such as:

_____   breathing independently
_____   intubated (tube type and size)_____
_____   clear breath sounds bilaterally
_____   abnormal breath sounds (describe)_____
         _____
_____   productive cough (describe sputum)_____
         _____

On a general surgical unit, an assessment form might contain categories for the incision, respiratory status, nutrition, elimination, pain, and ambulation. It is not necessary to develop these assessment guidelines as separate paper documents; for frequent assessments, a rubber stamp could be used on existing chart forms to assist the nurse with recording the appropriate information.

Another area where a specialized form can be useful is patient education.[19,20] Certain types of categorical information can be recorded easily and efficiently. A patient education form would include categories for the educational content, the teaching method, and the patient's response. While this type of form would be helpful in keeping track of patient teaching over time, a patient education form must be augmented with descriptive information about the patient's mastery of the content and responses to the teaching program in the patient record.

Flow sheets, specialized forms, or rubber stamps provide mechanisms for documentation

TABLE 7–5. GUIDELINES FOR DEVELOPING USEFUL FLOW SHEETS FOR NURSING DOCUMENTATION

1. *Find out what forms are needed*
   Review existing forms and documents
   Survey nursing staff and administration
   Consider existing policy and regulations in regard to documentation
2. *Consult with anyone who will be using the forms*
   Nursing staff
   Other departments/health care professionals who need or use the same information
   Medical records staff who have knowledge of forms creation, flow, and storage
3. *Consult those responsible for printing and storing forms*
4. *Design the flow sheet*
   Format the information in a way that is clear to users of the information
   Locate data on the flow sheet so that trends or patterns in the data can be easily identified
   Place similar types of data near each other (i.e. ventilator settings and arterial blood gas results together on an ICU flow sheet; intake and output near the section for test results of body fluids on med/surg forms)
   Avoid abbreviations that may be confusing or misinterpreted
   Use graphics for clarity
   lines, spaces, and boxes should be clearly labeled and of adequate size for the recording of the indicated data
5. *Develop guidelines for use of the flow sheet based on surveys and consultations in 1. and 2. above*
6. *Test the flow sheet*
   Survey users for ease of use and clarity of data found on the flow sheet
   Evaluate the flow sheet against existing policies and procedures
   Make any revisions indicated from the test
   Analyze results of test to assist in justifying this flow sheet to reviewing and approval bodies
7. *Submit flow sheet for approval through recognized channels*
   Administrative/policy review
   Mecdical records
   Information systems/data processing
8. *Introduce the flow sheet for general use in a systematic manner*
   How to use flow sheet as a document and how to interpret/analyze data as well as recording it
   When and when not to use flow sheet
   Where to obtain the flow sheet
   What to do with it

that use the nurse's time efficiently, contribute to consistency in data recording, and assist in organizing numerical, repetitive, or categorical data in a meaningful format. Other types of data may require another approach.

Principle #3: Descriptive data and information require an expository documentation format.

Although many clinical findings consist of numerical or categorical data, not all patient data lend themselves to documentation on flow sheets or specialized forms. Patient behaviors, statements made by the patient, the quality of respiration, the characteristics of drainage from a wound, and the resistance of joints to movement are but a few of the observations that nurses make. Such qualitative data must be recorded using a descriptive, expository approach.

The purpose of descriptive, expository documentation is to provide an accurate, precise representation of the facts and to support information derived from those facts. Consider the difference between "incision healing well" and "well-approximated, mid-line abdominal incision without redness, swelling, or drainage is healing well." While both of these statements are indicative of a wound that is healing without complications, the first statement consists of a conclusion, without any supporting data. In the second statement, a description of the wound provides the necessary supporting data for the clinical judgment about the progress of wound healing.

Certainly, it requires more words and more thought to record descriptions of clinical findings rather than isolated conclusions; however, this recommendation should not be construed to mean that voluminous notations are necessary. Only the descriptive data needed to support pertinent clinical information should be documented.

A descriptive, expository documentation strategy is very useful for data to support diagnostic conclusions, both nursing and medical. This approach can also be employed for the documentation of certain treatment activities. While the treatment activity itself may be recorded on a flow sheet or specialized form, these data must be interpreted to provide information about the patient's responses to treatment.

For the patient with a nursing diagnosis of Potential for Impaired Skin Integrity related to immobility, nursing interventions of turning and massage of bony prominences can be recorded on a treatment flow sheet as they are performed. A descriptive notation about the condition of the patient's skin is also needed, however, so that the effectiveness of these nursing interventions may be evaluated. Both the data on the treatment flow sheet and the descriptive notation are necessary to represent the clinical condition of the patient and the nurse's activities to address this.

The relationship between data and information, and strategies for recording these, have occupied this discussion thus far, and three principles for documentation have been presented. Nurses deal with a tremendous amount of data and have responsibilities for recording and interpreting patient data from both the human response and the disease perspectives. The determination of which data and information should be recorded in which format leads to the fourth principle for documentation of diagnosis-based nursing practice.

Principle #4: Determining which documentation format to use will depend upon which category of information is to be documented: Information about human responses, Disease-related information, or additional information.

In order to apply this fourth principle of documentation, the first step is to distinguish which category of information best suits the patient data and clinical findings to be recorded. This distinction is important both professionally and from a documentation perspective; however, the collaborative, interrelated nature of providing health care services for patients makes it difficult sometimes to clearly distinguish between nursing and medical information. Indeed, such a distinction may seem arbitrary to some nurses, but it is a useful one for examining documentation issues.

The discipline-specific perspective of nursing plays an important role in nursing documentation. While the nurse and physician collect and record similar data or clinical findings, this does not represent an inefficient duplication of efforts unless there is no difference in the use of the data. Accurate recording of the professional judgment and contributions of the nurse to the care of the patient is essential, and this is reflected in the documentation of information about human responses.

Nursing practice also includes carrying out aspects of medical therapy and making observations about the disease-related condition of the patient. These two types of information require different documentation strategies. For information about human responses, effective and professional documentation can be accomplished using the nursing process with nursing diagnosis, and this will be discussed in detail later in this chapter. Nursing documentation of disease-related information is best suited to a somewhat different approach.

Disease-Related Information.   The documentation of disease-related information includes observations about the signs and symptoms of diseases and medical conditions, the effects of medical therapeutics, and the execution of medical orders, and the issues here concern the use of medical terminology, distinctions between medical and nursing diagnoses, and the legal responsibilities of the nurse to carry out medical orders. It is the professional and legal responsibility of the physician to diagnose disease. Once this has been done it is incumbent upon the nurse to make pertinent observations, to carry out appropriate treatments, and to communicate these. Medical terminology is appropriate for the communication and documentation of these disease-related observations and treatments. Gordon states:

> There is no need to create new terms for diseases or pathophysiological processes in order to chart disease-related observations and treatments. The medical diagnoses provide the terminology. Use of those terms does not constitute medical diagnosis, provided that the physician has already identified them in his or her diagnostic judgment. If the medical diagnoses have not been recorded, either the symptoms were overlooked or new problems have occurred. In either case notification of the physician is appropriate.[21]

Clearly identifying disease-related information as such, and recording it in recognized medical terminology will prevent much of the confusion that can occur when beginning to use nursing diagnoses in documentation.

Nurses frequently make observations and judgments about disease-related conditions that are best described with medical terminology. In addition to these observations and judgments, the nurse must record the execution of delegated medical activities prescribed through physician orders. These two aspects of disease-related care require different documentation formats.

Documentation of the execution of medical orders can be indicated on a flow sheet or special form. The administration of medications, repetitive procedures or treatments, and specifically delegated observations that result in numerical data all lend themselves as well to documentation on flow sheets or specialized forms. The forms can make documentation easier and more efficient for the nurse, and they also provide a legal record of regularly scheduled nursing activities and contacts with the patient.

Recording of nursing observations and judgments about the disease-related condition of the patient will generally require a descriptive, expository format. For example, documentation of a critical change in the level of consciousness of a patient with cerebrovascular disease must contain descriptions of the patient's behaviors and responses, although numerical data such as heart rate and blood pressure will also be important. The need to record descriptive information, however, does not limit documentation format options to a narrative approach. It is also possible to include descriptive information in the problem-oriented record.

An example is helpful at this point. Consider an elderly patient with medical diagnoses of cerebrovascular disease, congestive heart failure, and diabetes mellitus. These medical conditions require careful observation by the nurse as well as professional nursing judgment about changes in the patient's condition and responses to medical therapeutics, such as diagnostic testing and medications. Some of these observations lend themselves to flow sheet documentation: vital signs, neurological checks, intake and output, and finger-stick blood glucose testing. Other observations and any judgments based on these observations will require a different format.

The development of confusion, disorientation, aphasia, and right-sided weakness would represent a critical and significant change in this patient's disease-related condition. Although data on the neurological flow sheet would reflect this change, a descriptive notation in the record is also indicated. This could be done in a chronological narrative format, or it could be handled through the problem-oriented approach. Examples of these notes are shown in Table 7–6.

In the examples, the same information about the patient is recorded accurately and concisely in the narrative, problem-oriented, Focus Charting formats. Rather than repeating information recorded on the neurological and vital sign flow sheet, only the significant data are repeated along with the nurse's judgment that these data reflected a critical change in the patient. Furthermore, a somewhat different approach to the problem-oriented notation is used than was discussed previously.

In the problem-oriented format example, notice that the problem heading was the *change in the condition* of the patient rather than a medical diagnosis. At this point it is not known whether this change is due to the patient's cerebrovascular disease, congestive heart failure, or diabetes, although the presence of a focal deficit makes a neurological cause most likely. As the medical diagnosis was not the problem heading, the Plan of the progress note was used to indicate the nurse's plan for the patient. If this had been a somewhat different clinical situation, where the disorientation was associated with an elevated blood glucose, then the medical diagnosis of diabetes mellitus could have been used; in that case, the plan for the medical diagnosis must come from the physician.

TABLE 7–6. PROGRESS NOTE FORMATS FOR DISEASE-RELATED INFORMATION

Chronological, Narrative Format
2/29/88 2:30 PM
  At 2:15 PM, Mr. Jones was noted to be disoriented to place and time, but not person. Motor exam shows right weakness which is a new finding (see flow sheet for motor testing results and vital signs). Speech is slow and thick, and he communicates ideas with difficulty. Speech change is also new. As this is a significant change, Dr. Smith was notified at 2:20 P.M., saw patient at that time.

Problem-Oriented Format
2/29/88 2:30 P.M.
Problem: Change in Neurologic Status
S: (in response to orientation questions) Why, I'm at home, aren't I? Who are you? It's January, or is it February? I don't feel right.
O: Unable to answer orientation questions correctly, new right-sided weakness noted, speech is slow and thick, and he communicates ideas with difficulty. (See flow sheet for complete neurocheck and vital signs)
A; Significant change in neurologic status, noted at 2:15 P.M.
P: Notify Dr. Smith immediately; monitor neurologic and general condition closely

---

Focus Charting Format

Date/Time	Focus	Notes
2/29/88 2:30 P.M.	Change in Neurological Status	**Data:** at 2:15 P.M. patient was disoriented to place and time, but not person. Motor exam shows right weakness which is a new finding (see flow sheet for motor testing results and vital signs). Speech is slow and thick, and he communicates ideas with difficulty. Speech change is also new. **Assessment:** Significant change in neurologic status, noted at 2:15 P.M.; Notify Dr. Smith immediately; monitor neurologic and general condition closely **Response:** NA

In this example, Focus Charting can be appropriately and effectively used. This format is organized in columns to emphasize the focus or topic of the descriptive information and its supporting data. The Data/Action/Response framework also structures data and information in a meaningful fashion; however it is not necessary for comments to be made in all three categories in every note.[22]

In recording disease-related information, strategies are necessary to 1) handle large volumes of repetitive, numerical data, 2) indicate that medical orders have been executed in a timely fashion, and 3) describe the observations and judgments that nurses make about the patients' disease-related conditions. The use of flow sheets can be highly effective for the first two areas of documentation. Recording observations and judgments requires descriptive documentation and narrative, problem-oriented, or Focus Charting formats, with some restrictions, can be used effectively for this.

One final point should be made about the nursing documentation of disease-related information: Beware of placing observations related to nursing diagnoses under medical problems.[23] This distinction is essential because of the unique perspective of each discipline:

> Each discipline functions more effectively because of the diagnosis and treatment of others. Each needs the diagnosis of the other. It is not enough to diagnose the neoplasm, the degenerative disease, the genetic anomaly. If the patient and those around him are to live effectively with the existing health situation, it is equally necessary to diagnose the disruptions in daily living, the adjustments in lifestyle, the changed relationships with people and the environment, and the new skills and knowledge needed in daily living.[24]

Often, it may be difficult to distinguish those patient data and clinical findings that are best related to the medical diagnosis and those that are more indicative of a human response that would require a nursing diagnosis.

As a general guideline, data and information that deal with the patient's *response* to the disease or medical condition indicate that a nursing diagnosis should be present. For example, the data and clinical findings from a patient with congestive heart failure indicate that the disease-related condition of the patient is stable; however, an increase in heart and respiratory rates, accompanied by a subjective sense of fatigue and slowness during ambulation and self-care activities would suggest a nursing diagnosis of Activity Intolerance related to imbalance of oxygen supply and demand. Using these data to arrive at this nursing diagnosis reflects the discipline-specific perspective of nursing, and they should be documented accordingly.

Additional Information. This category includes those data not directly linked to either the patient's disease condition or human responses, and it reflects information necessary to meet legal, regulatory, or organizational requirements. This category often consists of data and information that are necessary for the health care organization to record and maintain on all patients. Admission demographic data, risk-management analyses, and quality assurance monitoring needs can all contribute to documentation requirements for nurses. While the collection and recording of such data about patients is important, the determinations of the types and amounts of data that are necessary in this information category should be made carefully.

The nursing documentation requirements for additional information should include those essential items that only nurses could provide, and the documentation format should be easy and efficient to use. Documentation formats such as flow sheets and special forms should be utilized wherever possible; however, the critical aspect of this documentation category is the decisions about the types and amounts of data the nurse must record that are not linked to or the result of the patient's disease-related condition or human responses.

Information About Human Responses. This category of information reflects the responsibility of professional nurses to "diagnose and treat human responses to actual or potential health problems."[25] This definition of nursing by the American Nurses' Association clearly identifies the focus of nursing practice. Furthermore, verbal and written communications are an integral part of that practice, and the approaches and emphasis of documentation requirements for nursing practice must be congruent with this.

The practice of nursing is also a problem-solving process. In nursing, this is defined as the nursing process, consisting of steps for problem identification and problem solving. To document this, the problems that patients experience and that are amenable to nursing intervention must be named, consistently and accurately, and the efforts of nurses to solve these problems must be clearly linked with the identified problem. Nursing diagnosis, as a framework for naming the conditions of patients that require nursing care, and the nursing process, as a framework for the cognitive activities that nurses employ in their efforts to identify and solve patient problems, provide useful and effective strategies for the documentation of nursing practice.

Principle #5: Information about human responses can be effectively documented using the nursing process.

The nursing process is the recognized thinking model of the nursing profession; as such, it seems reasonable to use the nursing process as a framework for nursing documentation. Organizing the data and information that nurses collect and record in the framework of nursing process accomplishes a number of beneficial purposes. First, it contributes to congruence between the professional values of nursing and the clinical practice of nursing. Second, it provides the consistency and standardization of a recognized format. This second benefit is a crucial foundation for the third: nursing process, using nursing diagnosis, provides a framework for the computerization of nursing data and information.

The nursing process is the best known and most widely used scheme for organizing the collection, use, and storage of nursing data; furthermore, the data and information that nurses use and record in the course of delivering nursing services are a critical resource, and as such, these data must be organized, stored, and available for examination and analysis. In order to collect nursing data on a national scale and for purposes of computerizing nursing data, a set of limited and essential data must be identified. Such a data set has been proposed for nursing and is based on components of the nursing process. The Nursing Minimum Data Set (NMDS) consists of 16 data elements that could be considered to be national or international in scope and provide clues about trends in nursing and nursing resource allocation.[26] (See Table 7–7). The nursing care elements of the NMDS are based on the nursing process, and nursing diagnosis is the foundation of this set of elements. The nursing diagnosis describes the patient's condition, prescribes the required nursing interventions, and establishes parameters for outcome measures.

The potential benefits of the NMDS and a national nursing database include a analysis of nursing data at regional and national levels, projection of trends in the need for nursing care and nursing resources, costing of nursing services and evaluation of nursing care, and comparative nursing research on nursing diagnoses, nursing interventions, outcomes of nursing care, the effects of nursing care delivery systems, and the effects of computerized nursing information systems.[27]

TABLE 7–7. ELEMENTS OF THE NURSING MINIMUM DATA SET

Nursing Care Elements
1. *Nursing Diagnosis*
2. *Nursing Intervention*
3. *Nursing Outcome*
4. *Intensity of Nursing Care*

Patient Demographic Elements
5. *Personal Identification**
6. *Date of Birth**
7. *Sex**
8. *Race and Ethnicity**
9. *Residence**

Service Elements
10. *Unique Service Agency Number**
11. *Unique Health Record Number of Patient*
12. *Unique Number of Principle Registered Nurse Provider*
13. *Episode Admission or Encounter Date**
14. *Discharge or Termination Date**
15. *Disposition of Patient**
16. *Expected Payer for the Bill**

*Elements also included in the Uniform Hospital Discharge Data Set
Werley, H. Nursing diagnosis and the nursing minimum data set. In McLane, A.M. (Ed.), Classification of nursing diagnoses: Proceedings of the seventh conference. St. Louis.: C.V. Mosby, 1987, p.32

Another major benefit of the NMDS, is that the existence of a minimum data set for nursing offers a focus for the documentation of nursing practice. Nursing documentation at the health care organization level must include the elements of the NMDS if any of these benefits are to be realized. The development of the NMDS is an important step for nursing, with important implications for clinical nursing practice, nursing administration, nursing research, and nursing education.

The nursing process is usually taught to nursing students as a series or sequence of discrete steps consisting of assessment, nursing diagnosis, planning, intervention, and evaluation. This separation of activities is, however:

> an artificial separation of actions that in actual practice cannot be separated. To ensure a deliberateness and thoughtfulness in analysis of the process[,] however, it is necessary to label the phases and suggest that the practitioner name each action in terms of the phase of nursing being performed.[28]

This same artificial separation is useful for examining the documentation of nursing practice and for guiding the documentation process in a manner that is consistent with the professional thinking model of nursing.

The recommendation to use nursing diagnosis and the nursing process as a framework for nursing documentation is not new, but this approach does not appear to have provided any magical solution for the problems of nursing documentation. The use of nursing process for nursing documentation has been described in the following manner:

> Is it that the nursing process is so hard to understand? No. The problem seems to be that what nurses have always done now is being named and nurses have to slow down in midstride to identify what they are doing. The process isn't the problem, it's the writing it all down that most find frustrating.[29]

Perhaps an explanation for this frustration can be found in the clinical nursing practice culture. A predominant value of this culture is that providing nursing care is more important than documenting that care.[30] When this is combined with values and rewards for the accomplishment of tasks or simply recording raw data, then the nurse must simultaneously carry on two lines of thought in order to practice in a task-based manner while using nursing process to document that practice. One line of thought will be focused on the tasks to be accomplished or the data to be collected, and the rewards or sanctions for these activities. To translate this task-based practice into something that can be documented with the nursing process is no small challenge. This translation process, from task-based nursing practice to documentation of nursing care using the nursing process, does indeed require the nurse to slow down in mid-stride, and it can be very frustrating as well.

Another possible explanation for the frustration that many nurses experience in attempting to use nursing diagnosis and nursing process as a framework for nursing documentation may be found in the necessity of recording both nursing and medical information. Although there is often a great deal of overlap between these areas, the distinction between these types of information is an important one, both for clinical practice and for nursing documentation. Making this distinction is essential if nurses are to avoid feelings of frustration and confusion which can interfere with the recording of relevant information.

Once the distinctions between disease-related information and information about human responses are made, and appropriate documentation strategies to handle the volumes of data and the observations about the patient's disease-related condition have been identified, many of the issues about the documentation of nursing practice are clearer and easier to address. Issues of importance for nursing documentation then become the selection of a nursing framework for patient assessment, the role of the nursing care plan in nursing documentation, and the complexity of documenting a thinking process that handles large volumes of data and information without redundancy or double documentation. This last issue makes the use of a variety of documentation strategies desirable, and the remainder of this chapter will discuss documentation strategies for each step of the nursing process. (See Table 7–8).

ASSESSMENT

Assessment is the first step of the nursing process, and it consists of an organized method of collecting subjective and objective data from and about the patient. The purpose of assessment is to make a determination about the state of the patient. From a nursing perspective, this determination will be in the form of nursing diagnoses; however, it is useful to separate the assessment and nursing diagnosis steps of the nursing process for this discussion of documentation. Here the term assessment will be used to refer to data collection, while nursing diagnosis will refer to the clustering, interpreting, and labeling of those data.[31]

For the purposes of nursing documentation, it is helpful to think of assessment in two categories: 1) the initial assessment done at the time of the first nurse-patient interaction, and 2) reassessment or evaluation of changes or progress in the patient's condition. The initial assessment is concerned with obtaining baseline information about the patient that is used to initiate nursing care planning. These baseline data also play a role in the reassessment of the patient in that they serve as a basis of comparison with subsequent data for determination of patient progress and the evaluation of nursing care. In both of these categories there will be numerical, repetitive data that lend themselves to flow sheet documentation as well as data and information that require a more descriptive approach. This section will focus on the

TABLE 7–8. NURSING PROCESS: A FRAMEWORK FOR NURSING DOCUMENTATION

Step	Issues	Strategies
Assessment	*nursing focus*	*identify human responses and nursing diagnoses as focus of nursing assessment*
	assessment framework	*review existing nursing assessment frameworks:* • Functional Health Patterns[a] • Daily Living/Health Status[b] • specialty nursing frameworks • assessment frameworks based on nursing theories
		select nursing framework, design and implement assessment tool with emphasis on organizing data so that nursing diagnoses can be identified and supported
	flow sheets, special forms	*put repetitive or numerical data on flow sheets* *develop and implement special forms for categorical data (admission interview, post-op checks, patient teaching, etc.)*
Nursing Diagnosis	*format*	*review existing formats, such as P-E-S[c] and select* *determine how linkage between assessment data and nursing diagnosis will be documented*
	NANDA labels only or using others	*use NANDA labels as a starting point* *for patient situation for which there is no NANDA label, establish a format, approach, and clinical resources for identifying nursing diagnostic labels* *when using labels not on current NANDA list, collect data and compile; consider submitting new diagnostic label to NANDA*
	role of nursing diagnosis in care planning and charting	*establish guidelines for recording nursing diagnoses on the nursing care plan from the assessment tool and in progress note charting*
Planning *Expected Outcomes*	*format for outcome statements*	*establish format for outcomes: measurable, objective, realistic, and include a time frame* *record what the expected outcomes are in the nursing care plan, progress toward achieving outcomes in progress record*
	linkage with nursing diagnoses	*relate to the expected outcomes to the problem component of the nursing diagnosis*
Nursing Interventions	*format*	*start with action verb, include who, what, when, where, how much, and how often* *record what the interventions are in the nursing care plan* *record that interventions were executed on flow sheets, whenever possible (i.e. treatment record)* *describe patient's responses to interventions in progress record*
	linkage with nursing diagnosis	*relate the nursing interventions to the etiology component of the nursing diagnosis*
Implementation	*handling large volumes of data*	*use flow sheets for repetitive, numerical data* *design special forms for categorical data*

TABLE 7–8. **(Continued)**

Step	Issues	Strategies
	organizing narrative, descriptive documentation of implementation	*recognize that regularly recorded activities on flow sheets or special forms provide legal evidence of nursing actions and contacts; do not double document*
		when describing nursing interventions, identify the nursing diagnosis to which the interventions are directed
		data on flow sheets should be referred to, not repeated
		emphasize data analysis and clinical judgment
		supplement the use of a problem-oriented approach (Problem-oriented record, Focus, Outcome Charting) with a summary or overview of the patient periodically
Evaluation	*continuous assessment of the patient's condition*	*record reassessment data on flow sheets*
	accomplishment of expected outcomes	*identify the nursing diagnosis when recording data or information about progress toward outcomes; define the status of the nursing diagnosis (i.e. improving, resolved, stable, etc.)*
		record information about progress toward outcomes in descriptive terms rather than unsubstantiated conclusions (e.g. "ate well," "wound healing well")
		indicate any needed changes or modifications in the nursing care plan

[a] Gordon, M. *Nursing Diagnosis: Process and Application.* (New York: McGraw Hill, 1982), pp. 63–108.
[b] Carnevali, D.L. *Nursing Care Planning: Diagnosis and Management,* 3rd ed. (Philadelphia: J.B. Lippincott, 1983), pp. 11–29.
[c] Gordon, M. p. 8–10.

documentation issues of this initial assessment of the patient, and the issues of reassessment with be discussed in the evaluation section of this chapter.

The focus of data collection in nursing is the patient with a health problem; the nurse is interested in the patient's response to the health problem as manifested in daily living, lifestyle, and body function.[32] With the focus of nursing assessment clearly identified, the next step is to organize both data collection and recording in a manner that is logical and helpful. The biomedical systems model, traditionally used by medicine and nursing, is an assessment framework that is familiar and comfortable for most nurses; however, it is not an adequate model for nursing assessment because the focus of this model is physiology and pathophysiology. A nursing assessment framework should organize data in categories that reflect the focus of nursing: human responses to actual and potential health problems.

A popular nursing framework for patient assessment is the Functional Health Patterns established by Gordon. Eleven pattern areas organize basic nursing assessment data:

• Health-perception/health-management pattern
• Nutritional-metabolic pattern

- Elimination pattern
- Activity-exercise pattern
- Cognitive-perceptual pattern
- Sleep-rest pattern
- Self-perception/self-concept pattern
- Role-relationship pattern
- Sexuality-reproductive pattern
- Coping-stress-tolerance pattern
- Value-belief pattern[33]

These pattern areas represent a biopsychosocial expression of the whole person, making this an assessment framework that is consistent with nursing's values of wholeness and holism. Futhermore, organizing patient assessment data according to these patterns leads directly to nursing diagnoses.

Another framework for nursing assessment has been presented by Carnevali.[34] In this framework, the focus of nursing concern is identified as the relationship between the patient's pattern of daily living with health status and the immediate environment. Assessment data is organized around the requirements for daily living, including the patterns and demands of daily living, and the resources available to the patient, both internal and external.

In a slightly different approach, Kelly has proposed eight categories for nursing data collection: Activities of Daily Living, Comfort Level, Rest/Recreation/Activity, Basic Body Function, Illness/Health Promotion, Description of Self, Interpersonal Relationships, and Environment.[35] These categories are designed to elicit data which will assist in determining nursing diagnoses.

These three nursing assessment frameworks are presented here as a representative, but not exhaustive, example of ways to direct and organize data collection and documentation in nursing practice. Regardless of the assessment framework selected for a documentation system, it is critical that the information produced leads to the identification and support of nursing diagnoses. If the nursing assessment approach is limited to a biomedical systems review or restricted to disease history findings, it will be extremely difficult, if not impossible, for nurses to document accurate and meaningful nursing diagnoses. Furthermore, a documentation system that requires nursing diagnoses but provides no support in terms of data collection to make them will be frustrating for staff to use. The selection of an assessment framework that directs the types and amounts of data collected and recorded, organizes the data into meaningful patterns of information, and assists in identifying and supporting nursing diagnoses is a critical decision for the documentation of diagnosis-based nursing practice.

Once an organizing framework for nursing assessment is chosen, the next step is the development and implementation of an assessment tool. A useful tool should:

1. consist of information that will permit the nurse to develop nursing diagnoses and care plans quickly
2. provide the necessary baseline information to individualize nursing care in the particular setting
3. be concise and permit collection of the data in an appropriate period of time
4. avoid duplication of information gathered by other health care professionals[36]

Another consideration in developing an assessment tool includes the spacing and arrangement of headings so that it is easy to fill out and to locate information on the form. The assessment tool may be designed as a structured interview with the questions for interviewing the patient listed, or it may consist simply of headings or cue words to direct data gathering. If multiple pages are necessary, organizing the flow of information on the tool can help avoid paper shuffling to find the right space for recording information at different points in the patient interview.

In summary, the initial assessment of the patient can be documented effectively on a special form designed for that purpose. The choices of the types and amounts of data that are included on this assessment tool must be guided by the focus of professional nursing rather than the biomedical model. Finally, the data and information obtained in the initial assessment of the patient should identify and support nursing diagnoses, the second step of the nursing process.

NURSING DIAGNOSIS

The determination of nursing diagnoses reflects the clinical thinking of the nurse, in which patient assessment data is converted into information, the nursing diagnosis. Documentation issues for recording nursing diagnoses have to do with the format of the diagnostic statement: whether to limit the diagnostic labels used to only those nursing diagnoses approved by the North American Nursing Diagnosis Association (NANDA), and the necessity to record nursing diagnoses on both the nursing care plan and in the progress record. The discussion presented in this section will focus on the documentation issues of nursing diagnosis. For a discussion of the concept of nursing diagnosis, refer to Chapters 2, 3, and 4.

One of the first issues which must be decided about the documentation of nursing diagnosis is the format for the diagnostic statement. (See Chapter 2 for an extensive discussion of nursing diagnostic formats.) Several formats have been suggested for nursing diagnoses; one of the most popular is the Problem–Etiology–Signs and Symptoms (P–E–S) format.[37] In this format, the problem, the etiology, and the signs and symptoms that led to the determination of the problem are listed. This format can result in a somewhat lengthy diagnostic label, but it does provide both the supporting data and the nurse's judgment about the problem. An example of this format is:

Problem:
   Ineffective Airway Clearance
Etiology: (related to)
   respiratory muscle weakness
Signs and Symptoms: (as manifested by)
   weak cough
   crackles and rhonchi bilaterally
   thick greenish-yellow secretions
   inspirometer volumes of 900–1000 cc

This format offers a great deal of information about the patient, and it presents the supporting data for the nursing diagnosis clearly. In the busy world of clinical nursing practice, however, this format is lengthy and cumbersome at best and frustrating and time-consuming at worst.

For documentation purposes, the two-part nursing diagnostic format of problem and etiology statement is recommended for recording the diagnostic label. The necessity of supporting the nursing diagnosis with documentation of the appropriate signs and symptoms can be accomplished in many ways. Linking the pertinent assessment data with the nursing diagnosis can be accomplished by recording initial nursing diagnoses on the assessment tool with their supporting data. There are a number of other issues for documenting the nursing diagnoses that will be discussed throughout the remainder of the chapter.

A question that frequently arises in a discussion of nursing diagnosis is whether only those nursing diagnoses that have been approved by NANDA should be used, or can other nursing diagnostic labels be recorded? While the NANDA taxonomy is widely used, there is no universal agreement in nursing about diagnostic terminology. Furthermore, the NANDA taxonomy is not complete; in fact "black boxes" are included in Taxonomy I to demonstrate the provisional nature of this framework and to indicate areas where further examination and definition of nursing practice should occur.[38]

The nursing diagnoses approved by NANDA provide a useful starting point for documentation of nursing diagnoses. There are benefits to using the approved terminology whenever possible, including the greater ease of using an established diagnostic label rather than identifying a new label, and consistency of terminology between nurses. Using the approved nursing diagnoses can be less anxiety-provoking for nurses who are new to nursing diagnoses; however, limiting the choices to only the NANDA-approved labels can have unfortunate results.

When nurses are limited to the NANDA-approved labels, the incompleteness of Taxonomy I can lead to a great deal of frustration and, ultimately, resistance to the use of nursing diagnoses. The purpose of identifying a nursing diagnosis is to describe and communicate the state of the patient. When nurses are forced to select nursing diagnostic labels that do not accurately reflect the clinical condition of the patient because their options are limited, then nursing diagnosis becomes meaningless. Instead of clinical thinking and diagnostic reasoning, the process of reaching a nursing diagnosis is reduced to "picking something off the list."

Alternatives must be available for nurses who are struggling to identify the patient's condition, but find that there is no appropriate nursing diagnostic label in the NANDA taxonomy. One alternative is to permit use of nursing diagnostic labels developed by specialty organizations or published in the nursing literature. Oftentimes, a nursing diagnostic label may be proposed through these mechanisms and available for use before it can be submitted to NANDA. In fact, the clinical testing of nursing diagnostic labels must occur in nursing practice before the approval process.

It is also possible to make an approved nursing diagnosis more accurate or descriptive of a particular clinical situation by revising or identifying a new etiology statement for the problem statement. (See Chapter 3 for a detailed discussion of the role of the etiology statement in nursing diagnosis.) The etiology statement can improve the accuracy and precision of the diagnostic label, making the application of the recognized nursing diagnoses to individual patients and to specialty patient populations more meaningful.

Another alternative for clinical situations for which an approved nursing diagnosis is not available would be the development of a new diagnostic label. For example, a nursing unit that consistently encounters a patient condition for which no nursing diagnosis exists might decide to review the literature on this condition, collect data on a number of patients, and then develop a nursing diagnostic label that could be submitted to NANDA for addition to the taxonomy. This approach keeps the use of nursing diagnoses, and their documentation, focused on the needs and condition of patient rather than emphasizing a restrictive, task-based attitude about nursing diagnosis. If this alternative were widely used, it could also hasten the development of clinically useful nursing diagnostic labels.

A balance must be reached between encouraging the use of approved nursing diagnoses and restricting the description of patient conditions in nursing diagnostic terminology. On one hand, forcing an inaccurate diagnostic label on a clinical situation because only approved nursing diagnoses can be recorded is undesirable. On the other hand, every nurse creating a new label for every problem is equally undesirable.

As a general guideline, start with the approved nursing diagnoses in the NANDA taxonomy. If there is not an approved nursing diagnosis that accurately describes the patient condition, the next option is to explore possible etiology statements for an approved nursing diagnosis. If there is not an approved nursing diagnosis that even approximates the patient's condition, a review of the nursing literature, including specialty publications, is indicated. If there is nothing available in the nursing literature, then the development of a new diagnostic label may be necessary.

The nursing diagnosis, as a descriptive label for the condition of the patient, occupies a critically important role in the documentation of diagnosis-based nursing practice. The nursing diagnosis must be recorded so that the supporting data are clearly identified, the necessary treatment is prescribed, and the progress of the condition and responses to treatment can be evaluated. These requirements make it necessary to document the nursing dialogue as a discrete step of the nursing process and to refer to it in the documentation of other steps as well. While the determination of the nursing diagnosis usually occurs at the end of the assessment step, from a documentation perspective, it also serves as the beginning of the care planning step.

PLANNING

Planning is the third step of the nursing process. The importance and value of planning individualized nursing care is emphasized in nursing education and included in regulatory standards for nursing. In the JCAHO standards for nursing services, two standards specifically address nursing care planning. Standard NR. 5.3 states the expectation that "A registered nurse plans each patient's nursing care," while NR.5.5 indicates the concern that "The plan of care is documented and reflects current standards of nursing practice."[39]

In the clinical practice culture, however, providing nursing care is generally considered more important than the planning of that care. Nurses may indicate that they have a plan for their patients "in my head," but that a written plan is not necessary. The purpose of nursing care planning is to promote quality nursing care through the facilitation of individualized care, continuity of care, communication, and evaluation of care.[40] In view of these important reasons for nursing care planning,

> plans for nursing management cannot be kept in some nebulous state within the nurse's head but must be documented explicitly and publicly in a permanent form.[41]

Nursing care planning is a tangible indication of professional accountability in nursing.

In clinical practice, nurses are thinking ahead and planning for patient care. Benner has indicated that an outstanding characteristic of expert nurses is that "they spend a great deal of their nursing time thinking about the future course of a patient, anticipating what problems might arise and what they would do about them."[42] The challenge, then, is to capture on paper this "thinking ahead" that nurses do. Nursing diagnosis provides a way to focus the nursing care planning process on clearly identified problems, but this must be combined with a documentation format that is efficient and realistic.

As a document, the nursing care plan consists of the nursing diagnosis, the outcomes that can be expected from treatment of the nursing diagnosis, and the nursing interventions designed to achieve those outcomes. In the nursing care plan, the nursing diagnosis describes the current condition of the patient; outcomes reflect the desired health state of the patient. The expected outcomes are based on the problem component of the nursing diagnostic statement.[43] An examination of the discrepancy between the nursing diagnosis and the desired outcome leads to the identification of nursing interventions that will be most effective in narrowing the gap. These projected outcomes also play a critical role in evaluating the effectiveness of the nursing interventions.[44]

Expected Outcomes

Expected outcomes are measurable, observable behaviors or clinical findings. If they are to serve their dual purpose of guiding nursing intervention and determining the effectiveness of nursing care, then expected outcomes must be written in a way that can be easily understood. The following guidelines for writing expected outcomes have been recommended:

1. Outcomes should be patient-centered
2. Outcomes should be clear and concise
3. Outcomes should be observable and measurable
4. Outcomes should include a specific timeframe for monitoring progress toward their accomplishment
5. Outcomes should be realistic
6. Outcomes should be determined by the patient and nurse together whenever possible[45]

Expected outcomes for nursing diagnoses that are clear and specific offer prescriptive guidance in selecting nursing interventions and serve as evaluation criteria for the success of the nursing care plan. Furthermore, the determination of expected outcomes is dependent upon an accurate and precise nursing diagnosis of the patient's condition.

Nursing Interventions

The discrepancy between the current condition of the patient, the nursing diagnosis; and the desired state of the patient, the expected outcomes; is the focus for the next component of nursing care planning: nursing interventions. The terms "nursing intervention," "nursing action," "implementation," and "nursing order" have all been used to describe the treatment portion of the nursing process.[46] In this book, the term "nursing intervention" will refer to nursing activities to treat nursing diagnoses. The term "implementation" will indicate the execution of nursing interventions.

Nursing interventions are defined as:

> autonomous action based on scientific rationale that is executed to benefit the client in a predicted way related to the nursing diagnosis and stated goals. Nursing interventions are treatments for nursing diagnoses.[47]

For documentation purposes, several decisions must be made about nursing interventions, including the format for writing nursing interventions and strategies for individualizing nursing interventions.

Nursing interventions must be recorded with clarity and precision if they are to direct nursing activity effectively. To achieve this necessary clarity, nursing interventions must include:

1. The date
2. A precise action verb and appropriate modifiers

3. A content area indicating the what and where of the intervention
4. A time element specifying when, how often, and how long
5. The signature of the prescribing nurse[48]

Consider the difference between a nursing intervention written in the above format and one written in the usual nursing jargon. A favorite jargon phrase frequently seen on nursing care plans is:

Offer emotional support PRN.

Nurses know that most patients will need some type of emotional support at some point. The direction to offer emotional support, without any indication of reasons or strategies, is meaningless. A useful nursing intervention, however, would define strategies and opportunities so that any nurse reading the care plan could carry out the nursing intervention.

A nursing intervention for the same purpose, based on the guidelines listed above, might read:

2/29/88 Explore patient's feelings about the appearance of facial burns during grooming/self-care activities.

(signature)E. Miller, RN

Here, the nursing intervention begins with an action verb "explore" indicating the specific behavior that the nurse should use. The content of the intervention is specified as well: the patient's feelings about the appearance of facial burns. The timeframe is somewhat fluid, but linking an exploration of feelings about appearance with grooming and self-care activities is logical and practical. Finally, the date and signature are included.

Nursing interventions generally fall into three categories: assessment interventions, treatment interventions, and educational interventions. Assessment interventions are those observations of the patient that should be made in order to further define the patient's condition, to monitor the progression of the nursing diagnosis, and to evaluate responses to other nursing interventions. Treatment interventions are specific actions undertaken by the nurse to improve or to compensate for the condition of the patient as described in the nursing diagnosis. Educational interventions consist of teaching activities that the nurse uses to inform the patient about health, his or her present conditions, and self-care activities. Health promotion and the development of knowledge are important areas of independent nursing practice.[49]

Most patients will require nursing interventions from all three categories; however, the proportion from each category will be influenced by the current situation. For example, the nursing care plan for a newly admitted patient may have a higher proportion of assessment and treatment interventions, while a patient anticipating discharge will have nursing diagnoses and educational interventions to prepare the patient to assume health maintenance activities at home.

The purpose of the nursing care plan is to direct the nursing care of an individual patient over time. The registered nurse is responsible for developing the plan, but it may be executed by other levels of nursing personnel, such as LPNs or nursing assistants, under the direction of the RN. It is essential, then, that the nursing care plan contain clear and understandable statements about the patient's condition (the nursing diagnosis), what the plan should accomplish (the expected outcomes), and exactly how to go about achieving these changes in the patient's condition (the nursing interventions).

Planned nursing care, rather than spontaneous nursing activity, is considered to represent quality nursing care, and this is reflected in the JCAHO standards for nursing and in the education of nurses. Nursing care plans demonstrate the professional accountability of nurses, representing the willingness and the intent of nurses to alter or improve the condition of the patient. Furthermore, there is accountability inherent in the nursing care plan for both the nurse who identifies the nursing diagnosis and prescribes appropriate nursing interventions and for those nurses who carry out the plan.

The best nursing care plan form or automated care planning system will be for naught unless nurses are willing, able, and have the time to make directives for nursing care clear and explicit. A nursing care plan can accomplish none of its intended purposes—individualized nursing care, continuity and communication—if the information recorded on the plan is unclear, imprecise, or consists only of jargon. Documentation of nursing care planning, the actual writing aspect, is dependent upon the thinking processes and values of nurses, and the best documentation system in the world will not result in high-quality nursing care plans unless nurses actually develop and record them.

Developing nursing care plans which are clear, precise, and directive does require more words and more thought. Writing vague statements and jargon, however, is a waste of time for the nurses who write them as well as for those nurses who might read them. Indeed, one of the major reasons that nurses resist writing nursing care plans is the complaint that no one reads them; however, when the written plan consists of nebulous suggestions of things that the nurse would probably do anyway, then there is little point in reading that plan. A fundamental principle of nursing care planning is that the plan must be useful in directing patient care; otherwise, there is no point to it.

Types of Nursing Care Plans

The development of a useful, directive nursing care plan takes time, thought, and clinical knowledge. The development of a comprehensive nursing care plan for a newly admitted patient can consume one to two hours of professional nursing time.[50] In another study, registered nurses spent an average of 73 minutes per 8 hour shift on documentation for an average of 4.6 patients with 12 percent of that time spent on planning.[51]

Efforts to utilize nursing time effectively have resulted in several types of nursing care plans. In addition to the individualized plan that nurses learn in nursing school, there are standardized nursing care plans, modified standardized or generic nursing care plans, and automated nursing care plans. Each type of plan has advantages and disadvantages; furthermore, none of these alone can address the issues of nurses' valuing the care planning process and the administrative support that is essential for diagnosis-based nursing practice and its documentation.

The individualized nursing care plan generally consists of a blank form (or screen in an automated system) with headings for nursing diagnosis, expected outcomes, and nursing interventions. The advantages of this type of plan are that it can be highly individualized for a particular patient, and the nurse has essentially an open set of options in planning that allow creativity and flexibility. The major disadvantage of individualized nursing care plans is that they can be time-consuming to develop and record.

In order to minimize the time-consuming aspects of the individualized plan and to assure that nursing care plans were consistent with standards of care, the standardized care plan was created. A standard care plan is "a specific protocol of care that is appropriate for patients who are experiencing the usual or predictable problems associated with a given diagnosis or disease process."[52] Standard care plans include specific nursing diagnoses, expected outcomes, and nursing interventions in a printed or automated format, and they may be developed for a particular setting or found in the literature, such as journals and texts.

Standard care plans can be used in two ways. One approach is to use plan document as a part of the patient's record. The nurse would obtain a copy of the appropriate standard plan and place this in the patient's record. This approach minimizes the amount of actual writing that the nurse must do, and it does assure that the nursing care plans are consistent with the standards. An alternative approach makes the standard care plans available to nurses as a reference for developing individualized care plans. This addresses the concern that care plans reflect the standards of the organization, but it may not decrease the amount of writing involved.

The advantages of standard nursing care plans is that they are usually developed by clinical experts, who are familiar with the most current nursing practice issues, and that they reduce the time nurses must spend to write a nursing care plan. The disadvantages, however, are significant. The major disadvantage is that standard care plans are not designed for individual patients who may have similar conditions. While the nursing diagnosis on the standard plan may be appropriate, the predetermined expected outcomes and nursing interventions contained in the plan may not be useful or effective for a particular patient. Furthermore, standard plans restrict any participation in the care planning process by the patient.

Dissatisfaction with standard nursing care plans, which looked good on paper but never seemed to fit a real patient, led to the development of the modified standard plan. Here nursing diagnoses are identified, and expected outcomes and nursing interventions are listed; however, these are written with blank spaces, so that aspects of the plan can be modified to the particular needs of an individual patient. Expected outcomes or nursing interventions that are not appropriate for this patient may be crossed off (or in an automated system only the appropriate ones would be selected). This type of nursing care plan is also referred to as a generic plan.[53]

The advantages of the modified standard or generic nursing care plan include improved adherence to quality standards, the development of the plans by clinical experts, and a decrease in the amount of time required for documentation.[54] Failure to fill in the blank spaces, however, or to select and delete appropriate expected outcomes or nursing interventions can result in the same disadvantages for the modified standard or generic care plans as those found with standard plans. Lack of individualization of nursing care and lack of opportunity for the patient to participate in planning care can occur with this type of plan as well as with standard plans.

Automated nursing care plans are those plans that are developed and recorded in a computerized information system. Any type of nursing care plan can be automated: individualized, standardized, or the modified standard plan. The same advantages and disadvantages that are found with these types of plans in a manual system will occur in an automated system. The issues of nursing diagnosis and information systems are presented in Chapter 9.

In summary, the nursing care plan consists of the nursing diagnoses, the expected outcomes, and the nursing interventions. The purpose of recording these three components of the nursing process in the form of a plan is to direct nursing care activities. This direction is provided in two ways: by the nursing diagnosis, which clearly identifies the patient condition requiring nursing treatment, and by the clarity and precision of the written word. Remember, the practice of nursing is primarily a problem-solving activity; it is impossible to solve problems if you do not know what they are! Then, if vague, nebulous jargon is used to document nursing care planning, the plan will be ineffective in directing nursing care, at best; at worst, the plan will be meaningless and a waste of time.

Nursing care planning is generally not a popular topic in the clinical nursing practice culture. The negative perceptions about nursing care planning reflect the time-consuming aspects of writing care plans and the lack of usefulness of these plans for actual patient care. This perception must change. Yura and Walsh state:

> Failure to take the time to assess and plan before intervening contributes to the misuse of time and to wasted efforts and talents of nursing and health care personnel. The cost in economic, physical, and emotional terms can hardly be estimated. Economically and morally, the profession of nursing cannot permit this misuse of human and material resources.[55]

In this era of cost-containment, shortage of nurses, and increasing patient acuity, nurses cannot afford to waste valuable time rediscovering patient problems and strategies to deal with these in every nurse-patient interaction. Useful nursing care plans are essential, and guidelines have been presented in this chapter to promote clarity and precision of the plan, including formats for writing expected outcomes and nursing interventions.

IMPLEMENTATION

Implementation is the step in the nursing process in which the nursing interventions, specified on the nursing care plan, are put into effect. This definition of implementation assumes that a nursing care plan has been developed; however, in the clinical practice environment, planning and implementation often occur simultaneously. As the nurse identifies patient problems, actions to deal with these problems are immediately brought into play. Although the nursing process and documentation based on that process can be examined as a series of steps, in actuality the entire set of activities are always in mind, and each step influences the other.[56]

Documentation of the implementation of the nursing care plan includes recording both data and information. The implementation step requires documentation strategies to deal with large volumes of data, such as repetitive treatments and the times they were done. In addition, the observations about the patient's condition, behaviors, or responses to the nursing interventions must also be recorded. These two aspects of implementation require different documentation approaches. (See Table 7–8.)

Repetitive, numerical data can be effectively and efficiently recorded on flow sheets or special forms. A treatment record for the documentation of regularly scheduled nursing treatments can be used to indicate the intervention and the date and time that it was performed. This documentation strategy is useful for nursing interventions associated with nursing diagnoses and routine nursing activities, such as hygiene or safety checks. Furthermore, this type of documentation provides legal evidence of the quantity and nature of regularly scheduled nursing contacts and actions,[57] and it is unnecessary to repeat these data in the progress record.

Flow sheets or special forms are documentation strategies for recording that an intervention was done; however, these strategies do not provide a mechanism for recording observations of the patient's condition, behaviors, or responses to the interventions. These data are essential for monitoring the patient's responses and progress, and so a descriptive, narrative format is required for this aspect of the implementation of nursing care, which is usually recorded in the progress section of the patient record.

This descriptive aspect of the implementation phase can be accomplished using a traditional narrative format, the problem-oriented record, or a problem-oriented variation such as Focus Charting. In addition to the format selection, there are four key points regarding the content for documentation at this point. These points are:

1. The relationship between the nursing interventions and the nursing diagnosis
2. The relationship between the data on the flow sheet/treatment record and the descriptions in the progress record
3. The emphasis on clinical judgment and data *analysis* rather than simple data recording
4. The necessity of supplementing problem-focused documentation with a periodic summary or overview of the patient

Each of these points will be discussed further.

When nursing interventions are recorded on a flow sheet or treatment record, it is adequate to indicate that they were done; however, when descriptive data about the nursing interventions are recorded, the nursing diagnosis should also be recorded. This link between the nursing diagnosis and the nursing interventions will be critical in evaluating the effectiveness of the interventions in dealing with the problem. This determination cannot be made unless this linkage is clearly identified.

Consider a patient with a nursing diagnosis of Activity Intolerance related to imbalance between oxygen supply and demand. Nursing interventions on the nursing care plan include frequent rest periods, progressing the length of time for ambulation by 2 minutes each day, and consulting the physical therapist for energy conservation strategies. Notations on the treatment record indicate that this patient has ambulated in the hall at 10:15 A.M. and 8:00 P.M., bathed himself, and sat in the chair for all meals. Descriptive data in the progress record state that the patient has "had a good day, tolerating activity without complaint."

Based on the documentation in this example, it would not appear that the nursing care plan is directing this patient's care. In the absence of any linkage between the nursing diagnosis and associated care plan and the documentation of actual nursing care delivered, the question must be raised as to whether the patient received any of the nursing interventions identified on the care plan. It is also impossible to determine whether nursing care is successful in assisting this patient to deal with his problem of Activity Intolerance. In fact, from the progress record, even the existence of this nursing diagnosis for this patient could be questioned.

Consider an alternative progress note for this patient written in the traditional narrative format:

> (date/time): This 67-year-old male patient with a nursing diagnosis of Activity Intolerance related to imbalance of oxygen supply and demand has had a good day. Able to ambulate for an additional 2 minutes this morning without shortness of breath or chest pain although heart rate did increase from 88 to 104. Rest periods before and after meals seem effective in allowing him adequate energy to eat all of meals.
> (signature)

This note could also have been written in either the problem-oriented SOAP format or the Focus Charting format. The important point is that descriptive data about the nursing diagnosis and associated nursing interventions are recorded in such a way that the patient's progress and the effectiveness of the plan can be evaluated.

The second and third points about recording descriptive implementation data have to do with the relationship between the data on the flow sheet and the data documented in the progress record. It is helpful to think of the flow sheet data as raw, unstructured facts, while the progress record documentation reflects the processing and analysis of those raw data by the nurse's clinical judgment. From a documentation perspective, it is unnecessary to repeat the data on the flow sheet in progress record notations. What is necessary is to record the nurse's judgments and conclusions about the data.

Descriptive information in the progress record should demonstrate professional nursing judgment and interpretation. This may take the form of the detection of a change in the patient's condition or the status of the nursing diagnosis. The interpretation of data from the flow sheet, such as the recognition of trends of patterns, should also be recorded. Restating data from the flow sheet should only be done if it contributes to this analysis and interpretation.

A final point about recording descriptive information about the implementation of nursing interventions is the recommendation of a summary or overview of the general state of the patient at regular intervals. It is sometimes possible to lose track of the human being in a problem-focused documentation record, or as Turner suggests:

> the patient may get lost between the lines . . . On reading the progression of a patient problem record one can find out how a wound is healing or how a disease is progressing but not how the patient is doing.[58]

Supplementing problem-focused notations with a summary or overview of the patient's general state can do much to maintain the emphasis on the whole patient rather than reducing patients to simply a list of problems.

For the implementation step of the nursing process, the issues of format and content have been discussed. Another important issue has to do with the frequency requirements for nursing documentation, which can range from hourly notations in intensive care units to weekly summaries in the rehabilitation setting. Frequency determination must be guided by the clinical necessities of the patient population as well as legal and regulatory directives.

A few common sense guidelines are offered here for deciding upon the frequency requirements for documentation of the implementation step of the nursing process. First, the placement of flow sheets and treatment records at the patient's bedside makes it feasible for the nurse to document nursing activities as they are performed. The frequency requirement for documentation would be that nursing activities are recorded when they are performed.

Notations in the progress record of descriptive data and the nurse's clinical judgments are not quite so clear cut in terms of the frequency of documentation. Theoretically, progress notes should be written whenever there is a change observed in the status of the patient's problem or when there is no response, or an unexpected response, to treatment.[59] A minimal frequency requirement for acute care settings would be once every 24 hours; however, changes in the patient's condition or significant events should be recorded in a timely fashion. For example, on a general medical-surgical unit, a nursing note every 24 hours might be supplemented with a description of the patient's first time out of bed.

Determining the frequency of nursing notation in the progress record should reflect the clinical status of the patient population. When the clinical condition of the patients is changing rapidly, then frequent, brief notations focusing on specific problems may be required; however, a relatively stable population might be well-described with a more comprehensive, but less frequent, summary note. If flow sheets or treatment records are used to record nursing actions and contacts with the patient, then the frequency of progress notation can be decreased. In the event that the only documentation mechanism is a chronological, narrative format, then progress notes must be done more frequently, and they will probably be lengthy as there is no other mechanism for recording pertinent data.

In summary, the implementation step of the nursing process is where nursing interventions are put into effect. The documentation of this step requires strategies for recording the execution of the interventions as well as descriptive data and the nurses' judgments about the patient's responses and progress. Adequate, accurate documentation is essential at this step, both as a record of the nursing care provided for the patient and as clinical information about the patient's progress. This information about the patient's progress forms the basis for the next step of the nursing process, evaluation.

EVALUATION

Evaluation is the final step of the nursing process. The patient is reassessed in order to determine progress toward achieving the desired outcomes of care and to determine the effectiveness of the nursing care plan in accomplishing those outcomes. While the process of evaluation of nursing care is emphasized in nursing education and the professional standards of nursing, evaluation is not usually a strong point in nursing documentation. Carnevali states:

> Nurses have always been taught that it is important to chart action taken and client response. In practice, more emphasis seems to have been placed on what is done, than on how the client responds, unless the response is both dramatic and untoward.[60]

Again, the value of the clinical practice culture that holds that providing care is more important than documenting or evaluating that care seems to be the driving force.

Although evaluation is identified as the last step of the nursing process, it occurs at every point along the way. Nurses are continually assessing and evaluating their patients in the clinical practice environment; however, much of that thinking never makes it into the patient record. The evaluation phase of the nursing process is concerned with the continuous assessment and evaluation of the patient's condition and with the accomplishment of expected outcomes.

Documentation of the evaluation step is also concerned with the continuous assessment of the patient's condition and the accomplishment of the expected outcomes of treatment. In order to make evaluative judgments about the patient's progress, data must be collected and recorded in a way that lends itself to quantitative or qualitative measurement with some degree of reliability.[61] Vague, nebulous statements or jargon do not offer any way to evaluate the progress of the patient or the effectiveness of the nursing care provided to the patient.

The continuous assessment of the patient will be indicated through the collection of pertinent assessment data as recorded on appropriate flow sheets and special forms. Professional judgments about the meaning of these data will be documented in the progress record as a part of the implementation process. The nursing care plan also contributes important information for the evaluation process in the form of clearly stated outcomes and nursing interventions. The clarity of these statements is essential to determine if the outcome behaviors have been achieved and if nursing interventions have been properly executed.

Evaluation consist of three sequential steps:

1. Review of the expected outcomes of nursing intervention for the patient
2. Collection of data about the patient's current situation
3. Comparison of the expected outcomes with the patient's current situation

Evaluation can only be undertaken when specific goals have been set in advance and certain nursing interventions have been carried out. While assessment is concerned with arriving at the nursing diagnosis or a description of the patient, evaluation is concerned with the patient's progress toward defined outcomes.[62] Furthermore, that ability to make judgments about the patient's progress will depend, to a large degree, on the clarity and accuracy of the data and information in the patient record.

The evaluation phase of the nursing process is essentially one of judgment:

- Is the patient making progress?
- Have outcomes been achieved?
- Are the nursing interventions effective?
- Has the nursing diagnosis been successfully treated?
- Are there new nursing diagnoses present that require treatment?

These are the questions that must be answered at the evaluation step of the nursing process.

Documentation of evaluation of outcome accomplishment should be linked with the nursing diagnosis and nursing interventions whenever possible. Returning to the patient with Activity Intolerance related to imbalance between oxygen supply and demand, expected outcomes for this patient included a longer time period that he could ambulate without chest pain or shortness of breath, and the ability to eat most of his meals without feelings of fatigue. Nursing interventions on the nursing care plan include frequent rest periods as well as rest periods before and after meals, progressing the length of time for ambulation by 2 minutes each day, and consulting the physical therapist for energy conservation strategies. In the previous progress note, the implementation of these nursing interventions was documented. Now, add the evaluative component:

> (date/time): This 67-year-old male patient with a nursing diagnosis of Activity Intolerance related to imbalance of oxygen supply and demand has had a good day. Able to ambulate for an additional 2 minutes this morning without shortness of breath or chest pain although heart rate did increase from 88 to 104. Rest periods before and after meals seem effective in allowing him adequate energy to eat all of meals. Patient is making gradual improvement in tolerance of physical activity—now able to ambulate for 6 minutes, could only do about 30 seconds on admission. Current plan is working well, continue to monitor patient's cardiovascular condition and responses to activity.
>
> (signature)

This note is written in the narrative format. If it were written in the SOAP format, the addition of an I for the implementation of the plan, and an E for the evaluative component would be necessary.

This note includes a statement about the patient's progress (gradual improvement in tolerance of activity, now able to ambulate for six minutes) and a statement about the effectiveness of the plan (continue current plan). Both the patient's progress and the necessity to modify or change the plan of care for the patient are important in evaluating the patient's care. As this patient is making progress, albeit gradual, with the current plan, there is no indication to make modifications. On the other hand, if the patient was not making progress, then modification would be in order.

This example demonstrates the fundamental linkage between the nursing diagnosis, expected outcomes, and nursing interventions contained in the nursing care plan, and the implementation and evaluation of nursing care. The documentation of these components of the nursing process must also be linked. Evaluation of the effectiveness of nursing care can only take place if the information about the care provided and the patient's responses are available; in addition, it will be difficult, if not impossible, to evaluate the patient's progress in the absence of a clearly-defined nursing diagnosis and associated expected outcomes. Finally, it will be impossible to determine if the patient's progress is due to nursing care unless the required nursing interventions are specified and then executed.

CONCLUSION

The practice of nursing is not simple, nor can it be easily reduced into tasks and chores. Any approach to the documentation of nursing practice must reflect the complexity of nursing practice and the concerns of nurses for the whole patient. The use of nursing diagnosis, within the framework of the nursing process, offers a way to focus both clinical nursing practice and the documentation of that practice.

These issues and requirements are further complicated by the necessity for nurses to document disease-related information and additional information required by the health care organization, in addition to documenting nursing practice. Any system for nursing documentation must clearly distinguish these categories of information because the approaches for documenting these types of information can and should vary. There must be documentation strategies to record large volumes of data easily and effectively, as well as strategies for documenting descriptive information and the clinical judgments of the professional nurse.

A variety of strategies for documentation of nursing practice have been discussed in this chapter, and they are founded on five principles. (See Table 7–3). For a documentation system to be most useful, it should reflect the unique characteristics and requirements of the organization. These principles and the strategies suggested here are offered as a framework for developing an individualized system for documenting diagnosis-based nursing practice.

Finally, the documentation of nursing practice is different from nursing practice, but the realities of nursing practice are powerful determinants of what actually is documented in the patient record. The institution of a new documentation system will not solve clinical practice problems. If anything, documentation requirements that differ form the values and practices of the clinical practice culture may expose or create more problems than they solve.

A documentation system that includes nursing diagnosis cannot be effectively utilized in task-based nursing practice. Conversely, the efforts of nurses to practice in a diagnosis-based manner will be frustrated by documentation requirements that focus on tasks and chores rather than identifying patient problems and nursing treatment of these. The use of nursing diagnosis in clinical practice must proceed hand-in-hand with a documentation system for clinical practice for both to be successful.

REFERENCES

1. Saba, V.K. & McCormick, K. A. *Essentials of computers for nurses.* (Philadelphia: J.B. Lippincott, 1986, p. 105
2. Meade, C.D. & Kim, M.J. The effect of teaching on documentation of nursing diagnoses. In M.J. Kim, G.K. McFarland, & A.M. McLane, (Eds.), *Classification of nursing diagnoses: Proceedings of the fifth national conference.* St. Louis: C.V. Mosby, 1984, p. 241
3. Mundinger, M., & Jauron, G. Developing a nursing diagnosis. *Nursing Outlook,* 1975, *23,* 94
4. Meade & Kim
5. Lynnhoke, J.L. Charting for Dollars. *American Journal of Nursing,* 1985, *85,* 6, 685
6. Halloran, E.J., Patterson, C., & Kiley, M. Casemix: Matching patient need with nursing resources. *Nursing Management,* 1987, *18,* 3, 28
7. Iyer, P.W., Taptich, B.J., & Bernocchi-Losey, D. *Nursing process and nursing documentation.* Philadelphia: W.B. Saunders, 1986
8. *Ibid.*
9. Guzelaydin, S.K. & Pfoutz, S.K. Differences in documentation of nursing services according to recording format. In M.J. Kim, G.K. McFarland, & A.M. McLane, (Eds.), *Classification of nursing diagnoses: proceedings of the fifth national conference,* St. Louis: C.V. Mosby, 1984, p. 267
10. Turner, S.L. The nursing process for the very stubborn. *Nursing Management,* 1987, *18,* 6, 69
11. Lampe, S.S. Focus charting: Streamlining documentation. *Nursing Management,* 1985, *16,* 7, 43
12. *Ibid.*
13. Gamberg, D., Hushower, G., & Smith, N. Outcome charting. *Nursing Management,* 1981 *12,* 1, 37

14. Burke, L.J., & Murphy, J. *Charting by exception: A cost-effective, quality approach.* Somerset, NJ: John Wiley & Sons, 1988
15. Kim, M.J., McFarland, G.K., & McLane, A.M. *Pocket guide to nursing diagnoses,* 2nd ed. St. Louis: C.V. Mosby, 1987
16. Gordon, M. *Nursing diagnosis: Process and application.* New York: McGraw Hill, 1982
17. *Ibid.*
18. Kramer, J.D., & Notarangelo, P.L. Documentation: Designing forms that serve *you. Nursing Management,* 1986, *17,* 10, 72
19. Deane, D., McElroy, M.J., & Alden, S. Documentation: Meeting requirements while maximizing productivity. *Nursing Economics,* 1986, *4,* 4, p. 176
20. Miller, E. Computerized care planning. *Nursing Administration Quarterly,* 1986, *10,* 2, p.63
21. Gordon
22. Lampe
23. Gordon
24. Carnevali, D.L. *Nursing care planning: Diagnosis and management,* 3rd ed. Philadelphia: J.B. Lippincott, 1983, p. 159
25. American Nurses' Association. *Nursing: A social policy statement.* Kansas City: American Nurses' Association, 1980
26. Werley, H.H. Nursing diagnosis and the minimum data set. In A. M. McLane (Ed.), *Classification of nursing diagnoses: Proceedings of the seventh conference.* St. Louis: C.V. Mosby, 1987, 21
27. Werley, H.H. Status of the minimum data set and its relationship to nursing diagnoses. Paper presented at the meeting of the North American Nursing Diagnosis Association, St. Louis, March 1988
28. Yura, H. & Walsh, M. B. *The nursing process: Assessing, planning, implementing, evaluating,* 4th ed. Norwalk, CT: Appleton-Century-Crofts, 1983, p. 21
29. Turner
30. Meade & Kim
31. Gordon
32. Kelly, M. A. *Nursing diagnosis source book: Guidelines for clinical application.* Norwalk, CT: Appleton-Century-Crofts, 1985, p. 25
33. Gordon
34. Carnevali
35. Kelly
36. Carnevali
37. Gordon
38. A. M. McLane (Ed.). *Classification of nursing diagnoses: Proceedings of the seventh national conference.* St. Louis: C. V. Mosby, 1987, p. 469
39. Joint Commission on Accreditation of Health Organizations. *Accreditation manual for hospitals.* Chicago: JCAH, 1988, p. 146
40. Bower, F. *The process of planning nursing care,* 3rd ed. St. Louis: C. V. Mosby, 1982, p. 4
41. Carnevali
42. Brenner, P. *From novice to expert: Excellence and power in clinical nursing practice.* (Menlo Park, CA: Addison-Wesley, 1984, p. 102
43. Iyer, Taptich, & Bernocchi-Losey. *Nursing Process and Nursing Documentation,* p. 124.
44. Gordon, *Nursing Diagnosis: Process and Application,* p. 239.
45. Iyer, Taptich, & Bernocchi-Losey
46. Bulecheck, G. M. & McCloskey, J. C. *Nursing interventions: Treatments for nursing diagnoses.* Philadelphia: W.B. Saunders, 1985, p. 8
47. *Ibid.*
48. Carnevali
49. Kelly
50. Sovie, M.D. Managing resources in a constrained economic environment. *Nursing Economics* 1985, *3,* 3, 85
51. Deane, McElroy, & Alden
52. Mayers, M. *A systematic approach to the nursing care plan.* Norwalk, Ct: Appleton-Century-Crofts, 1983, p. 14
53. Deane, McElroy, & Alden
54. *Ibid.*
55. Yura & Walsh
56. Gordon
57. Carnevali
58. Turner
59. Gordon
60. Carnevali
61. *Ibid.*
62. *Ibid.*

CHAPTER 8

Quality Assurance in Diagnosis-based Nursing Practice

Dana Moriconi

Quality is an elusive but essential aspect of health care. While health care professionals, consumers, and those who pay for health care are all concerned about quality, there is also a great deal of concern about the cost of health care. These concerns about cost are particularly problematic because the concept of quality is not well defined or agreed upon in health care.

Quality may be defined as a peculiar and essential character, degree of excellence, high social status, or distinguishing attribute.[1] Another attempt to define quality views it as conformance to requirements, not as goodness.[2] Peters and Austin state that quality is about "care, people, passion, consistency, eyeball contact and gut reaction."[3] While all of these definitions provide some insight into the concept of quality, they fall short of a useful framework for defining and measuring the quality of health care in general, and nursing care in particular.

Another approach to quality consists of determining whether something meets or exceeds certain requirements or standards. For example, perfume and cologne are similiar in composition; however, a higher percentage of scented oils and aromatic products is a standard requirement for a fragrance to be labelled as perfume. Although cologne may smell as good, the perfume is less diluted with alcohol and water, has a higher percentage of scented oils, will cost more, and will last longer.

In a similiar vein, the quality of health care can be viewed as meeting certain requirements or standards. Unfortunately, exactly what these requirements or standards are or should be remains unclear. For example, mortality rates are used to evaluate the quality of medical care. While any health care professional recognizes that the quality of medical care is certainly a more complex issue, mortality rates do provide a measurable, objective, and comparable standard for evaluating care.

Determining the quality of nursing care is a complicated issue. A critical reason for this is that nursing care itself is not well defined. The American Nurses' Association (ANA) defines nursing as "the diagnosis and treatment of human responses to actual or potential health problems."[4] It contrast, another definition of nursing states that:

The nurse's place in the division of labor is essentially that of doing, in a responsible way, whatever necessary things are in danger of not being done at all.[5]

While this latter description of nursing is thirty years old, many nurses will recognize its fundamental accuracy to today's clinical practice environment. Efforts to assure that quality nursing practice occurs are constrained and confused by this lack of clarity and consensus about the practice of nursing.

In order to move forward and to capture the professional and cognitive aspects of the quality of nursing care, a strategy that both defines the practice of nursing and provides a measurable entity for determining the quality of care is needed. Nursing diagnosis offers such a strategy. The use of a consistent framework for identifying patient conditions, which then serves as the foundation for nursing intervention, guides the practice of nursing as well as the determination of the quality of that practice. This approach to standards of care for nursing practice has been used to develop process and outcome criteria for specific nursing diagnoses by the ANA in conjunction with four specialty nursing organizations: the American Association of Neuroscience Nurses,[6] the National Association of Orthopedic Nurses,[7] the National Nurses Society on Addictions,[8] and the Association of Rehabilitation Nurses.[9]

This chapter will define quality nursing care as that care in which accurate nursing diagnoses are identified and appropriate care plans are implemented and evaluated. By defining quality nursing care in this manner, emphasis is placed on the professional aspect of nursing practice, thus moving away from task-based nursing practice. Furthermore, this approach creates congruence between the practice of nursing and the efforts to measure the quality of that practice. In addition, this approach is consistent with the trend seen in the development of standards by some specialty organizations that are developing highly specific process and outcome criteria for selected nursing diagnoses.

While the nursing diagnoses and the related care plans are the foundation of quality nursing care, there are other aspects of nursing care that must be considered. Nursing practice also includes many activities that relate to the patient's medical condition and its management. The administration of medications is one such situation, and the observation of the patient's condition for significant symptoms or disease progression is another. These activities comprise an important part of nursing practice and, as such, must be considered in any approach to determining the quality of nursing care.

Historically, these medically-directed activities have been the focus of efforts to ascertain the quality of nursing care. The time has come to move beyond this limited perspective of nursing practice. Nursing diagnoses provide a mechanism for determining and measuring the quality of nursing care. This chapter will describe a strategy for a quality assurance process that uses nursing diagnoses as a framework for the standards against which nursing care can be measured and evaluated.

ESSENTIAL ELEMENTS OF THE QUALITY ASSURANCE PROCESS

Standards: The Foundation of Quality Assurance

Standards are the foundation of the quality assurance process because they are statements of accountability and define the requirements for quality nursing care. Standards are defined as something established and used by authority, custom, or general consent as a rule or basis of comparison in measuring quantity or quality.[10] Standards are based on the most current knowledge and are developed from actual practice, theory, expert opinion, and research. A standard is valid because it is "an agreed upon level of excellence."[11]

A nursing standard is a "valid definition of the quality of nursing care that includes the criteria by which the effectiveness of care can be evaluated."[12] A nursing standard is a guideline for a group of patients that have common characteristics. The standard is not a series of steps that must be followed for every patient; it is a general guideline for nursing practice. The standard should not limit or constrain the practitioner but should augment the delivery of care.

Standards must be derived from values. Values are the underlying reasons for acceptance of the standard. Values of nursing derive from many sources. Professional nursing values arise from nursing organizations such as the ANA and the National League for Nursing. Professional organizations outside of nursing such as the American Hospital Association and the American Medical Association can also exert an influence on the values of nurses.

While professional values play an important role in determining standards of nursing care, other influences are also present. Organizational values are described in the organization's philosophy, mission statement, policies, and goals. Societal values are stimulated by consumer expectations, and they are reflected in public policy and legal statutes such as nurse practice acts. Individual values are derived from the individual's previous experiences, education, background, interests, and unique skills. Values play an important, but as yet ill-defined, role in guiding and directing individual behavior.

The complex relationship between values and standards is represented in Figure 8–1. Professional nursing, organizational, societal, and individual values are translated into standards through the consensus of collective individuals. These influences on individual values make important contributions to the concept of quality held by individuals and groups of practitioners.[13]

The leaders of the organization must arrive at a definition of quality through discussion and consensus. This definition must then be communicated to all employees through philosophy statements, mission statements, policies, procedures, hiring decisions, reward systems, and day-to-day practice and it must be presented in clear and understandable terms so that every employee has the same operational definition of quality.

Only a strong commitment at all levels of management will assure an organizational culture that is committed to quality first. All employees must understand their individual roles in providing quality care. Nursing management's responsibility is to make sure everyone knows the requirements for quality patient care, provides the resources necessary for quality care, and encourages and helps employees to meet the quality requirements.[14]

The nursing quality assurance process is one part of the health care organization's quality process. The organization's definitions of excellence, as demonstrated by their mission, philosophy, policies, procedures, and standards, are applied to the nursing department through a formal written plan. The plan defines how nursing will determine excellence and how the information obtained will be integrated into the overall system.

Criteria for Evaluation of Standards

Many times the terms standards and criteria are used interchangeably but, in actuality, they describe different components. A criterion is a reflection of the standard through a measurable indicator.[15] Criteria describe critical components of the standard upon which a decision or judgment is made.[16] The difference can be shown by the perfume example used earlier. The standard for perfume would be a solution mix of high-proof alcohol and a high percent of scented oils and other aromatic products. The criteria for perfume would be 10 to 15 percent of scented oils and other aromatic products and 85 to 90 percent high–proof alcohol, while the criterion for cologne would be 3 to 5 percent of scented oils.

Another important aspect of criteria for the evaluation of standards is necessity of a

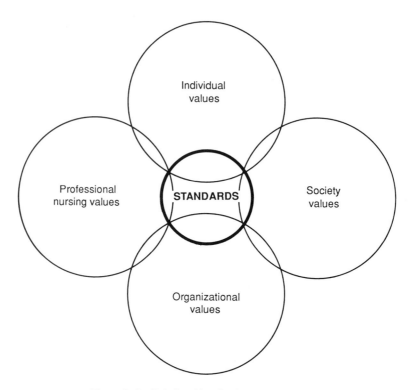

Figure 8—1. Relationship of values and standards

timeframe for the evaluation activity. Quality assurance monitoring activities are divided into two timeframes. Concurrent monitoring evaluates the care during the time the care is being rendered. In the concurrent approach the standards used to evaluate care consist of process standards or may include short-term outcome standards. The retrospective method of monitoring is done after the care has been rendered and the patient has been discharged or treatment has been stopped.

Structure, Process, and Outcome Standards

A widely used approach to the delineation of standards in health care is the structure, process, and outcome framework.[17] By examining these aspects of health care delivery separately and in conjunction with one another, a representation of the setting, activities, and results of health care delivery can be evaluated; however, the use of this approach must be grounded in the clinical and professional values of nursing.

A structure standard is a statement describing valued attributes of the setting that directly or indirectly influence care. Examples include the equipment and physical plant requirements, educational preparation of staff, annual review for CPR, staff mix, staff-patient ratios, the existence of specific policies and procedures, availability of teaching resources on the unit, and facility design. Many structure standards are mandated by regulatory agencies such as licensing boards, and external review boards such as the Joint Commission on Accreditation of Health Care Organizations (JCAHO).

Process standards are statements describing valued characteristics of care delivery within the context of the nursing process. Nurse activities that should be carried out are the process standards. The statements actually describe what nursing interventions will be done for patients. Turning the patient, teaching about the actions and side effects of specific medications, and discussing effective coping strategies are examples of process standards.

Standards that describe valued results for health characteristics, behaviors, or states of the patient are outcome standards. Examples of outcome standards would be the patient's knowledge of the actions and side effects of medications, intact skin, and self injection of insulin.

The types of standards discussed above are interrelated but look at different aspects of care delivery. At this point in time, a mix of the three types of standards is most frequently used for a comprehensive evaluation of quality care. The standard identifies the process needed to deliver safe care and includes the expected level and extent of care, the patient outcomes, the timeframes for process to occur and outcomes to be reached, and the criteria for evaluating delivery of care and the patient's response.

Nursing diagnoses provide a framework for the development of standards that offers consistent labels for grouping patients with similiar characteristics. Standards that are developed by nurses, based on nursing diagnoses, offer a mechanism for defining both the practice of nursing and the quality of that practice. A consensus approach to standard development in the nursing organization contributes to a definition of excellence that reflects the values of the clinical practice culture and serves as the standard of care for the organization.

CURRENT APPROACHES TO QUALITY ASSURANCE IN NURSING

Efforts to evaluate the quality of nursing care have been made since the time of Florence Nightingale. More recent efforts have used three approaches: structure, process, and outcome; however, many attempts at defining the quality of nursing care do not include the cognitive aspects of professional nursing practice, nor do they reflect the professional values of nurses. Methods for evaluating the quality of nursing care have been proposed in each of the three recognized approaches. This framework will be used to present a brief review of existing nursing quality assurance methodologies prior to the discussion of strategies based on nursing diagnosis.

Structure Approaches. The structure approach is essentially a review process of the existing structures of the nursing organization. The structure of the nursing organization and the documentation associated with that structure such as master staffing plans and job descriptions can be evaluated through a structure audit.

The structure approach cannot serve as the sole basis for determining quality. Although the supporting structure of care delivery is a critical aspect of quality, structure alone is not an adequate measure of the quality of care. The current focus of the structure approach is on the environment of the institution including both human and material resources, educational requirements, staffing, and support services.

In theory, the structure standards should exist for the processes to occur and the outcomes should not occur unless the processes are carried out; it cannot be assumed that because one type of standard occurs or exists, the other types will follow. An example of this would be a situation where the expected staff mix for a shift was present—a structure standard. This measure alone could not be used as an indicator that quality care was delivered. The correct staff mix alone does not indicate that the appropriate nursing interventions, representing process standards, were carried out or that patient outcomes were accomplished.

Process Approaches. Process, the second approach, was guided by the work of Maria Phaneuf in the 1960s with her development of a process audit based on the seven nursing functions established by Lesnik and Anderson.[18] The Phaneuf audit tool is a retrospective tool based on documentation. This audit assumes that good notes reflect quality care.

There are three additional process audits that are frequently referenced in the literature. The Rush–Medicus System is a comprehensive process review tool.[19] The processes that are supported by the structures and obtain the desired outcome are highlighted. The data is obtained by review of nursing documentation, observations of the patient and nurse, and interviews of the patient, nurse care giver, and charge nurse.

The Quality Patient Care Scale (Qual PACs) is a process audit that measures the quality of nursing care given to one patient as care is being rendered.[20] The Slater Competency Scale, the third example, focuses on the nurse's performance to identify quality care.[21] Both the Qual PACs and Slater Scale use direct observations for data collection.

The process approach is the foundation of the ANA's Model of Quality Assurance.[22] In the early 1970s, the ANA adopted a quality assurance model based on the original work of Norma Lang, which was developed to assist nurses in the implementation of a quality assurance program. The ANA model is based upon the standards for nursing practice developed by the Division of Practice in 1973 that reflect the steps of the nursing process. It is interesting to note that in Standard II it is stated that: "Nursing Diagnoses are derived from health status data."[23] It would seem that the use of nursing diagnoses for the purposes of quality assurance is not a new idea.

The ANA Model is divided into six components as shown in Table 8–1. A cyclic pattern is outlined beginning with the first component and advancing through each component. The process then starts anew. The first component identifies values of the nursing organization. The practice of nursing is dynamic and the scientific foundation of the practice is evolving; therefore, any approach to evaluating the quality of nursing practice must be responsive and flexible.

Standard identification is the second component of the model. The standards define what is acceptable, not optimal, for quality care. Since the measure of quality is dependent on the quality of the criteria, this is a very difficult but important step.

The third component determines the reality of actual practice in comparison to the predetermined standard. There are many methods that can be used to determine the level of actual practice, including observations, interviews, tests, surveys, appraisals, and record reviews to name just a few. Judgments comprise the fourth component. These judgments, weighing the strengths and weaknesses of the practice, are based on the data collected in the

TABLE 8–1. COMPONENTS OF THE ANA MODEL FOR QUALITY ASSURANCE

- *Identify Values*
- *Identify Structure, Process, and Outcome Standards and Criteria*
- *Secure measurements needed to determine degree of attainment of standards and criteria*
- *Make interpretations about strengths and weaknesses based on measurements*
- *Identify possible courses of actions*
- *Choose course of action*

previous step. These are necessary for the fifth component: identifying the appropriate actions that will encourage the strengths of the practice to continue as well as modifying any weaknesses prevent conformance to the standard.

The final component is to choose a course of action. Actions taken based on these judgments include rewards, education, administrative or environmental changes, and in extreme cases, punitive measures. The alternatives should be evaluated carefully to determine the most effective and efficient course of action. Planning for implementation of the best alternative, implementation of the selected strategy, and documentation of the results of the new strategy are the last step. The process then starts again.

Outcome Approaches. The third approach is the outcome audit which is retrospective. This approach compares the state of the patient at a defined period of time, usually at the time of discharge, to a predetermined standard. This approach has been controversial for a number of reasons.

Outcome evaluation is fraught with difficulties. A primary factor in these difficulties is that outcomes are not always associated with processes. The old adage, "The operation was a success, but the patient died," is an example of the lack of absolute linkage between process and outcome. Another confounding factor is the difficulty in ascribing the achievement of outcomes to specific processes or to a particular provider group. Furthermore, the only outcomes examined tend to be outcomes of disease treatment, and this approach does not reflect the independent, professional contributions of nursing.

Traditionally, disease entities were the usual focus of the outcome audit and nursing care was only a part of the multidisciplinary approach in the treatment of the patient, therefore, the contributions of nursing to the patient's outcome were difficult if not impossible to determine. The question must be raised, however, of the appropriateness of nursing outcome criteria that are focused exclusively on a disease model.

The use of nursing diagnosis makes an outcome methodology less controversial for nursing quality assurance because a consistent language for naming the patient conditions that nurses treat provides a mechanism for identifying outcomes for nursing care rather than medical care; however, the diagnostic language of nursing is in its early development and the cause-and-effect relationship between nursing interventions and outcomes remains to be demonstrated through research. This clinical and administrative nursing research on nursing diagnoses can only be done if nursing diagnoses are used in clinical practice and for the evaluation of that practice.

The New JCAHO Quality Assurance Standard

JCAHO sets standards for the purpose of assuring that the organization is functioning within specific guidelines. Changes in JCAHO standards reflect the changing economic environment of nursing and health care in general, but they are also concerned with the quality of care. Recent changes in JCAHO standards on quality assurance have significantly changed the focus of quality assurance activities.[24] A diagnosis-based nursing process provides a useful framework for meeting these standards.

In 1979 the focus of the standards was on review activities that would identify problems and assist in determining solutions to those problems. The process involved problem identification, prioritization of the problem, use of criteria to evaluate the extent of the problem, implementation of a plan to address problems that existed, and follow-up activities to ensure resolution. In many hospitals the focus of these activities was limited to one-time problem identification and resolution. Long-term monitoring was not a part of the process.

The 1984 revisions refocused the activities to continuous monitoring. The nursing services standard was changed to:

> As part of the hospital's quality assurance program, the quality and appropriateness of patient care provided by the nursing department/service are monitored and evaluated, and identified problems are resolved.[25]

The standard further describes the required characteristics of a quality assurance program. The standard states that monitoring and evaluation are accomplished through:

> routine collection . . . of information about important aspects of nursing care; and periodic assessment of collected information . . . in order to identify important problems in patient care and opportunities to improve care.[26]

The standard also requires the use of objective criteria that reflect current knowledge and clinical expertise. The criteria must be reviewed and agreed upon by the nursing department. Nursing diagnoses can form the basic framework for the standard and criteria used in the process.

The specifics of the quality assurance process are left up to the organization. By not defining the specifics in the standard, JCAHO has allowed and encouraged each facility to develop a program that best fits the unique characteristics of the organization; however, nursing diagnosis can provide a framework for standardization of nursing monitoring activities through the use of standards and criteria that are based on specific nursing diagnoses.

The characteristics of monitoring and evaluation activities are summarized in Table 8–2. The specific characteristics for a planned, systematic, and continuous program include a repeated pattern for the procedure, schedule, method, and frequency of the reviews, and they would vary depending on the clinical setting or the type of patient.

The development of quality assurance programs that improve care rather than meet bureaucratic requirements is the primary motivator for the JCAHO standard changes. A nursing diagnosis-based model for quality assurance activities provides the framework for standard development and meets the characteristics of the ANA model for quality assurance and the changing JCAHO requirements.

NURSING DIAGNOSIS, NURSING PROCESS, AND STANDARDS OF CARE

The nursing process is the recognized thinking model of the nursing profession. The addition of nursing diagnosis as a discrete step offers two advantages. From the clinical perspective, nursing diagnosis clearly identifies the patient's problem or the condition that must be treated with nursing care, thus providing guidance for the planning, intervention, and evaluation steps

TABLE 8–2. CHARACTERISTICS OF MONITORING AND EVALUATION ACTIVITIES

- *Planned, systematic, and continous*
- *Based on indicators and criteria that are agreed upon by the staff*
- *Comprehensive*
- *Accomplished by regular data collection and periodic assessment to evaluate the data*
- *Appropriate actions are identified to resolve problems and improve care*
- *Integrated with information throughout the facility*
- *Annual reappraisal of nursing quality assurance activities*

of the nursing process. From the perspective of quality assurance, this clear, precise definition of patient problems serves as a useful framework for the development and monitoring of standards of several important aspects of nursing practice. The usefulness of nursing diagnosis for quality assurance purposes is reflected in the work of several professional nursing organizations that have used nursing diagnosis as the framework for the development of specialty nursing standards, including the American Association of Neuroscience Nurses, the Association of Rehabilitation Nurses, and the Orthopedic Nurses Association.

The relationship of nursing process and nursing diagnosis to quality can be summarized in three key points: (1) nursing process is a way of defining quality for nursing care based on standard problem names, the nursing diagnosis; (2) nursing process specifies the process for delivering the quality of care; and (3) the use of nursing diagnosis, within the nursing process, provides a framework for evaluating the quality of care.

The underlying principle of quality assurance is accountability. Webster defines accountability as "answerable, responsible, or liable to be called for reckoning."[27] Accountability for nursing care means taking responsibility for the provision of care and the outcome of that care.

Since accountability is the underlying principle of quality assurance, nursing care should be evaluated for the problems that nurses can identify and treat. Nursing diagnoses describe those patient situations that comprise the practice of nursing. Therefore, nurses are accountable for the nursing diagnoses they make and the interventions they prescribe. Quality nursing care is nursing care in which accurate nursing diagnoses are identified and appropriate care plans are implemented and evaluated. By defining quality nursing care in this manner, emphasis is placed on the professional aspect of nursing practice, thus moving away from task-based nursing practice.

Nurses are accountable to the public for the standards of care they develop. Nursing diagnosis-based standards define, both to peers and consumers, what the nurse will treat and what the nurse will contribute to the patient's care. In addition to nursing diagnosis-based standards for nursing practice, those aspects of nursing practice that deal with disease-related situations under medical order also must be included in the standards of care for nursing practice. The standards of care for all aspects of nursing practice become reality-based when practicing nurses are involved directly in reviewing, developing, and then implementing them.

In the past, nursing quality assurance activities have been based in the functional aspects of nursing and delegated medical practice activities. Since nursing diagnoses can be used to define the patient conditions that are the focus of nursing practice, they provide a framework for evaluating the quality of nursing care, based on the processes and outcomes of that care. The disease-related medical activities cannot be ignored and must be a part of the evaluation process, but they must not be the sole focus or main component of the quality assurance process for nursing because they do not reflect professional nursing practice.

A quality assurance process, based on the ANA model and using nursing diagnosis, should have indicators for each step of the nursing process. This would include the determination of the accuracy of the nursing diagnoses and the corresponding interventions through additional assessments and evaluations. The link between nursing process and the measurement of the quality of nursing practice based on nursing diagnosis is then clearly established.

Nursing diagnosis describes patient conditions that can serve as a basis for standards development, and the work of the North American Nursing Diagnosis Association (NANDA) has resulted in a recognized taxonomy of nursing diagnostic labels. This has a number of important implications for the quality assurance process. No longer might the nursing diagnosis vary according to the facility or health care setting. With consistent nursing diagnostic terminology, it will be possible to begin collecting and analyzing nursing data on regional and national levels. A consistent language also facilitates the development of national standards for nursing practice, standards that are measurable and specific to professional nursing practice rather than focusing on dependent medical functions or the unique characteristics of particular health care organizations.

The Relationship Between the Nursing Care Plan and Standards of Nursing Care

While the nursing care plan may be considered to represent the standard of care for an individual patient at a particular point in time, the nursing care plan and standard of care are not interchangable, nor does one replace the other. The standard and the nursing care plan are linked to each other, but they are different in that each serves a distinct and separate purpose. The nursing care plan is the statement of outcomes (goals) and nursing interventions (processes) that reflect the needs of the *individual* patient; however, it should be remembered that accurate nursing diagnoses, reflecting the unique situation of the patient, are essential for a nursing care plan to have the necessary specificity to direct nursing care in this way.

The standard of care, on the other hand, describes quality care for a *group* of patients. Since standards focus on groups of patients, they must be broader than the types of statements used for individual patients, but standards must also be measurable. The care plan reflects the nurse's professional judgment and specialized knowledge in applying the broad standard to a unique situation for particular patients. In order to accomplish this individualized nursing care, based on the unique needs of particular patients, standards of care must be clearly defined for groups of patients, yet broad and flexible enough to cover a range of patient situations.

An example illustrates the roles of the standard of care and nursing care plan. For the nursing diagnosis Potential for Altered Skin Integrity related to immobility, the desired outcome is implicit in the diagnostic label; if the patient condition indicates the possible development of skin breakdown, then the desired outcome is that the skin will remain intact. This statement then serves as an outcome criterion that can be used to evaluate the effectiveness of nursing care for this individual patient as well as a standard of care for any patient with the nursing diagnosis Potential for Altered Skin Integrity.

In this example, the next step is the selection of nursing interventions that will be most effective in accomplishing the desired outcome for the patient. An example from the standard of care for all patients with a nursing diagnosis of Potential for Altered Skin Integrity would be: patient will be turned at scheduled intervals. For a patient with an area of reddened skin on her left hip who is at high risk for developing additional breakdown, the care plan would state: turn the patient to the right side at 1 A.M., 7 A.M., 1 P.M., and 7 P.M., on her back at 3 A.M., 9 A.M., 3 P.M., and 9 P.M., and on her abdomen at 5 A.M., 11 A.M., 5 P.M., and 11 P.M. Here the nursing care plan has applied the broad standard to a specific patient.

The addition of nursing diagnosis into the quality assurance process is both challenging and overwhelming. While the potential applications of nursing diagnosis in defining and evaluating nursing care are exciting, the realities at this time are somewhat daunting. The lack of nursing diagnostic labels for many clinical situations and the development of necessary diagnostic skills for many nurses are just two issues to be addressed; however, it is possible to work with existing nursing diagnoses, within the context of the quality assurance process, to create a strategy for evaluating professional nursing practice.

Incorporating Nursing Diagnosis into the Quality Assurance Process

The ANA model for quality assurance and nursing diagnoses can be used as the foundation of a diagnosis-based quality assurance strategy. In addition to these two elements, a third component is required to define and measure the quality of those aspects of nursing care that are focused on the disease-related condition and those medically-delegated activities that nurses perform. Finally, the characteristics of nursing care quality has certain unique aspects based on the clinical setting where nursing care is delivered. This four-component structure contains two components that focus on professional nursing care (the ANA model and nursing diagnosis), one element concerned with delegated medical activities, and one element that takes the characteristics of the setting into account.

As an example of these four components consider the patient with a nursing diagnosis of Activity Intolerance related to prolonged bedrest. While patients with a medical diagnosis of congestive heart failure or a malignancy are often candidates for this nursing diagnostic label, this nursing diagnosis may be seen in a variety of patients. Furthermore, they may receive health care in an acute care center or in the home, but the nursing diagnosis and etiology that directs the nursing interventions for the activity intolerance may often be very similiar.

The problem statement of Activity Intolerance indicates the state of the patient. By clearly defining the patient's condition in consistent language, desired outcomes can be identified that can serve as outcome standards. An example might be: "the patient will have increased tolerance for activity." The etiology of prolonged bedrest guides the nurse to the necessary interventions, which could be considered process standards for this particular patient. "Increase the time periods for sitting in the chair by 10 minutes each day; monitor heart rate and respiratory rate before and after sitting" would be examples of nursing interventions to accomplish the desired outcome.

In addition to the diagnosis-based quality criteria, additional standards for the administration of medications, performance of procedures, and other delegated medical activities would be required, and the unique characteristics of the health care setting should be considered. These issues are important and should be carefully and thoughtfully considered in the quality assurance process; however, the evaluation of the quality of nursing care must be focused on professional nursing practice. The remainder of this chapter will focus on the issues of diagnosis-based quality standards and criteria and their implications for the quality of nursing care.

Quality Assurance and Clinical Practice Reality. Before nursing diagnosis can serve as a framework for the quality assurance process in a particular organization, diagnosis-based nursing practice must be present. Only if nurses in clinical practice are using nursing diagnoses as *the* way in which patient conditions are described and recorded will there be documentation to review for the quality assurance process. While the implementation of nursing diagnosis as a clinical practice change and the incorporation of nursing diagnosis into the quality assurance process can occur simultaneously, the critical linkage between these two activities must not be forgotten.

After the decision has been made to incorporate nursing diagnosis into the quality assurance process, several steps must follow. The focus of data collection for the quality assurance process needs to be defined. This choice might be organized around data about a particular nursing diagnosis, nursing diagnoses within a particular diagnosis-related group (DRG), or an individual caregiver or groups of caregivers. Although the focus on caregivers is a somewhat recent development in the quality assurance area, it reflects critical concerns about performance because accreditation groups are beginning to look at the issue of individual competence.

Other data collection methods include a random sample review of patient records, a research study on a defined topic, or a generic criteria review for all units. (See Table 8–3). In reality it may be that more than one of these approaches may be necessary or useful for the quality assurance process in a certain organization. The choices about the focus and type of

TABLE 8–3. A QUALITY ASSURANCE MODEL USING NURSING DIAGNOSIS

1. *Determination of the type of monitoring*
   Focus
   - *Specific nursing diagnosis*
   - *Caregiver*
   - *Specific nursing diagnosis for a particular DRG*
   - *Random sample review*
   - *Special study*
   - *Generic criteria for all units*
   Approach Process
   - *The assessment data for this patient supports the diagnosis*
   - *The patient's care plan is reviewed to determine if the planning of care was consistent with the standard*
   - *The interventions were carried out within the timeframes or exceptions were noted*
   - *Progress towards the expected outcomes was evaluated and appropriate changes were made*
   - *Clinical problems were referred to the appropriate resource*
   Outcome
   - *Accurate nursing diagnosis is identified*
   - *Outcomes were met*
   Criteria for patient selection
   - *Number of patients*
   - *Required length of stay on unit*
2. *Development of indicators*
3. *Review of compliance with the standard*
4. *Review of strengths and weaknesses of the care provided*
5. *Review of trends*
6. *Review of the goals and action plan*
7. *Evaluation of the plan*

data collection for quality review should be based in the unique characteristics of the organization and the clinical issues in the practice culture.

After the focus for quality review has been decided, the next step is to determine the type of monitoring to be done: concurrent or retrospective, process or outcome. If concurrent monitoring is selected, a process criteria framework is most useful, while outcome criteria are evaluated more readily with a retrospective review process. This decision may have been defined in the yearly quality assurance plan; however, this plan may require changes as a result of previous findings or a more specific definition at this time. A nursing diagnosis framework is a flexible framework that will support changes in the focus of the monitoring. The yearly plan should support but not constrain the process.

A useful starting point for carrying out these decisions would be to begin with a particular nursing diagnosis and an identified group of patients for quality monitoring. Standards must be written and the appropriate indicators developed for the selected nursing diagnosis. When more nursing diagnoses have associated standards and indicators developed, then a random review of patients can be done. Special studies can be done as issues or problems are identified. While professional nursing groups are pursuing this work of standard development, the testing of those standards, as well as further development of others, must occur in the clinical practice areas.

There are also quality issues pertinent for *all* patients. Standards and indicators that reflect these concerns are called generic criteria. These generic criteria will apply to the entire patient population and must be reviewed on a periodic basis. Many of the generic criteria will involve delegated medical functions of nursing such as medication administration, or they may focus on issues of concern to the institution such as patient identification and safety. A decision must be made on the criteria to review and the frequency of the review.

Developing Nursing Diagnosis-Based Standards and Criteria

The development of nursing diagnosis-based standards and criteria is a critical and essential component of a quality assurance process for diagnosis-based nursing practice. The development of standards and criteria, based on nursing diagnoses, will be discussed for each step of the nursing process. This focus is not meant to minimize the importance of the generic criteria mentioned earlier; however, shifting to a diagnosis-based approach of quality assurance is the goal.

Establishing nursing diagnosis-based standards and criteria will depend on the nursing diagnoses themselves. In fact these standards and criteria will be unique for each nursing diagnosis and etiology. A model for writing standards and criteria for nursing diagnoses has been described by McCourt;[28] that model has been modified and expanded here.

The first step is to review the current literature on the nursing diagnosis in question. From this review and clinical practice knowledge, standards and criteria can be developed that can be used, through review of patient records, to determine if the documented nursing diagnosis accurately describes the health state of the individual, if appropriate nursing interventions were used to treat it, and if desired outcomes were accomplished. This may be determined by the assessment data, observations, interview of the patient, and other pertinent information in the patient's record.

Making an accurate nursing diagnosis may be considered to be an outcome standard; the outcome of concern is the nursing diagnostic label, and the quality issue rests in the accuracy and correctness of that nursing diagnosis. In order to determine if the correct nursing diagnosis was made, actual patient data should be compared to the defining characteristics for that nursing diagnosis in the established criteria. This step is very important because if the nursing diagnosis is not accurate, the nursing interventions, which would reflect process criteria, may be to no avail and the outcomes standards are not likely to be met. It also must be determined if the nursing diagnoses that reflect high priority problems for this patient have been identified.

Nursing interventions represent the processes of nursing care; therefore, a process approach to a quality evaluation is appropriate for this step of the nursing process. At this point standards and criteria that describe the essential and effective nursing interventions for the nursing diagnosis must be determined. These can then be used to measure the quality of the plan of care. Additionally, indicators for the follow-through of orders and progress towards expected outcomes need to be developed.

While standards and criteria are necessary to measure the quality of nursing care, another aspect of quality that must be remembered is the individualization of nursing care for the patient. In fact, individualization of the nursing interventions can be considered a process criteria. This strategy represents a combination of those nursing interventions recognized to be effective for a nursing diagnosis, the "standard" interventions as it were; moreover, the use of these "standard" interventions that have been adapted or modified for the unique needs of the patient represents the highest quality of nursing care.

The purpose of nursing interventions is to accomplish certain desired outcomes in the patient's condition. Outcome standards and criteria reflect this intent. The general outcome for the patient in a particular diagnostic category is defined within the nursing diagnosis-based standard. The specific patient outcome is identified in the nursing care plan.

Standards and criteria at this point should describe realistic, measurable, and objective patient behaviors or clinical findings, based on the nursing diagnosis. These standards and criteria can then be used at two points: in the nursing care plan, expected outcomes should be indicated, while the patient record should contain information about the patient's condition to indicate progress toward or accomplishment of these outcomes.

If an outcome approach is used, it is necessary to determine if the outcome was met;

however, accomplishment of the outcome is not always possible, and exceptions may occur. The exceptions could include inability to accomplish the outcome within the specified timeframe or extenuating circumstances that made achievement of the outcome impossible. When exceptions are found in the quality assurance process, note should be made of these. For consistently occuring exceptions, it may be useful to develop exclusionary criteria within the standard for that nursing diagnosis.

The reason for the exception should be explored, and this information should be directed to the most appropriate group. The administrative team may need to review their structure standards such as staff mix if the current staff mix does not allow for completion of the necessary workload. The lack of a nursing diagnosis for a certain clinical population or problem may be forwarded to the group responsible for future development of nursing diagnoses.

When the appropriate standards and criteria have been developed for the nursing diagnoses, an evaluation tool should be based on these, and it should be designed for ease of use, as well as accurate data collection. In addition, the quality review process is most effective if completed at the nursing unit level. The summary of nursing unit and department findings, trends, goals, and action plans should be recorded, discussed, and an evaluation of the process must be completed. The process then starts again.

All of this evaluation and standard activity is fruitless unless the nurses at the patient's bedside are aware, invested, and supportive of the use of nursing diagnosis in their clinical practice and the specific standards and criteria used in the quality assurance process. One way to create a clinical environment that meets these requirements is through shared governance and unit-based quality assurance programs. The concept of shared governance is attractive to many nurses because it places clinical decision making in the hands of the clinical practitioners; unit-based quality assurance programs accomplish the same goal and, indeed, are an important aspect of a shared governance model.

A SHARED GOVERNANCE MODEL FOR THE QUALITY ASSURANCE PROCESS

The concept of participation is especially important to the quality assurance process because clinical practitioners must define and then meet certain predetermined standards. Furthermore, judgments made about the quality of care provided by these practitioners are based on these same predetermined standards. Clinical practitioners must be part of the process from the beginning step of standard development to the end, the evaluation of the quality of nursing care.

Organizational structure is the framework for accomplishing the organization's purpose. In nursing this includes the model of practice at the unit level and the structure of the nursing department at the nursing service level. The structure should facilitate information flow from all the people in the organization that perform the work so that decisions are made by the "grass roots," that is, the people that have to carry out the decisions in their day-to-day work.

Participatory management is a frequently identified characteristic of successful organizations and that concept has been a consistent theme in most of the recent nursing management literature. Staff members at the lowest appropriate level of the organizational structure can make the decisions that affect their work life in a participatory management environment. This is the most frequently mentioned management style of magnet hospitals.[30]

Successful organizations of the future will consider processes more than structure and will focus on function and self-governance. Employees that are accountable for their work will be central to the organization. The movement toward participatory management and the strong theoretical movement away from the traditional bureaucratic structures have set the stage for the development of shared governance or self-governance structures. These suggested structures shift from the traditional structure by encouraging staff to make recommendations to management for change in an organization.

In shared governance, policies, procedures, and solutions to problems are suggested by front-line practitioners, making these changes more likely to be in the best interests, of the individual and the organization. The shared governance structure supports the professional need for autonomy and professional practice in organizations that are tied to the bureaucratic structure; however, the shared governance structure will work if, and only if, the decisions and recommendations made by the employees are supported and implemented by management.

Quality Assurance at the Nursing Unit Level

One aspect of a shared governance approach to quality assurance is to locate the activity and responsibility for quality assurance at the nursing unit level with those clinical practitioners. In order to use nursing diagnosis-based standards and criteria effectively, the actual review of patient records must be done by clinicians who are knowledgeable about the patient, the specialty, and the nursing diagnosis in question. In fact, with diagnosis-based standards, it is very difficult for someone unfamiliar with the clinical situation to make appropriate judgments about whether the standards were met or not.

When the quality assurance process occurs at the unit level in a consistent manner, the information from the unit's quality assurance process can also be organized and summarized for groups of nursing units and the nursing organization. (See Table 8–4.) This organizing and summarizing can be handled by the Quality Assurance Committee. A strategy in keeping with a philosophy of shared governance is to designate a unit staff member as liaison to the Nursing Quality Assurance Committee. The integration of quality assurance into a shared governance organizational structure will be discussed further at the end of this chapter.

One of the most important responsibilities of the unit quality assurance staff member is the selection of patients for review. The selection will be directed by the generic criteria of the organization and the unique characteristics of the patient population. For example, the generic criteria of the organization might specify that all patients will be reviewed only after a specified period of time such as 24 hours. An example of patient selection based on unique characteristics might be that all patients who experience falls will be reviewed for indicators of the nursing diagnosis Potential for Injury.

Once the patients are selected, the next step is the review of the patient record. The nursing diagnoses and nursing documentation are the primary focus. The nursing care plan is reviewed for specific application of the indicators for each step of the nursing process with particular attention to the particular patient situation, the accuracy of the nursing diagnoses, the appropriateness and individualization of nursing interventions, and the achievement of desired outcomes.

The second step in the model involves comparing the information in the patient record

---

TABLE 8–4. QUALITY ASSURANCE AT THE NURSING UNIT LEVEL

The model has eight stages:
1. *Selection of the patient for review*
2. *Determination of compliance with the standard*
3. *Identification of the strengths and weaknesses of the care provided*
4. *Review of trends*
5. *Discussion of alternatives*
6. *Identification of the goals and action plan*
7. *Implementation of the plan*
8. *Evaluation of the plan*

with the appropriate indicators in order to determine if the standards of process and outcome were met. Although the standard and criteria statements are designed to be clear and measurable, the review will be enhanced by the insights of an experienced, knowledgeable, professional practitioner. Specific, measurable criteria attempt to eliminate most of the judgment calls, but clinical practice will always have some grey areas. A clinical expert is the key element in this step. Specific or measurable feedback to the quality assurance coordinator will help in evaluating the quality of nursing care delivery for the nursing unit, and it would improve the quality of the indicators used in this process.

The information regarding compliance with the standard should be summarized and answer the following questions:

- What were the strengths in the care this patient received?
- What were the weaknesses in the care this patient received?

The summary is based on the following considerations:

- Were the nursing diagnoses accurate?
- Were the priority diagnoses identified?
- Were the standards of outcome and/or process met in regard to nursing interventions and desired outcomes for the patient?

The summary should be short and concise. The summary also should explain any unusual circumstances such as that a particular nursing diagnosis was not formulated or documented on the chart.

The nursing unit management team, unit quality assurance staff member, and nursing quality assurance coordinator should meet periodically to review the current summaries with the past summaries and identify the trends. The identification of some trends can take months to determine. Periodic discussions of strengths and weaknesses will give indications for changes that should be considered.

The source of any problems must be identified in order to determine appropriate alternatives. The problems identified may have numerous causes including performance as well as educational or management issues. An appropriate diagnosis may not be available for the patient, and certainly as the development of the classification system is continued, nursing diagnoses will be added and revised to describe accurately the health states of the patients.

Educational issues for the staff nurses need to be referred to those responsible for staff education. The group may determine that structural standards might need to be reviewed and revised, such as the staff mix, staffing pattern, or nurse-patient ratio. Unit staff may be the best source of information because the perceptions of the managers can sometimes differ from the realities faced by the frontline practitioners.

Staff meetings should be used to update unit staff on the findings and to identify the goals and plans for change. Action plans that reinforce the strengths and eliminate the weaknesses can be generated. Creativity and brainstorming, as well as the airing of problems, should be encouraged.

From these activities, a course of action will be decided upon and implemented. The regular quality monitoring activities can be used to determine the success of the plan and whether additional actions are necessary. The summary of findings will be forwarded to the quality assurance coordinator and will include: strengths, weaknesses, trends, goals, action plans, and evaluation of the previous goals and action plans.

The more involved the nursing unit staff is in the entire process, the more valued the process becomes, and the more likely that improvements in patient care will be seen. Every staff member should be involved in the process. The involvement might include data collection providing input into the potential source of the problem or helping to problem solve. Novice practitioners that may want to help with data collection might become involved in special follow-up studies for which their level of expertise is appropriate.

The approach presented here supports the evaluation of professional nursing practice in determining the quality of care. Nursing diagnoses are used to develop standards that are defined for groups of patients having common characteristics or defining characteristics represented by the nursing diagnosis. The standards are agreed upon by representatives of the nursing department and are known to all practitioners. The evaluation of the independent practice is realistic because it is based on the problems that nurses can treat and links the nursing process to nursing practice.

A Shared Governance Model For A Nursing Service

The shared governance approach to quality assurance and the placement of the quality assurance process at the nursing unit level is only one portion of a shared governance model. Shared governance is a management philosophy supported by organizational structure in which relationships and roles are designed to position the organization and its members in a more direct relationship with accountability for determining policy, goals, and responses to consumer demand. The philosophy and approach of shared governance have particular importance in the area of quality assurance, which must be founded in shared goals and values to be effective; however, other aspects of a shared governance model have a role in diagnosis-based nursing practice and a diagnosis–based quality model.

A shared governance model for nursing, based on a number of reports in the literature, is shown in Figure 8–2.[30-33] The model shows the relationship of the formal management positions to the representatives of the shared governance bodies. All representatives are unit and department staff members who have been chosen by their peers to represent their concerns to the committees. The key formal manager, the chief nursing officer, is central in the model.

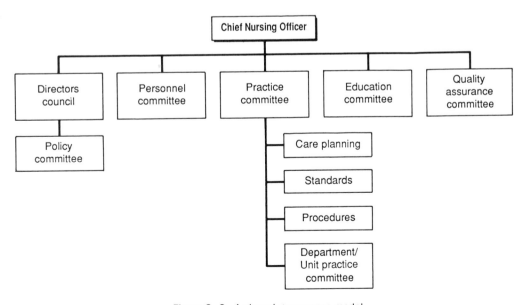

Figure 8–2. A shared governance model

The Director's Council is the forum of top managers that report to the chief nursing officer. While this group is responsible for the policy of the nursing department, this responsibility is shared with the policy committee. The policy committee writes policies that are forwarded to the Director's Council for formal adoption. Negotiation may be necessary between these two groups since the policies developed by the staff must be administratively sound. Additional feedback, when needed, can be obtained from the frontline practitioners on the Nursing Practice Committee.

The Personnel and Education Committees have representatives from the nursing units or, in the case of large nursing organization, there may be departmental representatives to these groups. The Personnel Committee will deal with recruitment, retention, and quality of work-life issues. The Education Council will organize and direct patient and staff education programs that meet overall needs of the environment.

The Nursing Practice Committee reviews issues that affect the delivery of nursing care. The Standards, Procedures, and Care Planning Committees are key components of the structure. The Standards Committee will develop the standards of care. The Care Planning Committee will develop standard care plans with open-ended statements that allow for patient specific information to be recorded.

The Nursing Practice Committee will have subcommittees that support the major functions. These groups could be *ad hoc* committees for specific projects, or they could become formal entities. Examples of these subcommittees could include discharge planning, case mix, practice models, scheduling, or computerization.

The Quality Assurance Committee is made up of members appointed from each unit or department. The members should be selected carefully. Potential members must have an interest in and commitment to quality assurance. The members need to be clinical experts and knowledgeable about quality assurance. The development of future members of this committee will take place at the unit level.

The Quality Assurance Committee is chaired by the director or coordinator of quality assurance, who also serves as a member of the Nursing Practice Committee. The committee will develop the quality assurance yearly plan and submit this to the Director's Council. The council will make technical decisions about the details of the quality assurance process and direct the specific quality assurance activities based on the model. Subgroups that focus on the component of the process can be an effective strategy for developing the process in a timely fashion. The subgroups might be divided into an indicator-development group, a methodology group, and a findings-and-recommendations group.

The work of the Quality Assurance Committee is supported by the Standards Committee, a subgroup of the Nursing Quality Assurance Committee and the Care Planning Committee. The subgroup structure encourages maximum integration of standards, care planning, and evaluation through quality monitoring throughout the practice environment. The Standards Committee develops standards from which quality will be judged. The Practice Committee makes recommendations as it reviews the information obtained from the monitoring, discusses and adopts the necessary changes, and the representatives will model changes in the practice setting. The Education Committee can provide specific interventions for resolution if the cause of the problem is an educational one.

The governance model supports the quality assurance process by making it a dynamic, peer-controlled system that has input from all departments and all levels of staff. The commitment to the shared governance model and the quality assurance process must be evident in all aspects of the organization's culture. The process will be successful only if the nurses believe their input will be processed and changes that improve patient care will result.

CONCLUSION

Quality is an important issue for the health care industry. The cost containment incentives of the present reimbursement system have caused a great deal of concern about the future of quality health care. Many health care providers believe that resource reduction for cost effective care and quality care are mutually exclusive concepts, yet legislation has mandated the concepts be compatible.

External demands place increasing pressure on nursing to prove that quality care is given. Quality care has become an important issue to numerous groups outside the profession such as consumer groups, the government, regulatory agencies, and accreditation boards. Within the profession, concern about quality care has escalated in light of constrained or declining resources in the health care environment.

Consumer demand for quality services was the driving force for beginning quality assurance programs. Consumer demand continues to be a driving force in view of escalating costs of health services. The consistent labeling of nursing problems through nursing diagnosis nomenclature will help nurses articulate to the public the practice of nursing. The articulation of nursing practice will contribute to the demise of the handmaiden image and will clarify what nurses legally can treat and what consumers can expect from a nurse provider.

Within the profession of nursing, there also have been efforts by nurses to focus on the issue of quality care. The commitment of professional nursing organizations to establish standards that define nursing practice has been influential in refining the quality assurance process. The issues of professional accountability and autonomy become a reality to the individual practitioner when linked to a process that measures quality of care. In addition, the focus on productivity, in light of the declining supply of nurses, has renewed interest in establishing the qualitative aspects of quantified goals.

The demands of external groups and internal, professional forces place increasing pressure to prove that quality care is given. A nursing diagnosis-based model for quality assurance provides a means of determining the quality of nursing care through the link of nursing process and nursing practice. With the use of nursing diagnosis, nursing practice can be defined, assessed, implemented in a planned and systematic manner, and evaluated.

REFERENCES

1. *The Merriam-Webster dictionary.* New York: Pocket Books, 1974
2. Crosby, P.B. *Quality without tears.* New York: New American Library, 1984, p. 64
3. Peters, T. & Austin, N. *A passion for excellence.* New York: Random House, 1985, p. 98
4. American Nurses' Association, *Quality assurance workbook.* Kansas City: American Nurses' Association, 1976, p. 7
5. Hughes, E. C. *Men and their work.* IL: The Free Press, 1958, p. 74
6. American Association of Neuroscience Nurses & American Nurses' Association. *Neuroscience nursing practice: Process and outcome criteria for selected diagnosis.* Kansas City: American Nurses' Association, pub no. MS-13, 1985
7. National Association of Orthopedic Nurses & American Nurses' Association. *Orthopedic nursing practice: Process and outcome criteria for selected diagnoses.* Kansas City: American Nurses' Association, pub no. MS-14, 1986
8. National Nurses Society on Addictions & American Nurses' Association. *Standards of addictions nursing practice with selected diagnoses and criteria.* Kansas City: American Nurses' Association, pub no. PMH-10, 1988
9. Association of Rehabilitation Nurses & American Nurses' Association. *Rehabilitation nursing practice: Process and outcome criteria for selected nursing diagnoses.* Kansas City: American Nurses' Association, in press
10. *Webster's new collegiate dictionary.* (Boston: G. & C. Merriam Co., 1961

11. American Nurses' Association. *Quality assurance workbook*

12. Shroeder, P. & Maibusch, R. *Nursing quality assurance.* Rockville, MD: Aspen, 1984, p. 72

13. Meisenheimer, C. *Quality assurance.* Rockville, MD: Aspen, 1985, p. 47

14. Crosby

15. Meisenheimer

16. Schroeder & Maisbusch

17. Donabedian, A. Evaluating the quality of medical care. *Milbank Memorial Fund Quarterly,* 1966, 44, 2, 166

18. Phaneuf, M. *The nursing audit: Self-regulation in nursing practice.* New York: Appleton-Century-Crofts, 1976

19. Medicus Systems Corporation. A methodology for monitoring quality of nursing care. Washington DC: USDHEW Publication no. 76-25, 1976

20. Wandelt M. & Ager, J. *Quality patient care scale* New York: Appleton-Century-Crofts, 1974

21. Wandelt M. & Stewart, D. *Slater nursing competencies rating scale* New York: Appleton-Century-Crofts, 1975

22. American Nurses' Association. *Quality assurance workbook*

23. *Ibid*

24. JCAH's new standard calls for more deliberate QA activities. *Hospital Peer Review,* 1983, *8,* 12, 155

25. Joint Commission on Accreditation of Health Organizations. *Accreditation manual for hospitals.* Chicago: JCAHO, 1984, p. 149

26. *Ibid*

27. *Webster's dictionary*

28. McCourt, A. Nursing diagnoses: Key to quality assurance. In M. E. Hurley (ed.), *Classification of nursing diagnoses: proceedings of the sixth conference.* St. Louis: C.V. Mosby, 1986

29. McClure, M., Poulin, M., Sovie, M., & Wandelt, M. *Magnet hospitals.* Kansas City: American Nurses' Association, 1983

30. Porter-O'Grady, T. & Finnigan, S. *Shared governance for nursing.* Rockville, MD: Aspen, 1984

31. York, C. & Fecteau, D.L. Innovative models for professional nursing practice. *Nursing Economics,* 1987, 5, 4, 162

32. Ortiz, M.E., Gehring, P., & Sovie, M. Moving to shared governance. *American Journal of Nursing,* 1987, *87,* 7, 923

33. Becker, J., Mercier, B., & Nussbaum, K. *Manager's Resource Manual.* Richmond, VA: Virginia Commonwealth University/Medical College of Virginia Hospitals, Nursing Services, 1985

CHAPTER 9

Supporting Diagnosis-based Nursing Practice with Information Systems

John A. Horton and Emmy Miller

Nursing can be viewed as an information processing activity. In the clinical setting, the nurse obtains data about the patient and then processes this data into nursing diagnoses and associated nursing interventions, as well as recognizing and responding to significant medical symptoms and other disease-related findings. The issues of data collection, storage, and processing are critical ones in nursing; however, nurses in the clinical setting usually refer to these issues as assessment, documentation, and clinical thinking, while in nursing administration, aggregated information from patient assessments and nursing documentation is described as quality assurance monitoring and determining nursing resource allocation.

Many nurses have not yet assimilated the language of information systems, and automated information systems remain a relatively untapped resource. The possible benefits and efficiencies of automating nursing documentation remain to be seen. In a recent study of inpatient health care agencies, only 7 percent of those health care agencies with automated systems used these systems for nursing care planning, while only 4 percent documented nursing care in their information system.[1]

The purpose of this chapter is to examine data collection, processing, and storage in diagnosis-based nursing practice and to reconcile nursing language and the terminology of information systems so that nurses can become knowledgeable consumers of information systems as well as communicating effectively with information systems professionals. In order for two specialized groups—nurses and information systems professionals—to communicate effectively, there must be a shared understanding about which data are essential, ways that these data are collected and recorded, and the information and operational flows within the organization.

Nurses must be able to articulate the unique aspects of nursing practice and define their data processing requirements in terms that are meaningful to the information systems professional. Conversely, information systems professionals must be able to analyze the practice of nursing and its data and information processing requirements so that the resulting automated system is useful to nurses. While information systems analysts are skilled at identifying the information needs of organizations, the evolution of information systems has occurred primarily in the business world. The information needs of clinical and administrative nursing practice are not yet well-defined, and nurses must take an active and informed role in establishing these requirements through collaboration with information systems professionals.

Another requirement for successful communication and collaboration between nurses and information systems professionals is the ability to describe and analyze nursing practice, at clinical and administrative levels, as an information processing activity. This presents a number of interesting challenges. Nurses are concerned with "wholeness and health of humans, recognizing that humans are in continuous interaction with their environments for health."[2] Information systems are concerned with data processing, in which raw data are changed into information; moreover, this processing is always done in the same manner, based on instructions from the applications program, and it is usually logical and linear in nature.[3] In order to obtain the benefits of information systems for nursing, the holistic concerns of nursing must be described in a manner compatible with data processing concepts.

NURSING AS INFORMATION PROCESSING

Most of the tasks of nursing and other health professions involve the handling of information;[4] however, in nursing practice, the responsibilities and requirements for handling data and information seem to take a secondary role to the delivery of nursing care. Yet, this direct care delivery aspect of nursing is fundamentally concerned with collecting and analyzing data about the patient and about nursing care activities, documenting judgments based on these data, and communicating information about the patient's condition.

Nursing is defined as "the diagnosis and treatment of human responses to actual or potential health problems."[5] The diagnosis and treatment of human responses consists of both information processing activities and the execution of nursing care. It is the information processing activities, however, that determine which patient conditions the nurse identifies for treatment and the types of treatments selected. The recognized framework of the nursing profession for these information processing activities is the nursing process.

The nursing process consists of a series of steps: assessment, diagnosis, planning, intervention, and evaluation.[6-8] It represents the recognized thinking model of professional nursing. Information from biological, social, medical, and nursing fields are used by the nurse, but this information is used within the context of the nursing process and focused on the patient's human response. The nursing process is also the best known and most widely used scheme for organizing the collection, use, and storage of nursing data.[9]

Within the context of the nursing process, the information processing activities of the nurse are directed toward two areas: diagnostic decisions and treatment decisions. Diagnostic decisions are reached through an information processing activity described as the diagnostic reasoning process. Treatment decisions are contingent upon the clinical accuracy and precision of the nursing diagnosis; once the nursing diagnosis is identified, treatment decisions are guided by this. Nurses must also process information and make decisions about disease-related symptoms, responses to medical therapy, and execution of medical orders. (See Chapter 4 for further discussion of diagnostic and treatment decision making in clinical nursing practice.)

Nurse administrators are also confronted with information processing activities. While nursing process is recognized as a framework for organizing nursing data in clinical nursing practice, a corresponding framework for nursing administration has not been identified. Managers use data and information primarily for controlling their operations and for planning. This information may be in the form of lists, grouped information, and descriptive statistics.[10]

Examples of this use of information in nursing administration include determining patient acuity and allocating appropriate nursing resources, evaluating the clinical performance of nurses based on documentation of their practice, and planning for the delivery of nursing services by using clinical data to forecast the anticipated demand for nursing resources. These, and other administrative strategies, depend upon the availability and accessibility of data and information from clinical nursing practice.

Information processing in nursing can be examined at three levels. At the first level are data and information used in individual nurse–patient interactions, such as nursing diagnoses and associated nursing interventions for a particular patient, and execution of nursing interventions and medical orders. When information is aggregated, for a specific nursing unit or nursing organization, this represents a second level of information processing. An analysis of data about nursing care and resources on local, regional, and national levels represents the third level of information processing for nursing. This permits the analysis and projection of trends in the needs for nursing care and the required nursing resources that goes beyond a single nursing organization.

COMPUTERIZING NURSING DATA

In order to process large amounts of information computerization can be used to facilitate and standardize the collection, storage, and analysis of data and information. A nursing information system (NIS)[11] is defined as:

> a computer system that collects, stores, processes, retrieves, displays, and communicates timely information needed to do the following:
> - administer the nursing services and resources in a health care facility
> - manage standardized patient care information for the delivery of nursing care
> - link the research resources and the educational applications to nursing practice

Nursing information systems may be a part of a larger hospital information system, or they may be free-standing systems, sometimes referred to as dedicated systems. A dedicated system is concerned with a single application or function; patient classification systems, nurse scheduling systems, and documentation systems are examples of dedicated systems.[12]

Benefits and Uses of Computerization

Computerization offers a number of benefits for recording, storing, and analyzing the data and information for clinical and administrative nursing practice, particularly the ability to process large volumes of data and quickly produce useful information. Computers process data by selection of data items to meet certain criteria, summarizing data into a manageable form, sorting data into a desired order, and performing mathematical calculations. Query processing is another approach to data processing, where users can extract information from a computerized database with a series of questions entered at a keyboard.[13]

Nursing information systems are used in four major areas: nursing administration, nursing practice, nursing research, and nursing education.[14] In nursing administration, NIS are often subsystems, dedicated to functions such as quality assurance, personnel files, communication, budgeting, and payroll. Other administrative uses of NIS include special purpose dedicated systems for patient classification, nurse staffing and scheduling, incident reporting and risk management, and shift summary reports.

A number of roles for computerization are found in the clinical practice areas. Computerized physiological monitoring systems and specialized stand-alone systems are found in a variety of clinical settings. These include ventilators, blood gas analyzers, pulmonary function systems, intracranial pressure monitors, cardiac/diagnostic systems, and drug administrations systems. Larger information systems, as a part of online, integrated hospital information systems, may be used for order entry, charting of vital signs, care planning, nursing notes, and other types of patient care documentation.[15]

Another type of computer technology appearing in the clinical setting is optical character recognition. This technology uses optical scanners to recognize marks, characters, and codes. These symbols are transformed into digital form for storage in the computer.[16] For example, selected point of care systems use bar code readers to automate nurse charting and medication administration, monitoring both the correct identification of the patient and the drug.[17] Technology is also available to scan and recognize handwriting, and it has been tested in one hospital emergency room.[18]

Nursing research is an area where computers are routinely used, including literature search programs, statistical analysis programs, database management systems, and word processing programs. In nursing education, computer assisted instruction is being used for students in schools of nursing, continuing education, and even patient education programs. Other resources, such as expert systems, are also in use or in development.[19]

Considerations for Computerizing Nursing Data

The process of computerizing nursing data must be guided by a number of important considerations. First, the decisions necessary for nursing practice, administration, and research must be specified. In the next step, a set of limited and essential data for making those decisions must be identified and an algorithm or model of each decision must be developed. This process must also be supported with the necessary resources. Finally, an appropriate evaluation program should be developed and implemented.[20]

Three key issues for computerization will be discussed in this section: defining a data set for nursing, the use of nursing process as a framework for computerizing nursing data, and role of nursing diagnosis.

The Nursing Minimum Data Set. A critical component of computerization of nursing information is the identification of a limited and essential data set. A Nursing Minimum Data Set (NMDS) has been proposed for collecting, storing, and analyzing nursing data. The concept of a NMDS is based upon the concept of uniform minimum health data sets, defined as "a minimum set of items of information with uniform definitions and categories, concerning a specific aspect of health or dimension of the health care system, which meets the essential needs of multiple data users."[21] Using this definition as a guide, the NMDS may be defined as:

> a minimum set of items of information with uniform definitions and categories concerning the specific dimension of nursing, which meets the information needs of multiple data users in the health care system . . . [including] those specific items of information that are used on a regular basis by the majority of nurses across all types of settings in the delivery of care.[22]

The NMDS is concerned with those data elements that could be considered to be national or international in scope and to provide clues about trends in nursing and nursing resources allocation.[23]

The purposes of the NMDS are to:

1. establish comparability of nursing data across clinical populations, settings, geographic areas, and time

2. describe the nursing care of patients and their families in a variety of settings, both institutional and non-institutional
3. demonstrate or project trends regarding nursing care needs and allocation of nursing resources to patients or clients according to their health problems or nursing diagnoses
4. stimulate nursing research through links to the detailed data existing in nursing information systems (NIS) and other health care information systems (HCISs) in both institutional and non-institutional settings.[24]

The 16 elements of the proposed NMDS cover three broad categories: nursing care elements, patient demographic elements, and service elements. There are four nursing care elements: nursing diagnosis, nursing intervention, nursing outcome, and intensity of nursing care. The demographic elements consist of a personal identification element, date of birth, sex, race or ethnicity, and residence. Service elements include the unique facility or service agency number, the unique health record number of the patient, the unique number of the principle registered nurse provider, the episode admission or encounter date, the discharge or transfer date, the disposition of the patient, and the expected payer of the bill.[25]

Ten of the NMDS elements are also found in the Uniform Hospital Discharge Data Set,[26] while six of the NMDS elements are specified for nursing. These specific elements are the four nursing care elements and two service elements, the unique health record number of the patient and the unique number of the principle RN provider.

The Nursing Process. The nursing care elements of the NMDS are nursing diagnosis, nursing intervention, nursing outcome, and intensity of nursing care. The nursing process was described earlier as the most widely used scheme for organizing nursing data, but in the NMDS the nursing process is reflected rather than reproduced. In NMDS the action steps of the nursing process—assessment, implementation, and evaluation—are converted into data elements, also referred to as entities. Assessment is subsumed into the diagnostic step, represented by nursing diagnosis. Planning and implementation are represented by nursing interventions. The process of evaluation is represented by the nursing outcome data element. For the purposes of NMDS, the action-oriented steps of the nursing process have been converted into entities that have known attributes that can be collected, stored, and analyzed as data elements.

While the nursing process serves as a foundation for the elements of the NMDS, there are several problems associated with the use of nursing process as a framework for organizing nursing data. The first is the necessity for nurses to record data and information about the patient's disease-related condition as well as nursing conditions. The vast amounts of patient data available in today's health care organization can be overwhelming, and the nurse may opt for simply recording data rather than attempting to organize and analyze it in either manual or automated form. This situation is exacerbated by a second issue, the perception of many nurses that nursing process is an educational activity rather than a thinking tool for clinical practice. As a result, nursing process may not be a viable part of the clinical practice culture, and so it offers little guidance for the nurse attempting to organize and record large volumes of data.

A third issue is the emergence of nursing diagnoses as a standardized framework for naming patient problems. The addition of nursing diagnoses has a dual impact on the usefulness of nursing process as a framework for organizing nursing data. While nursing diagnoses can be used to describe the basic data set for nursing in consistent terminology, problems with this approach include ascertaining the reliability and validity of diagnostic labels, analyzing nursing data when there is more than one nursing diagnosis, and determining accurate patient descriptors for the diagnostic labels.[27]

Nursing Diagnosis. The introduction of nursing diagnosis raises questions about the terminology used by nurses, the need for nursing care planning, and ultimately the scope of nursing practice. Despite the challenges presented by the evolving nursing diagnostic terminology, the consistency and standardization offered by a diagnostic language for nursing is an essential aspect of organizing the collection, storage, and analysis of nursing data.

Nursing diagnosis is the foundation of the nursing care elements of the NMDS; it describes the patient's condition, directs the types of nursing interventions that should be used, establishes parameters for outcome measures, and can serve as an indicator of nursing intensity. A critical aspect of any minimum data set is the existence of uniform definitions and categories. The need for uniform definitions and categories in order to computerize nursing data and the concerns about the uniqueness of human beings, wholeness, and health as the focus of nursing represent two critical viewpoints in nursing. Both are important, and, in some way, both must be reflected in an approach to organizing, collecting, and storing nursing data and information. These concerns about uniqueness and wholeness, however, must not be used as a crutch to avoid the issues of patterning and order that are fundamental considerations of theory and science[28] as well as essential aspects for computerizing nursing data.

Computerizing nursing data requires an explicit description of the thinking processes used by nurses to process patient information into nursing diagnoses and associated nursing care plans. In view of the holistic concerns of nurses and the often intuitive means of knowing used in expert nursing practice,[29] discovering and describing these processes presents exciting and challenging areas for examination and research. However, computerizing nursing data cannot wait until this knowledge is available. Today, the nursing process offers a useful starting point for organizing nursing data, and nursing diagnoses provide a beginning framework for naming patient conditions of concern to nurses. Let us now shift this discussion to the area of information systems.

INFORMATION SYSTEMS

In all scientific or professional disciplines, the basic foundation of the discipline is formed by a common understanding of concepts, terminology, symbols, and analytical techniques. This is particularly true in information systems, where much of what goes on cannot be seen or touched by the user. Information systems are often viewed with great awe because many people lack understanding of these systems. This is seen in the common perception of many individuals that computers, or information systems, are mystical black boxes. Problems are frequently blamed on "the computer" as though it were somehow operating with a mind of its own. Computerized information systems are designed, developed, implemented, and controlled by people; these machines only do what they have been programmed to do.

In this section, an effort will be made to remove some of the mystical qualities of computerized information systems by defining some commonly used terminology and describing the ways that computers accomplish their "magic." This discussion also presents the process of developing an information system in the hopes that the reader will be able to participate in this process as a collaborative partner with information systems professionals rather than a hesitant or fearful one.

Relevant Concepts and Terminology

A number of key concepts from the information systems area are defined and examples from diagnosis-based nursing practice are presented here to assist the novice in information systems. An understanding of these terms is essential for nurses to participate in any analysis, design, development, or implementation of information systems. The interested reader may also wish to investigate the wide variety of resources available in the information systems areas, including texts, journal articles, and workshops.

A **system** is defined as a set of components that are interrelated and function together to perform a task or to serve a purpose. The human body is a familiar and excellent example of a system.

An **algorithm** is a procedure for solving a problem that frequently involves repetition of an operation. An **information system** is defined as a set of interrelated algorithms that function together to receive defined inputs, in the form of raw data, and then processes those inputs to produce certain desired outputs, in the form of information, to meet the identified needs of the user. From a nursing perspective, assessment is analogous to the data collection procedure that produces inputs for the nursing process. When assessment data are subjected to clinical thinking processes, such as clustering data and recognizing patterns in the data, a nursing diagnosis represents the output of this information processing activity.

Data are the raw materials, including individual facts and figures gathered from various sources, that serve as inputs for some thinking or decision-making processes. **Information** is the product resulting from subjecting raw data to some type of analytical process. Such a process consists of predefined conventions and algorithms that convert raw datum inputs into information by giving these data form and structure according to some recognized framework.

Typically, data may be only loosely related prior to processing, yet they must be organized in some meaningful fashion if the data are to be converted to information. A clinical example of this is a patient's temperature. When a nurse is presented with a single fact that Mr. Jones has a temperature of 102°, the conclusion is that this patient has fever; therefore, this solitary fact is considered by the nurse to be information that has meaning rather than data. In reality, however, this solitary fact has meaning only because the nurse has processed this input by comparing the observed temperature to known normal values for body temperature and the patient's previous temperature readings. The result of this process of comparison was information: the patient has fever.

The diagnostic reasoning process is another way that nurses convert data into information. Consider the following data collected by the nurse in an initial patient assessment: shallow respirations, respiratory rate of 32 breaths per minute, bilateral rhonchi or auscultation, productive cough, and history of cigarette smoking for 10 years. When these data are clustered and compared with known defining characteristics of respiratory nursing diagnosis, this processing results in a diagnostic conclusion of Ineffective Airway Clearance. This nursing diagnosis has meaning and is information, and it serves as further input into the diagnostic reasoning process; now, the nurse continues to collect and to process pertinent data to determine an etiology statement for this problem, such as thick tenacious pulmonary secretions. These two diagnostic conclusions, the nursing diagnosis and the etiology statement, are the result of processing patient assessment data to provide information that can be used in the nursing care planning process.

The distinction between data and information may seem insignificant, but it is a crucial one in the world of information systems. Defining essential data inputs, the resulting outputs, and the place of those outputs in further information processing activity is a critical aspect of system analysis and design. The clinical thinking processes of nurses can play an important role in designing meaningful systems for nursing practice. As a nurse progresses through the process of caring for an individual patient, information developed at one stage will serve as input data to the next step of the nursing process, and this process must be reflected in information systems to support diagnosis-based nursing practice.

Input is the raw, incoming data that are subjected to some process. A **process** is a logical structure that performs predefined operations to transform incoming data into some form of output that has meaning to the user. **Output** is information that results from the application of some process to the incoming data. In the preceding example, the nursing diagnosis of Ineffective Airway Clearance related to thick tenacious pulmonary secretions is the output resulting from the process of clinical thinking by the nurse on the patient assessment data.

These three components—input, process, and output—form the basic foundation of all information systems. Any system, regardless of its complexity or scope, can be reduced to a finite set of individual processes with specific input requirements and desired output. Therein lies the beauty of information systems; once developed and fully tested, systems are known, predictable, and controllable by the user and systems analyst.

A **database** is defined as a grouping of data, related to some common subject, that is structured or organized in a manner to meet the information processing needs of one or more users without unnecessarily duplicating those elements that are common to the needs of all users. **Data management** is concerned with managing the facts and the meanings of those facts stored in computerized systems, including all the activities necessary to ensure that high quality data are available to produce needed information and knowledge.[30] For example, all users of a hospital information system require access to patient demographic data, such as name, age, hospital record number, and date of admission. The concepts of database and data management are important ones for nurses as this approach to information processing offers many advantages for nursing.

The concept of data management and the database approach are relevant to the practice of nursing from both clinical and administrative perspectives. Indeed, it has been suggested that "one of the projects that the entire nursing profession needs to be concentrating on has to do with the establishment of a national database."[31] The existence of a national nursing database would create exciting opportunities for clinical and administrative nursing research, for the analysis of trends in nursing care requirements and resource utilization, and for linkage with other health care databases.

Important Attributes of Information. In addition to the concepts defined thus far, there are several attributes of information and information systems that are important to consider in analyzing and designing these systems. Definitions will be presented here, and the role of these attributes in system development will be discussed later in this chapter.

The term **online** describes input devices that are in direct communication with, or controlled by, the central processing unit, the "brain" of the computer. This type of input device usually refers to workstations or terminals. In the early days of information systems most input data were submitted to the system using punched cards; today the two most common types of system input are user keyboard entry and data transfer from other systems.

Real-time refers to *when* the processing of input takes place. Real-time processing is the capability of a fast-response online system to access and process data so that output is provided rapidly enough to affect the outcome of an activity or process. A familiar example is an automatic bank teller, where the account balance is adjusted at the time that a withdrawal is made; however, deposits are not immediately credited to the account. Instead, all deposits made that day are accumulated and processed together, and this is called **batch-mode** processing.

The term **accuracy** describes the extent to which data processed for specific outcome requirements actually represent reality. For example, a nurse caring for an unstable postoperative patient in the intensive care unit may want to know the patient's urine output during a certain time period. Greater accuracy is achieved if the nurse measures urine volumes with a graduated container rather than "eyeballing" the amount in the urinary drainage bag. Different types of data often require differing degrees of accuracy; low, moderate, and high degrees of anxiety provides a reasonable estimate of that concept, while physiological measurements may require very precise numerical measurement. Accuracy requirements of the data are an important consideration for structuring data collection and analysis components of an information system.

The **relevance** of information is concerned with the concept of collecting, storing, analyzing, displaying, and reporting *only* data and information that are applicable or necessary for the intended uses of the system or the process currently being executed. For example, there are certain demographic data elements that are collected during the hospital admission process, such as admitting physician, employer, previous visit dates, and admitting medical diagnosis. An information system to support diagnosis-based nursing practice should permit nurses to access these admitting department data, where appropriate, rather than requiring the nurse to repeat data collection and entry processes for data that may not be relevant for nursing care.

Determining which data are relevant and which are not is a crucial decision in information systems design. Including irrelevant data in a system results in cluttered screens and reports, as well as providing distractions from pertinent data collection and analysis. The costs of collecting, storing, and processing data must be weighed against the value of having those data. This sometimes means making hard choices about "need to have" data as opposed to "nice to have" data.

Freshness refers to the age of the data or information that the information system makes available to the user. This may be through an online terminal display, printed report, or as input to subsequent data processing. Freshness is a particularly important attribute for information systems that provide data and information for clinical decision making about patient conditions.

Consider a patient with a nursing diagnosis of Ineffective Airway Clearance related to thick tenacious secretions. A desired outcome for this patient is that arterial blood gas (ABG) measurements remain within normal limits. The patient is presently stable, and blood gas measurements every four hours are adequate to monitor this patient. For another patient where the differential nursing diagnoses are Ineffective Airway Clearance or Impaired Gas Exchange and respiratory status is highly unstable, more frequent ABG measurements are needed. When patient conditions are changing rapidly, freshness of the data assumes critical importance.

The **flexibility** of an information system is a measure of the system's ability to meet changing requirements for data input, processing procedures, or user needs for specific outputs. The greater the degree of flexibility, the more support the system can offer for the needs of the user. Flexibility is usually desired in areas such as input formats, data storage, output design options, and definition of parameters.

An example of flexibility in an information system to support diagnosis-based nursing practice can be seen in documentation pathways for nursing interventions. For the nursing diagnosis of Ineffective Airway Clearance related to thick tenacious secretions, the nurse has the option to select a variety of nursing interventions on the screen. In addition, the flexibility of the system can be seen in the presence of type-in spaces so that the nurse can adapt specific strategies and timeframes for the patient. Rather than a standardized nursing intervention such as:

Turn, Cough, and Deep Breath

a flexible system would permit the nurse to type in the positions for turning and a timeframe:

Turn to _____ (position) q____hours.

Flexibility can enhance both the acceptance of a computerized information system and the usefulness of the information that it produces; however, a word of caution is in order. Building unnecessary flexibility into an information system is a waste of design and development time, and therefore undesirable. Nurses involved in the design and development processes should choose points for flexibility that enhance the usefulness of the system for clinical nursing practice and for producing requisite information for managing nursing services.

Fundamental Principles of Information Systems.   Nine fundamental principles for computerized information systems have been suggested by Hodge and Clements:[32]

1. Data should be recorded when and where they occur.
2. Data should be placed in a form that can be read, processed, and stored automatically at the earliest possible stage.
3. Every practical method for verifying, balancing, and controlling the data entering the system should be used.
4. Data should be classified so that they can be readily retrieved and associated with other data elements as necessary.
5. Only data with a reasonable likelihood of being used should be kept permanently in the database or file.
6. Duplication among files should be avoided.
7. Reports produced by the system should focus on information of value in decision making; concise summaries, reporting exceptions and variations, and statistical analyses are a few examples.
8. No datum should be in the system that does not have a "pay-off" for it being there.
9. No system can be devised that is foolproof against personnel who do not know or care enough to make it work properly.

These principles represent general guidelines for decisions in the analysis and design of information systems; however, situations arise that do not always fit general guidelines, and, in those cases, unique solutions are required.

The terms, attributes, and principles presented here provide a basic knowledge base about information systems. In the next section, this information is placed within the systems development framework, and the process of designing and implementing an information system is discussed. The issues of supporting diagnosis-based nursing practice with information systems are discussed within the context of the system development process.

SYSTEMS DEVELOPMENT: FRAMEWORK, SYMBOLS, AND TECHNIQUES

In the recent past, the information systems industry has adopted a general framework or structure for the process of creating and implementing an information system: the Systems Development Life Cycle. A variety of life cycle structures are described in the information systems literature and used in the industry; however, all versions deal with the same basic phases: analysis, design, development, and implementation.

Analysis

The analysis phase serves as the initial point of contact between the users requesting an information system and the information systems professionals. In organizations that have an information systems department, representatives of the department provide their services to other groups and departments in the organization. Those organizations without such resources may work with information systems consultants or vendors of information systems. Many of the issues and questions in the analysis phase are the same whether an information system is to be developed or an existing system is to be purchased.

In the analysis phase, the user and the information systems professionals work together to define the proposed system. This is the initial stage where the determination of the user's objectives as well as the scope and complexity of the proposed system occur. Based on this information, the feasibility of the project must be evaluated and the requirements for such a system must be defined. A conceptual model or framework for the system is developed and the logical flow of data is established. The products, also referred to as deliverables, of this phase are a summary feasibility report and a detailed definition of system requirements. The result of this is an overview of the proposed information system and an estimation of the potential costs and benefits of the system. An important purpose of the analysis phase is to examine and evaluate requests for information systems at a preliminary level, without major commitments of personnel or money.

The analysis phase consists of three components: initial assessment, feasibility study, and requirements definition. In the initial assessment, the objective is to identify the purpose of the proposed system and methods for accomplishing this purpose. Often, a request for an information system arises out of a particular situation such as the need to solve a specific problem or to improve data collection or increase consistency or output information; however, a system may be requested to meet requirements from regulatory groups or external agencies that require certain information from the organization. The main concern of the initial assessment is defining the objectives to be achieved with the implementation of the proposed system; furthermore, these objectives must be clearly stated and agreed upon by both the information systems professionals and the users.

In order to establish the objectives of the system, factfinding and information gathering occurs. A number of strategies are used to obtain information from potential users of the system. Interviews, surveys, direct observation of information and product flow, and review of documents and reports are used to analyze and evaluate the current method for dealing with the situation as well as strengths and weaknesses of these methods, the needs and perceptions of potential users, the potential benefits of using an information system for the situation, any relationship between the proposed system and long-range plans for the organization, and a preliminary identification of costs where possible.

The second component of the analysis phase is a feasibility determination for the proposed system. This consists of three aspects: technological feasibility, financial feasibility, and operational feasibility.

The technological feasibility of the proposed system depends upon the ability of currently available technology, both hardware and software, to meet the needs of the user requesting the system. For example, nurses might request a system that interacts with the hospital's laboratory information system to provide rapid access to test results. Such an interaction would require a real-time interface between the nursing information system and the lab's information system. Technical incompatibility could prevent this type of online, real-time interaction from being possible.

The financial feasibility determination is essentially a cost–benefit analysis. The organization must consider the costs associated with developing the proposed system, and those costs must be weighed against both the anticipated benefits or savings associated with the system and the financial risk associated with not developing the system. In the case of nursing systems requests, a cost–benefit analysis may be difficult to support of the benefits of the system cannot be stated in quantifiable terms, such as improved nursing resource allocation and productivity or enhanced monitoring of nursing data for quality assurance purposes. As the development of information systems is often costly and time-consuming, nurses must strive to identify all benefits for nurses, patients, and the organization that an automated information system might produce.

The assessment of operational feasibility is directed toward the capacity of the users to operate the proposed information system as planned, in order to realize the benefits of having such a system. This area of assessment includes a preliminary analysis of the human, technical, and environmental resources required by the proposed system, and it is basically concerned with the practicality of the project, in operational terms. The objective of this assessment is to identify the probable characteristics of the proposed system and how such a system would fit into the operations of the organization.

Requirements definition is the third component of the analysis phase. Here, the information systems professionals and the intended users work closely together to establish a thorough understanding of the activities of the proposed system. As part of this detailed investigation, answers to the following questions will be sought:

- Who are the intended users?
- What activities are included in the domain of the function to be supported with this information system?
- Exactly how are each of these activities performed?
- What is the frequency and volume of each activity?
- What data are required for input?
- How are these data to be processed?
- What is the nature and the format of the required output?
- What other personnel, departments, systems, or processes are affected by the implementation of this system or by the absence of such as system?

The answers to these questions provide essential information about the inputs, processes, and outputs of the proposed system.

To find answers to these and other questions during the requirements definition process for a nursing information system, factfinding and information gathering is necessary. Interviews with selected nurses in clinical practice and administration, solicitation of ideas from the nursing staff through questionaires or group meetings, direct observations of day-to-day patient care activities, and inspection of existing documentation and information-handling systems are useful strategies. Nurses must provide direction and assistance in the selection of interviewees, setting up group meetings, drafting questions for surveys, and choosing documents for review and activities for observation. Participation of nurses from all levels of the nursing organization permits the assessment of the needs and perceptions of the broad user group, and clinical and administrative issues should be examined in a pragmatic, operational manner. In this way, information that is relevant both to nursing practice and systems development can be obtained for the systems development process.

Requirements definition for the proposed system is the last step of the analysis phase. The initial assessment, feasibility study, and requirements definition are then combined into an end product: a comprehensive written document that contains all of the user's requirements for the proposed information system. This document serves as proposal and master plan for the new system, including descriptions of and recommendations for:[33]

1. data input functions described as close to the source of data as is practical and alternative sources of data entry
2. user experience or lack of experience with considerations for developing the necessary user skills and attitudes
3. descriptions of the outputs and reports to be generated by the system, including purpose, frequency, and distribution
4. identification and description of the data elements necessary to produce the desired outputs and to support automated functions of the system
5. definition of all inputs within the system and the data elements contained in each input, including the source of the input, data elements contained in the input, methods of data collection, manual processing, and required manual and automated controls
6. definition of data structures to facilitate processing of inputs to generate outputs and to satisfy other necessary computational requirements
7. estimation of the peak and average volumes of activity for the system and the anticipated areas for growth in these areas
8. description of operating constraints such as report deadlines, operating schedules, or space and staffing limitation
9. description of external constraints such as data security and regulatory requirements
10. identification of areas where the proposed system conflicts with existing organization policy and the impact of such conflicts
11. definition of controls for the quality of input data, processing of transactions, and the system-generated outputs
12. determination of organizational requirements for system development and implementation, such as the need to create new positions, changes in staffing levels, or modifications of job description criteria, as well as concomitant financial implications
13. identification of the criteria for evaluating the proposed system after its implementation.

The system proposal is a detailed summary of information obtained in the analysis phase and highlights the major issues and opportunities for the development of the proposed system. This report serves as the basis for a management decision to proceed or not to proceed with the development of an information system.

Design
In the design phase, the recommendations in the systems proposal are translated into a detailed set of specifications. At the conclusion of this phase, a series of specifications is produced that describes the system's output and the data necessary to generate the desired output, including data entry procedures and file structure. The processing requirements to accomplish transformation of input data into outputs must also be specified.

The product, or deliverable, of this phase is a detailed design document that can be used by information systems professionals to develop the proposed information system. The logical design document is much like the architectural drawings for a building. While actual, logical, design decisions are the responsibility of the information systems professional, the user is involved in reviewing and approving the structure of system outputs and the logical flow of the system.

For nursing information systems, identifying the essential information for clinical and administrative nursing practice must be done so that the unique requirements of nurses are reflected in the design specifications. The ability to aggregate patient data by nursing unit as well as medical service, to retrieve clinical data for quality monitoring and nursing resource decisions, and to identify cost and billing data for nursing services are just a few areas where output from an computerized system would be very useful. Flexibility in nursing documentation aspects of the system should be included to permit the nurse to individualize patient care plans and to record data accurately and precisely. At this point, nurses must be able to clearly describe and define their information needs, the purposes for which this information is required, and the ways in which the information is produced. Designing and developing information systems is time-consuming and costly; nurses must present their information needs in a way that is readily understood by information systems professionals and the administrators who ultimately give approval for the system.

Output. Designing the content and format of the output for the proposed system is a big step toward the final system specifications. The decisions made about the output of the system are critically important; all subsequent decisions in the design phase will be based on these decisions.

Much of the output from the proposed system will be in the form of screens and printed reports. The informational elements, the type of characters (alphabetic, numeric, or alphanumeric), the number of characters, and any special characteristics must be identified and defined for each screen and report that will be generated by the system. Existing reports may provide a useful starting point; however, this opportunity should be used to improve and enhance documents so that they are as informative and helpful as possible.

The output of the system may be produced in the batch-mode or from interactive query from the user. Examples of batch process reports include detailed exception reports, based on the principle of management by exception, and summary reports of accumulated information at varying levels. Interactive processing permits the development of a variety of report formats to meet specific operating information needs.

Another important decision about output has to do with the distribution of the output from the system. Basically, there are two types of output reports: reports for internal use that assist employees in the performance of their duties and reports for external use that focus on satisfying information demands originating outside the organization.

A final consideration is the layout of output reports. The assistance of a specialist can be invaluable in deciding issues such as the size and shape of the report, filing procedures, the placement of items on the page, the use of color, typography, titles and heading, page numbering, and sequence and spacing of data that play a role in the visual presentation, the usefulness, and the user acceptance of the reports.

Input. The input design process is concerned with identifying the required input data to generate the desired outputs and determining the most effective ways for entering, organizing, and coding the input date. While much of the information needed at this point is identified during the analysis phase, at this point it is important to examine any alternatives that might improve the quality of the output, facilitate input procedures, and also take into consideration the human element. It is essential that inputs are compatible with their final use in generating outputs.

In specifying the input requirements, the data element, its source, its specific format, and any unique characteristics must be defined for each input. Then the most efficient and active methods of data entry must be determined. Common methods include input terminals, punched cards, and various key entry devices. Important questions are: *who* enters data, *when* and *where* does data entry occur, *how often* must data be entered, and *what* is the likely volume of data entry?

Decisions regarding the entry of nursing data into an information system should reflect the realities of the clinical practice environment and the resources of the information system.

For example, if there are only two data entry terminals on a 35-bed nursing unit and if nurses are required to enter large volumes of patient data, such as vital signs and routine nursing treatments, then it is very likely that such requirements will be frustrating to nurses struggling for access to a terminal and that data may be of lower quality with many missing data. The decisions about nursing input must reflect the lack of access to the terminals, and the use of manual documentation for bedside charting of vital signs and nursing treatments may result in less frustration and improved quality of documentation. This choice, however, means that a great deal of clinical data is unavailable for aggregation and analysis except through manual chart review but, on the other hand, a point of care system makes it easy and efficient for nurses to enter large volumes of patient data accurately and easily. This does not mean that nurses should not enter data into automated systems; it does mean that decisions about which data nurses are required to enter should be made carefully and based on clearly defined needs for nursing information.

Processing. After identifying the desired outputs and the necessary inputs to produce those outputs, the final part of the design procedure is to specify the processing requirements to transform the inputs into outputs. Here, the specific operations to be performed on the input data are defined.

The specification of outputs, inputs, and processing requirements is the product, or deliverable, of the design phase, and this specification takes the form of a logical design model. To facilitate both decision making and presentation of the logical design of the proposed system, a number of representational techniques are used in the information systems industry.

Activity Diagramming

Efforts to identify all of the activities and functions of a proposed information system can be challenging or even overwhelming. A technique for presenting the activities of the system is activity diagramming. This technique is based on the premise that all endeavors are hierarchial in nature. In developing activity diagrams, the highest level of abstraction is the starting point, and lower levels represent successively more concrete operations. This approach forces consideration of major issues before less important ones, helping to keep the system design phase focused on the overall goals as well as addressing the specific issues.

An activity diagram is a chart that identifies activities at each level to be included in the system. The hierarchy and sequence of activities on the diagram is indicated through a numbering scheme and through the placement of the activity on the diagram. The mission of the nursing department in a hospital provides an example of an activity diagram in Figure 9–1. At the highest level of abstraction is the mission statement: Provide Professional Nursing Services. In the next level of the activity diagram, three aspects of this broad mission statement are identified and numbered: care for individual patients (1.0), manage nursing operations (2.0), and establish strategic direction for nursing practice (3.0).

The activities presented in Figure 9–1 are a more explicit representation of Providing Professional Nursing Services, and these activities can be used to define the information needs of the nursing organization. Information about caring for individual patients is necessary for the nurses and other health care providers involved in that patient's care; furthermore, this information serves as input data for managing nursing services. These data can be aggregated and analyzed, in conjunction with other data, to provide information about patient requirements for nursing care, resource allocation, and compliance with quality standards. This information can then be used as input data for strategic planning by the nursing department.

In Figures 9–2 through 9–5, activity 1.0 Care for Individual Patients, is examined and activities at the next level are presented. Indeed, it is possible to define additional levels of

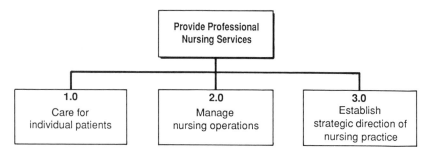

Figure 9–1. Level 1 Activity Diagram: Nursing service operations, at the highest level of abstraction

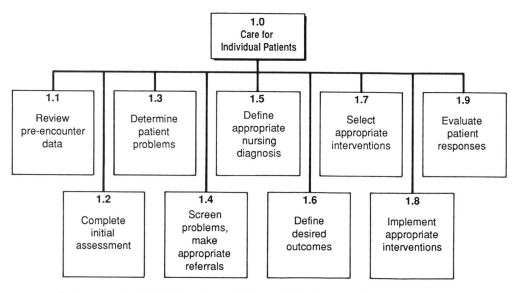

Figure 9–2. Level 2 Activity Diagram: Major activities in caring for individual patients

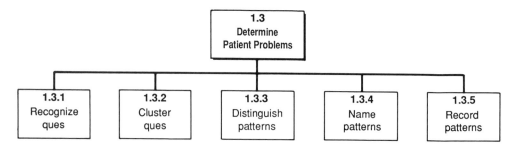

Figure 9–3. Level 3 Activity Diagram: Activities in determining health problems of individual patients

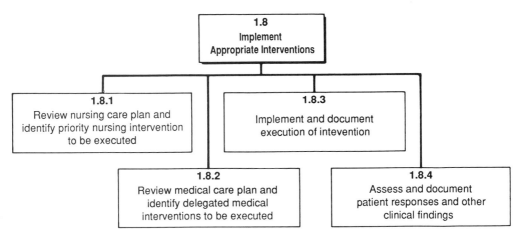

Figure 9–4. Level 3 Activity Diagram: Activities in implementing selected nursing interventions

detail for the activities outlined in these figures; the figures should be considered representative of a nursing information system rather than exhaustive. In Figure 9–2, nine activities associated with Care for Individual Patients are defined. These activities are similar to the decision points of the nursing process, described in Chapter 4. Using this activity diagram to design a nursing information system would support diagnosis-based nursing practice because the thinking processes of the nurse and the data processing procedures of the information system are congruent.

An important step in the nursing process is identifying patient conditions that indicate a need for treatment. This activity is represented in Figure 9–3. Here the term "patient problems" is used, making it possible for the nurse to identify nursing diagnoses as well as other types of problems. If this diagram were taken to the next level at Activity 1.3.4, Name Patterns, activities might include Identify Nursing Diagnoses (1.3.4.1), Identify Significant Changes in Medical Condition (1.3.4.2), and Identify Other Problems (1.3.4.3). In this way, identifying nursing diagnoses would lead to development of nursing care plans, identifying significant changes in medical conditions would lead to execution of standing orders or notifica-

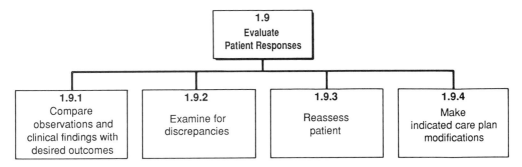

Figure 9–5. Level 3 Activity Diagram: Activities in evaluating patient responses to selected nursing interventions

tion of physician, and identification of other problems would lead to an appropriate referral. A similar procedure is seen in Figure 9–4, representing the activities associated with Activity 1.8, Implement Appropriate Interventions. Here both nursing interventions and delegated medical responsibilities are included. In Figure 9–5, another example is presented, describing the next level of activity associated with Activity 1.9, Evaluate Patient Responses.

Activity diagrams are a useful technique for defining and organizing hierarchically the operations of an information system. The next step is to identify the specific data inputs and decisions associated with each activity or group of activities. A useful technique for this process is Decision Structure Diagramming.

Decision Structure Diagramming

Defining the decisions in clinical and administrative nursing practice is an undertaking of immense scope and complexity. A useful starting point is the decision points in the nursing process (see Chapter 4). These decision points can be examined with the technique of decision structure diagramming with decision trees.

The nursing process is essentially a decision-making process, containing a number of decision points. At each of these points, direction for subsequent decisions is provided; this direction is clearly demonstrated through the influence of the diagnostic decision on the selection of etiological statements and expected outcomes. In Figure 9–6, this decision process is represented for the three respiratory nursing diagnoses: Ineffective Breathing Pattern, Ineffective Airway Clearance, and Impaired Gas Exchange. These three nursing diagnoses are choices in this decision process. For the selection Ineffective Airway Clearance there are three choices for the etiological component of the diagnostic statement, and for the diagnosis/etiology combination Ineffective Airway Clearance related to respiratory muscle weakness, a choice of three expected outcomes are presented. This decision tree must be considered as representative of the decision structure in identifying a nursing diagnosis, etiology, and expected outcomes, rather than as an exhaustive representation of all possibilities.

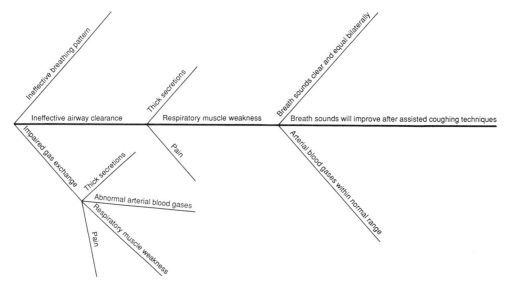

Figure 9–6. Decision Tree: The decision paths for etiology statements and expected outcomes based on the nursing diagnosis Ineffective Airway Clearance

The decision process in Figure 9–6 demonstrates an important issue for computerizing nursing information. Notice that two of the nursing diagnoses share etiology statements: for both Ineffective Airway Clearance and Impaired Gas Exchange there are three etiology statements that are exactly the same. To an information system professional this might seem like an inappropriate duplication; however, for a nursing diagnosis decision structure, this duplication is appropriate and necessary. Nurses participating in the design process must be able to describe, demonstrate, and defend pertinent duplications of data as well as the inclusion of those data necessary to support and document clinical and administrative decision making by nurses.

In Figure 9–7, another example of decision diagramming is presented. Continuing the clinical example of Ineffective Airway Clearance related to respiratory muscle weakness, this decision tree represents decisions about nursing interventions associated with the expected outcome state of breath sounds clear and equal bilaterally. Decision options for the selection of nursing interventions include three categories: assessment interventions, treatment interventions, and teaching interventions. After selecting an intervention category, specific nursing intervention choices are made.

The decision tree can define and simplify the various decision structures contained in an information system. Once this task is complete, nurses and information systems professionals can review the activity diagrams and decision trees for the purpose of identifying and cataloging the necessary inputs and outputs for each decision. The results of this effort enables the information systems professional to proceed to the next technique of system design, the data flow diagram.

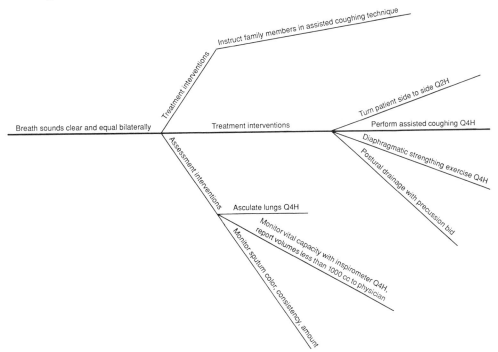

Figure 9–7. Decision Tree: The decision paths for nursing interventions based on the expected outcome of breath sounds clear and equal bilaterally

Data Flow Diagramming

In most information systems, data is collected and stored to meet a variety of needs. Typically, much of the same data is used by multiple processes to support decisions and to direct actions, with data flowing from multiple points to multiple points. To ensure that the final data structure allows each process or each user to access all data necessary for his or her particular needs, a logical model of the flow or movement of data within the system is required.

Data flow diagramming is a technique that has been adopted by the information systems industry to build logical models of data flow. One of the most widely used techniques was developed by Gane and Sarson[34] and uses four basic symbols to represent data flow in diagrammatic fashion.

An **external entity** is symbolized by a square block, and it represents a source of data that the information system can process. It may also represent a destination of output from the system. As the name implies, external entities are outside the bounds of the system. Each unique external entity is identified by a lowercase letter in the upper left corner of the square block. The label or name of the external entity is placed in the center of the block. Figure 9–8 shows a data flow diagram for an information system to support diagnosis-based nursing practice. An example of an external entity is seen in the upper right hand corner of the figure; physicians recording data in the progress record section of the system are a data source external to the system. Other external entities, not represented in Figure 9–8, might include the Admissions Department, which provides data for the system, and the Quality Assurance Department, which uses output from the system for quality monitoring purposes.

A **process** is symbolized by a vertically oriented rectangle with rounded corners. This symbol depicts activities or functions within the system that accept input data and apply defined conventions to produce output to meet the needs of the user. Each unique process is assigned an identification number when it is placed on the diagram; this identification number is placed at the top of the rectangle, and it has no relationship to the place of the process in the sequence of the data flow.

A description of the process is placed in the center of the rectangle. This description should begin with an active verb and describe the essential purpose of the process succinctly. In the lower section of the rectangle, a notation may be used to indicate the location where the process takes place; alternatively, this lower section may be used to identify the user responsible for completing the activity or interacting with the system at that point. In Figure 9–8, a number of processes are present. Process 5.0 is described as Define Nursing Diagnoses, and a notation in the lower section of the rectangle indicates that the RN is responsible for this activity.

A **data store** is symbolized by a horizontally oriented rectangle with square corners and an open right side. This symbol represents the storage, or holding area, for data in the system. Data are considered to be at rest when they are not in route to or from a process or when they are not being processed. Data stores are resting points for data when those data are not actually in use. Each data store is identified by a unique number shown in the left side of the rectangle and by a label that describes the subject matter of the data. Data stores represent conceptual groupings of data; they do not imply any of the physical representations of the data, such as file structure or storage devices. For example, a data store named Pre-Encounter Data includes data collected and entered in the Admitting Department, prior to nurse–patient contact; however, this data store is available to the diagnosis-based nursing information system so that nurses need not repeat this data collection and entry process.

A **data flow** is symbolized by a simple arrow, and it represents movement of group of data between a data store and a process. Data can flow in both directions, as both an input to a process and as an output from that process. The label assigned to a data flow should describe

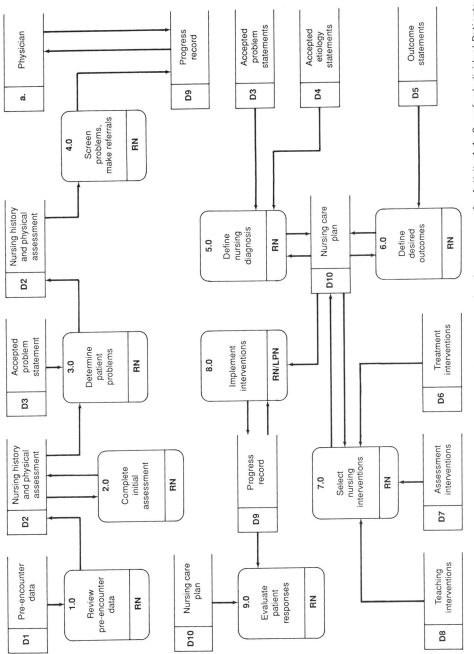

Figure 9–8. Data Flow Diagram: Overview of the required data stores and major processes for Activity 1.1. Care for Individual Patients

215

the data contained in the data flow, not the nature of the transport media such as chart forms or magnetic tape. Once the logical design of the system is completed, decisions about the types of storage and transport media are made. For the purposes of data flow diagramming, it is the data and their movement that are important.

A data flow diagram of a system for diagnosis-based nursing practice contains data stores, processes, and data flows that link those processes. Examples of data stores, shown in Figure 9–8, have to do with data that nurses collect and enter into the system, and these data stores are linked with specific processes by certain data flows. Data stores representing Nursing History and Physical Assessment data (D2), are linked with four processes in this system: Process 2.0, Complete Initial Assessment; Process 3.0, Determine Patient Problems; Process 4.0, Screen Problems, Make Referrals; and Process 5.0, Define Nursing Diagnoses. Additional data stores also provide data for these processes The Accepted Problem Statements data store (D3) and the Accepted Etiology Statements (D4) also provide data for Processes 3.0 and 5.0.

If this seems complicated, recall the decision points of the nursing process and the types of data used in those decisions. (See Chapter 4.) Data stores, in the data flow diagramming technique, are simply groups of data that are needed for a particular process. A nurse must have data from patient assessment in order to identify nursing diagnoses. A nurse must also know about nursing diagnoses, including the diagnostic labels and etiology statements, to formulate a nursing diagnosis. Through the diagnostic reasoning process, data are collected and clustered, patterns are named and recognized, and a diagnosis/etiology label is assigned.

This same diagnostic process is represented in the data flow diagram in the form of data store D2 of patient assessment data obtained during the nursing history and physical, and data stores D3 and D4 containing nursing diagnoses and etiology statements. Data from these stores are processed (Processes 2.0, 3.0, 5.0) to produce output to another data store, D10, the Nursing Care Plan. The identified nursing diagnoses are output from Process 5.0 and stored in D10, Nursing Care Plans; however the nursing diagnoses are also input into nursing care planning, represented in Process 6.0, Define Desired Outcomes, and Process 7.0, Select Nursing Interventions. Further data for these processes are found in data store D5, Outcome Statements, and data stores D6, D7, and D8, for three types of nursing interventions. Implementation and evaluation of the nursing care plan uses data from data stores D10, the Nursing Care Plan, and D9, the Progress Record, as well as Processes 8.0, Implement Interventions, and 9.0, Evaluate Patient Responses.

Data flow diagrams are a useful technique for information systems design. Figure 9–8 represents the data flow of a system analogous to Activity Level 1.0 in Figure 9–2, and it can be considered as an overview of the system. As such, it represents the highest level at which the system can be modelled and still reflect the scope of activity and information processing requirements that must be supported by the system. Similar diagrams for activity 2.0, Manage Nursing Operations, and Activity 3.0, Establish Strategic Direction of Nursing Practice, would be necessary to design a comprehensive nursing information system for diagnosis-based nursing practice. The data collected, processed, and stored in the system presented in Figure 9–8 would provide important data inputs for this additional work.

The data flow diagram in Figure 9–8 is based on the decision points of the nursing process and nursing diagnosis as the organizing logic for the data stores and processes of a logical design for a diagnosis-based nursing information system. Such an approach has the advantage of congruence with the professional values of nurses, and it is consistent with recommendations for computerizing nursing data, including the specification of decisions for clinical practice and the use of the elements of the Nursing Minimum Data Set. Nurses must participate in the systems design phase by providing this type of information to information systems professionals and assisting in the delineation of the activities of nursing services and the decisions in those activities. Only if nurses are knowledgeable and informative about information systems and able to examine nursing as an information processing activity will this collaborative participation be possible.

Development

In the development phase, the logical model produced in the design phase is actually developed. This activity consists of writing and testing all of the application programs as well as developing the file and database structures. The technical procedures are created and refined through the generation and testing of a prototype of the proposed system. Other aspects of this process include developing the procedures and manuals necessary to train the intended users of the system and planning for the conversion and installation of the system.

The development phase is a complex one, and responsibility for it lies almost solely with the information systems professionals. Involvement of the user is minimal: meeting with information systems personnel to discuss the progress of the project, assisting with identifying data for use in testing the prototype, and reviewing user documentation for clarity and usefulness. The deliverable for this phase is the proposed information system, ready for implementation.

Implementation

In this phase, the user returns to a role of central prominence. Hardware is installed in accessible locations, user personnel are trained to use the system, and the required input data are loaded into the system. Once these tasks are completed and reviewed, the system is ready to "go live."

While implementation is an exciting time, a word of caution is in order. The entire implementation process must be carefully and thoroughly planned. Without comprehensive planning, for both the expected and the unexpected, the implementation process can result in chaos—manual systems no longer available and the computerized system not yet working. The results of a poorly planned and executed implementation phase include lost productivity, increased costs, and, most importantly, user resistance to the system. The old adage, "Failing to plan is planning to fail," might have been written for this situation.

Five focus areas of the implementation phase have been identified: assessing, training, activating, supporting, and evaluating.[35]

Assessment. During the implementation phase, assessment of policies and procedures for needed changes should be determined and developed. Departmental and unit level procedures for manual back up systems are an important part of this phase. Other important areas for assessment and policy/procedure development include user access and responsibility, protection of patient confidentiality, the work environment and work patterns of various areas and departments, and any changes needed in the system. While some of these issues were addressed in the analysis and design phases, in the implementation phase these preliminary plans are expanded to detailed procedures and those procedures are put into effect.

Training. A critical area for successful implementation of an information system is user training. Plans for an effective training program must consider available human resources to conduct the training program, the accessibility of training facilities, timeframes for the project, and the number and types of users to be trained. The training program should cover familiarization with the hardware, location of terminals on the patient units, and supervised practice sessions using the system.

Another vital aspect of the training process is the examination of the effects of the new system on the work environment. In many instances, shifting from manual systems to automated systems influences the way the work is done, the timing of work activities, and the results of the activity. Consider the implementation of an automated information system for physician order entry, patient billing, pharmacy services, and nursing documentation in a busy intensive care unit. A task as seemingly simple as ordering and administering intravenous fluids becomes fraught with problems and frustrations when the usual patterns and routines are changed. Prior to the automated system, when a patient required a change in the type or amount of IV fluids, the nurse could obtain the new fluid with a phone call to the pharmacy. The written order could be dealt with later; particularly for rapidly changing patient conditions, this was often the case and the nurses found this mechanism extremely helpful. With the automated system, however, new IV fluid orders are not filled until the order is entered into the computer, either by the physician or by the nurse through a verbal order pathway.

While entering the IV fluid order into the automated system might appear to be easier than making a phone call to the pharmacist, it represents a significant change in the usual work pattern of the unit. Instead of calling a person, the pharmacist, on a familiar technology, the telephone, the nurse must deal with "The Computer," an unfamiliar technology that does not provide immediate feedback in a human form. If this and other changes in work routine are not considered in the implementation phase, a great deal of time and energy can be diverted into anxiety, resistance, and frustration about the new information system.

Changes or modifications in the work activities for nurses resulting from the introduction of an automated system can include changes in the availability of information and supplies, changes in the timing or sequencing of activities, and changes in the scrutiny of nursing documentation. These changes may occur because of issues with access to terminals, user skill, and clinical issues. For example, the nurse used to receiving calls from the laboratory about abnormal test results may find it difficult to remember that now the lab print-out box must be checked for test results that are reported to the nursing unit via the information system, rather than depending upon a phone call. In another situation, nurses who are used to sitting down at the end of their shift to document nursing care activities may find that terminals are unavailable at that time, because *everyone* is waiting till the end of the shift to chart. Changing work patterns to enter nursing documentation data earlier or more frequently during their shift represents a significant change for many nurses.

These are just a few examples of the changes in work habits and patterns that should be anticipated and addressed in the implementation phase. These issues may be subtle ones, and sometimes they may be more apparent to the unit nursing staff, while other problems may be better detected by individuals outside the work group. Either way, it is invaluable to examine the work routines and patterns, as well as the nurses perceptions about these. Strategies to prevent problems with changes in work patterns and routines involve thoughtful assessment of work patterns, identification of important system applications for a particular unit and patient population, an examination of assumptions about their work patterns, and participation by nurses in the development of procedures and policies for the implementation of the system.

It is essential that the assumptions underlying system implementation are validated with nurse-users on the nursing unit. In the earlier example, one assumption might be that entering an order into the computer for a new IV fluid is easier than making a phone call; however, if the nurses perceive that a phone call gets a better response that a computer order entry, then this reality must be considered in the implementation process. This does not mean that the automated system should not be used to obtain IV fluids from the pharmacy; it does mean that the differences in the procedure should be anticipated, made clear to nurses using the system, and that this aspect of the system should be emphasized in the training and implementation phase.

Emphasizing *how* to get things done with the automated system, rather than *what* the system does is a very useful implementation strategy. This is a major concern of nurses, who often pride themselves on their ability to accomplish things rapidly and effectively for their patients. Presenting the automated system, in practical terms, as a way to assist in these efforts can be very effective. This strategy, however, depends upon a thorough analysis of the work patterns, routines, and rituals of the nursing unit, and, for best results, differing aspects of the system will require emphasis on different units. In the critical care unit, for example, obtaining needed IV fluids rapidly is a key concern, so emphasis on IV order and charting pathways is an important strategy to enhance acceptance of the system. On a nursing unit with complex medical patients, a great deal of nursing time and energy is occupied with administration of medications. Ensuring that nurses are knowledgeable and skilled in using that aspect of the system can promote acceptance of the system.

The implementation of a system for diagnosis-based nursing practice will contain an emphasis on the nursing care planning and documentation. Here again, the role of assumptions, existing work routines, and availability of resources play important roles. If nursing care planning is not currently occurring in a nursing organization, the assumption should not be made that the introduction of an automated system containing nursing diagnoses will reverse that trend. Similarly, if nurses are in the habit of sitting in the nurses' lounge or conference room so that nursing care plans can be developed in a quiet environment, it can be anticipated that nursing care plan development at terminals located in noisy, busy areas may occur with less frequency than previously.

An automated system for diagnosis-based nursing practice must support and facilitate the use of nursing diagnoses in care planning and other documentation; however, an automated system cannot accomplish diagnosis-based nursing practice alone. Such a system must be based on a clinical practice foundation that uses nursing diagnoses as the framework for nurses to describe patient conditions and that offers the necessary structure to the clinical practice environment so that nursing practice is diagnosis-based rather than task-based. (See Chapter 5 for an overview of the diagnosis-based nursing practice environment.)

Activating and Supporting. Activation is the point at which the ownership of the system transfers from the information systems professionals to the users. Activation refers to the actual initiation of the automated system, or "turning on the computer." This may be accomplished by activating nursing units in a sequential fashion, one after the other, or all units may be activated together.

The decision to proceed with activation of the system sequentially or en masse is based on the availability of resources to support users in the initial activation period and the particular issues with data and information processing. An important issue for nursing units is the availability of resources to support nurses as they make their first attempts in using the new system. This supporting role encompasses on-the-spot education, problem solving, and analytical assistance in using the system; however, a critical aspect of this support is emotional.

Staff responses to the automated system may range from amazement, anxiety, fear, and unrealistic expectations to resistance or overt hostility. One nursing unit responded to the activation of a hospital information system by making a doll named HIS for Hate Information Systems and hanging the doll in effigy at a staff meeting. While this response may sound extreme, it did accomplish a useful purpose in expending some of the frustration that nurses were feeling about the system, and it introduced an element of humor into a stressful situation. In fact, this was a turning point for the staff, and the implementation proceeded much more smoothly after this staff meeting. The individuals in a resource role during the activation period must be able to provide emotional support, diffuse anxieties, and maintain a sense of equilibrium with the staff during this period.

Evaluation. The evaluation of an automated information system is a continuous process; however, an evaluation of the implementation process and the initial use of the system is essential. Two aspects are of concern: the technical functioning of the system and the products of the system, including the users' involvement with the system. The technical concerns have to do with the operations of the hardware and software, including setting of priorities, analysis, specification, programming, and debugging.

A post-implementation review of products of the system and the user's involvement is done to evaluate the successes and shortcomings of the system in meeting the objectives of the system. Issues to consider here are the performance of the system in producing the desired information, the acceptance of the system by the users, a preliminary cost–benefit analysis, and the continued validity of the original objectives of the system.[36]

In order to accomplish this evaluation, surveys, questionnaires, interviews, and observations of users are all useful techniques. An examination of quality assurance audits, standard reports, and other documentation from the system is also helpful. All of the information obtained in the evaluation process can then be used to determine if the system is meeting its objectives and what measures are required to maintain or to enhance both technical and product performance.

In evaluating the technical and product performance of an information system for diagnosis-based nursing practice, two areas are important. The first is the support that the system provides for diagnosis-based nursing practice at the nurse–patient interaction level. The second area is the ability of the system to aggregate and analyze nursing data so that it provides meaningful information for nurse administrators in managing operations and strategic planning, and for nursing research as well.

An information system that supports diagnosis-based nursing practice organizes nursing data according to a nursing model and facilitates the identification and documentation of nursing diagnoses and associated interventions. Such a system also provides efficient mechanisms for nurses to record data about their delegated medical responsibilities, including administration of medications, observations about significant symptoms and responses to medical therapies, and the execution of treatments. Data and information about both of these aspects of nursing care should be accessible for retrieval and analysis of nursing practice.

An information system that supports diagnosis-based nursing practice includes the elements of the Nursing Minimum Data Set, and it reflects the clinical thinking processes of the nurse. The use of the decision points from nursing process offers a structure for a system to document clinical nursing practice activities, and this is presented in Figure 9–8. Congruency between clinical thinking nursing practice and the information systems used to collect, store, and analyze nursing data is the desired goal. Such congruence supports professional nursing values and enhances the acceptance and ease of use of the system.

Finally, an information system that supports diagnosis-based nursing practice is one in which knowledgeable and informed nurses have participated in the analysis, design, development, and implementation process. Nurses must describe the clinical and administrative practice of nursing as an information process activity and articulate this in the language of information systems. The information systems industry only knows about nursing what it hears; therefore, nurses must be able to participate in the creation of information systems that meet the unique and particular needs of nurses.

CONCLUSION

It has been suggested that there is "beginning support for a science of nursing based on information processing."[37] The opportunities that this approach and the use of computerized information systems offers for nursing practice are exciting and challenging. Nurses cannot wait, however, for information systems professionals or vendors of information systems technology to provide them with systems that will meet the needs of professional nursing practice. Rather, nurses must become informed and knowledgeable partners in this process.

This chapter has presented an introduction to the purposes and design of computerized information systems in diagnosis-based nursing practice. Much of the knowledge necessary for the development of such systems is available, but there is a great deal that remains to be discovered, from both nursing and information systems perspectives.

In order to gain the knowledge and skills to participate in developing and using information systems, the following recommendations are offered:

- Learn about information systems, Contact colleagues that work with information systems, explore the literature, and attend conferences, workshops, or courses.
- Do not rush the process of analysis and design of a new information system, or the selection process if a system is to be purchased. Clearly identifying *what* is needed, *who* or *where* it will come from, *how* it will be used, and the *technical requirements* to accomplish this take time, energy, and commitment. The results, however, are worth it.
- Be an advocate for nursing. Represent the data and information processing issues of clinical and administrative nursing practice accurately and with a sense of conviction. Information systems professionals cannot design systems to meet the needs of nurses unless those needs are defined in precise and concrete terms.
- Do not be stubborn. Refusal to learn about information systems or to participate in their development and use in health care organizations is self-defeating. Alternatively, insistence on "nice to have" information or applications may interfere with the ability of the system to provide the "need to have" things.
- Explore the possibilities of information systems for clinical and administrative nursing practice with an open mind and an inquiring spirit. While computerized information systems can accomplish many wonderful and useful things, they will not solve all the problems of the world. Realistic expectations and a sense of the possible are important tools for nurses working with information systems.
- Use the professional knowledge of nursing, including the nursing process as an organizing framework, and the Nursing Minimum Data Set. Find out what has been done in the area of information systems and nursing, then use that knowledge as a foundation. There is no point in re-designing the wheel, particularly in an area as specialized and complex as information systems.

These suggestions are offered with hope and optimism. Computerized information systems present effective and important opportunities for the collection, storage, and analysis of nursing data. These systems can process raw data elements from nursing practice into information to generate new knowledge about nurses, patients, and health care organizations; this must be a concern of all nurses.

REFERENCES

1. Ratliff, C., Summers, S., Resler, M., & Becker, A. Computerized nursing diagnosis and documentation of nursing care in inpatient health care agencies. Paper presented at the meeting of the North American Nursing Diagnosis Association, St. Louis, March 1988
2. Donaldson, S.K. & Crowley, D.M. The discipline of nursing. *Nursing Outlook,* 1978, *26,* 2, 113
3. Saba, V.K. & McCormick, K.A. *Essentials of computers for nursing.* Philadelphia: J.B. Lippincott, 1986
4. Naisbit, J. *Megatrends.* New York: Warner Books, 1982
5. American Nurses' Association. *Nursing: A social policy statement.* Kansas City: American Nurses' Association, 1980, p.9
6. Yura, H. & Walsh, M.B. *The nursing process* 4th ed. Norwalk, Ct: Appleton-Century-Crofts, 1983
7. Mundinger, M. & Jauron, G. Developing a nursing Diagnosis. *Nursing Outlook,* 1975, *23,* p.94
8. American Nurses' Association, p. 12
9. Grier, M.R. Information processing in nursing practice. In H.H. Werley & J. J. Fitzpatrick (Eds.), *Annual review of nursing research,* vol. 2. New York: Springer Publishing Company, 1984, p. 265
10. McHugh, M.L. Information access: A basis for strategic planning and control of operations. *Nursing Administration Quarterly,* 1986, *10,* 2, 10
11. Saba & McCormick
12. *Ibid*
13. Parker, C.S. *Understanding computers and data processing: Today and tomorrow.* New York: Holt, Rhinehart and Winston, 1987, p. 58
14. Saba & McCormick
15. *Ibid*
16. Parker
17. Yerow, M. St. Francis Hospital goes bedside and beyond, *Health Care and Computing,* 1988, 48
18. Hallisey, J. Write on! *PC Computing,* 1988, 1, 4, 62
19. Saba & McCormick
20. Grier, M.R. Health information systems: Toward computerization of nursing diagnosis. In M.E. Hurley (Ed.), *Classification of nursing diagnoses: Proceedings of the sixth conference.* St. Louis: C.V. Mosby, 1986, p.168
21. Health Information Policy Council. *Background paper: Uniform minimum health data sets.* Washington, DC: U.S. Department of Health and Human Services, 1983
22. Werley, H.H. Status of the nursing minimum data set and its relationship to nursing diagnoses. Paper presented at the meeting of the North American Nursing Diagnosis Association, St. Louis, March 1988
23. Werley. Status of the nursing minimum data set.
24. *Ibid*
25. Werley, H.H. Nursing diagnosis and the minimum data set. In A.M. McLane (Ed.), *Classification of nursing diagnoses: Proceedings of the seventh national conference.* St. Louis; C.V. Mosby, 1987, p.21
26. Health Information Policy Council. *1984 revision of the uniform hospital discharge data set.* Washington, DC: Federal Register, 50:31038, July 1985
27. Grier, Health information systems
28. Meleis, A.I. *Theoretical nursing: Development and progress.* Philadelphia: J.B. Lippincott, 1985
29. Benner, P. *From novice to expert: Excellence and power in clinical nursing practice.* Menlo Park, CA: Addison-Wesley, 1984
30. Loomis, M.E.S. *The database book.* New York: Macmillan, 1987
31. Grier, M.R. Discussion following paper presentation. In M.E. Hurley (Ed.), *Classification of nursing diagnoses: Proceedings of the sixth Conference.* St. Louis: C.V. Mosby, 1986, p. 177
32. Hodge, B. & Clements, J.P. *Business systems analysis.* Englewood Cliffs, NJ: Prentice-Hall, 1986
33. *Ibid*
34. Gane, C. & Sarson, T. *Structured systems analysis: Tools and techniques.* Englewood Cliffs, NJ: Prentice-Hall, 1979
35. Mitchell, N.M., Cappaglia, J.A., and Taylor-Loughran, A. Selecting automation to support human resources management activities. In E.M. Lewis and J.G. Spicer (Eds.), *Human resource management handbook: Contemporary strategies for nursing managers.* Rockville, MD: Aspen Publishers, Inc., 1987 p.53
36. Hodge & Clements
37. Grier, 1984

Educating the Diagnostician: Issues and Strategies for Teaching Clinical Thinking

Pamela H. Shurett

Nursing education is faced with the challenge of preparing nurses for the role of diagnostician. Preparation takes place in the school or college of nursing and in the health care organizations that must prepare experienced nurses for diagnosis-based practice. This chapter will approach diagnosing as an issue of skill acquisition that requires a clinical knowledge base of nursing practice.

Nurses have been dealing with the issues of *if* nurses diagnose, *what* nurses diagnose, and *how* nurses diagnose for years. Today, nurse educators recognize that accurate diagnosis of patient conditions is essential to good nursing practice. What to teach and how to teach it remains the challenge. To novice nurses, educators must teach the art of diagnosing—the diagnostic process. For experienced nurses, the task is to teach a nursing framework for nursing problems.

In the course of nursing practice, many different types of patient conditions or problems occur. Many times these problems are the result of the patient's disease and its associated medical or surgical treatment. The ability to recognize those medical problems or changes in the patient that require medical interventions is an important function of the nurse. This aspect of nursing practice requires a sound theoretical background in the sciences, as well as expertise obtained from seeing patients with similar conditions over and over again.

The use of nursing diagnosis enables the nurse to go beyond the medical diagnosis and to identify conditions that must be treated with nursing interventions rather than medical therapy. Indeed, these conditions identified with nursing diagnoses may not be related to the medical problem. For example, a young mother with asthma may be far more concerned about her children at home than she is about her breathing. The experienced nurse will diagnose and treat this patient's anxiety as well as offering interventions to ease breathing. Clearly and accurately identifying the nursing diagnosis permits consistency and continuity of intervention; it also provides a mechanism for the treatment efforts of the nurse to be documented and recognized.

It is important to remember that nursing diagnosis terminology is in an evolving state at this time. The endorsement of Taxonomy I in 1986 provided a starting point for a diagnostic framework for nursing practice. In order to add to this taxonomy and to improve the clinical usefulness of the diagnoses, they must be tested in clinical practice. Classification systems for other professionals have developed over many years, and for nursing this process has just begun. Taxonomy I offers assistance to the nurse educator in focusing on nursing problems and interventions rather than medical ones. The use of nursing diagnosis will challenge novice diagnosticians to *think* rather than to assume that a patient's problems are found only in the medical diagnosis.

INFORMATION AND SKILLS NEEDED TO FORMULATE A NURSING DIAGNOSIS

Certain information is needed in order to formulate an accurate nursing diagnosis. First, information from and about the patient must be collected. Second, the meaning of this information must be recognized. Third, knowledge of nursing science and what the nurse can do for the patient is necessary. And finally, critical thinking skills are essential in order to derive a nursing diagnosis.

In order to obtain this information, the diagnostician needs a number of assessment skills. Interviewing skills, including the ability to use open–ended questions and to be non-judgmental, are essential. Rapport skills must be developed so the nurse compiles accurate, honest information. The diagnostician must be able to collect data from the physical exam so basic skills in physical assessment are necessary. The ability to gather data from the patient's medical record and other health care professionals that have contributed to the care of that patient completes the information-gathering or assessment process.

Determining the meaning of all the information gathered during the assessment process requires the diagnostician to draw on knowledge and principles from biology, psychology, and sociology as well as other disciplines. The information collected from the patient is compared to a wide range of norms that exist for various patient populations. The diagnostician must have knowledge of nursing science and the treatment options for diagnostic categories.

The development of critical-thinking skills are the foundation of diagnostic thinking, and as such they are essential to accurate diagnosing. Critical thinking represents the thought process that accompanies problem solving and decision making. There are a number of important attributes of critical thinkers. Critical thinkers and learners ask questions, consider alternatives offered by others, and evaluate reasons for accepting one idea or another. Critical thinkers are non-judgmental and do not make decisions on the basis of subjective or arbitrary data.

The nature of nursing practice requires nurses to be critical thinkers because nurses are constantly called upon to make decisions about and with their patient. Nurses must determine the nature of the patient condition, if additional data collection or validation is needed, and if action is actually necessary. Carefully developed problem-solving ability and critical-thinking skills assist the nurse in making correct diagnoses.[1]

Despite the need for accurate nursing diagnosis in clinical practice and the need for critical-thinking skills to accomplish this, studies of the diagnostic abilities of nurses and nursing students show a different picture. Nurses are not diagnosing with accuracy or utilizing a theoretical approach to diagnosing. Aspinall[2] found that nurses were unable to state the patient's problem and seemed to lack the theoretical knowledge of what might be responsible for the dysfunction. Matthews and Gaul[3] reported that there was no overall relationship between critical thinking as defined by scores on the Watson–Glaser Critical Thinking appraisal and the ability of nursing students to make a nursing diagnosis. Frederickson and Mayer[4] evaluated the ability of AD and BS degree nursing students to problem-solve, and they found no significant difference in the ability of the students problem-solving ability, although the BS students scored significantly higher on a standardized test for critical-thinking skills. Lee and Strong[5] found that AD and BS students achieved similar scores in their perceptions of competence in identifying nursing diagnosis.

Development of the cognitive skills necessary to make a nursing diagnosis is a critical concern to nurse educators in both schools of nursing and in staff development because of the importance of nursing diagnosis in clinical nursing practice. What the nurse, student or not, does with the data is just as important as how the data is collected. In this chapter the educational principles and teaching skills essential to prepare nurses to formulate nursing diagnoses in clinical practice will be discussed. An approach to diagnostic thinking, within the context of the nursing process, will be presented that can be used with students of nursing and with those experienced nurses who may be learning the diagnostic process and nursing diagnosis for the first time.

Prerequisite Considerations

There are several factors that must be taken into consideration by the educator before beginning the process of teaching nursing diagnosis. There are differences in the population of learners to be taught nursing diagnosis. Also the organizations in which the learners are encountered are different. These differences require flexibility on the part of the nurse educator so that teaching strategies are meaningful to each situation.

The problem for the educator, regardless of the setting, is to make material regarding nursing diagnosis relevant to various levels of experience. The process of skill acquisition, which Benner[6] has generalized to nursing, assumes that learners pass through five levels of proficiency in the development of a skill: novice, advanced beginner, competent, proficient, and expert. Progression through these levels reflects a movement from reliance on abstract principles to the use of past concrete experiences as models and the ability to view the situation as a whole regarding which data are relevant.[7] The descriptions of the phases experienced during the acquisition of a skill provide a unifying framework for the nurse educator to teach nursing diagnosis and diagnostic reasoning. This approach views the ability to use nursing diagnosis as a skill. Specific educational strategies for learners at different skill levels will be presented later in the chapter.

The organization in which concepts about nursing diagnosis are taught may be the school of nursing, the hospital, or other practice setting. These organizations share some common qualities such as the diverse student (learner) population, but there are some important differences. These differences should influence the choices of educational strategies used in teaching nursing diagnosis and diagnostic thinking.

Educational Settings

The student population in nursing programs is widely diverse. In addition to the traditional student, many enter nursing programs as returnees after long absences from formal educational programs. RNs return for BS and MS degrees; others have previous education in the military or LPN/LVN programs.

Every school of nursing has a philosophy and curriculum. These should be examined for clear expression of the faculty's belief and commitment to the role of the nurse as a diagnostician. While the philosophy is a composite reflecting the philosophies of individual faculty members, the faculty should endeavor to reach some consensus on a number of issues. The definition of nursing diagnosis, the use of the NANDA taxonomy, the importance of the diagnostic role to the profession of nursing, and the incorporation of nursing diagnostic content into didactic and clinical courses are key areas for faculty consensus. In the absence of such consensus or congruence between the written and enacted philosophy of the school, conflict and confusion can occur.

The curriculum should include content and instructional methodologies designed to direct the behavior of the learner after the course of study is completed.[8] While the entire curriculum will not require change, the curriculum should incorporate nursing diagnosis content. Nursing diagnostic labels work well with most curriculum content outlines. After working with nursing diagnoses, faculty may become even more committed to a curriculum emphasizing nursing diagnosis. The best written curriculum, however, is only as effective as the individual faculty members who operate it.

One common goal of any nursing curriculum is to teach the use of the nursing process. This problem-solving process is taught universally by nurse educators, although the complexity of the diagnostic steps may vary. Nursing diagnoses made by the learner may vary with the type of program—technical, professional, master's, or continuing education. The terminal objectives or exit behaviors identified by the faculty for the graduate will have an influence on diagnostic sophistication by the graduate. These exit behaviors must consider the role the graduate is going to assume in community agencies as a practicing nurse. For example, a nurse with an associate degree practicing in a community in which there are few baccalaureate prepared nurses must have diagnostic ability. This ability is best begun in the formal educational process and continued in the practice setting.

The faculty also must consider the time commitment of including nursing diagnosis content in nursing courses. Nursing diagnosis cannot be introduced in one course and forgotten. Rather, it must be introduced and then reinforced throughout the curriculum in every course. Workshop and conference time to develop the diagnostic skill of individual faculty members is necessary, as well as inclusion of nursing diagnosis in the orientation of new faculty members.

Clinical Settings

These differences in educational background and clinical experience also occur in the hospital or institution contemplating introducing nursing diagnosis. In the hospital there are new graduates, nurses with many years of experience, and experienced nurses in new practice settings. Also there are LPNs and perhaps nurses' aides, who do not make nursing diagnoses but participate in data collection and ongoing assessment of patients. Therefore, educational programs about nursing diagnosis must be meaningful to all levels of personnel.

In the health care organization, the nursing service philosophy provides guidance and can lend support when dealing with the issues relating to nursing diagnosis, including tasks, time, and money necessary for the implementation of a new educational project. Most philosophies speak of providing excellent patient care and the inclusion of nursing care plans for patients. Using nursing diagnosis certainly will help meet those goals.

Time is also an issue in the clinical practice culture. There are often time restrictions in a hospital. The issue of time may be a particular concern when nursing diagnosis is new and extensive educational activities are planned. Nursing time away from patient care is expensive, and compensation for the time commitment required must be resolved before beginning an inservice program, particularly a cognitive task endeavor that may be perceived as unnecessary by some.

The nurse educator in the hospital setting must be thoroughly familiar with nursing diagnosis and how it relates to clinical practice. This requires the educator to attend conferences and have collaboration time with other educators for support and validation of operating methods.

Nurse educators in hospitals or other health care settings encounter additional problems when contemplating the educational issues about nursing diagnosis. Many institutions place more value on the technical skills of the nurse rather than cognitive tasks, such as assessment and diagnosis. The nurse who can quickly set up for insertion of a pulmonary artery catheter and calibrate the monitors may be valued more than the nurse who diagnoses Alteration in Family Process related to critical illness of spouse. The values of the clinical practice culture must be considered carefully when making choices about educational programs on nursing diagnosis or any other topic.

Also, the educator must be thoroughly familiar with the documentation system in place at the institution. The documentation system must allow and promote documentation of the diagnostic process. If the documentation system needs revision, the educator must then deal with the committee responsible for this. A change in the documentation format, in conjunction with the introduction of nursing diagnosis, requires even more change for nursing personnel. (See Chapter 7 for a discussion of documentation issues and nursing diagnosis.)

The philosophy and curriculum are very personal issues to nursing educators involved in their design and implementation. Changes are often based on the value judgments of individual educators and organizations. Issues of time, the institution's values, and the educators' commitment are among the issues to be considered before teaching nursing diagnosis. Planned changes must occur to keep curricula relevant to professional nursing practice.

PRINCIPLES OF TEACHING AND LEARNING RELEVANT TO TEACHING NURSING DIAGNOSIS

Psychologists and educators have struggled for years to understand how learning occurs. Nursing educators must examine principles of teaching and learning carefully as there are cognitive, affective, and psychomotor aspects within the body of nursing knowledge.

Many theories of learning have been proposed and evaluated, primarily in laboratories using animal subjects. There is doubt regarding the usefulness of such learning theories as practical guidelines for teaching.[9] The reader is referred to references on learning theories for additional information in this area. For purposes of this discussion, emphasis will be on basic principles of adult learning and generalizations from learning theories that have particular relevance for teaching nurses to make diagnoses. Because of the complexity of diagnosing and the cognitive processes involved, the educator must use a variety of creative and thoughtful techniques based on sound educational principles. Five learning principles particularly relevant to teaching nursing diagnosis are discussed here, and their application in both the school of nursing and the health care organization is described.

The learner should be involved in decisions about what is to be taught.

Learning is a personal process and the ultimate responsibility rests with the learner. Students should be involved in curriculum development as participants on the committee. Student input into courses occurs as a result of student evaluations. The content and process of learning should be individualized as much as possible.

Staff nurses in hospitals should be involved in decisions about professional developments within the institutions. They should serve on committees that make decisions about information, new skills, and policies. Clear lines of communication should be available for the staff nurse to contribute input and suggestions. The expertise of staff nurses should be utilized in teaching classes when possible.

The implementation of nursing diagnosis in a hospital can be threatening to many nurses. The terminology is new, the thinking process seems different, and it may involve changes in the clinical practice systems. Also, diagnosing and the resulting care plan may be viewed as unnecessary and unrealistic by many staff members—*and it will take more time!* The more the staff is involved in the decision making, planning, and implementation of the project, the less resistance will be encountered.

The experienced learner needs autonomy in educational experiences; therefore, an authoritarian manner is ineffective when teaching adults.

The learner should be an active participant in utilizing educational experiences. Examples from previous experiences should be encouraged for discussion in the classroom or clinical setting.

Writings on adult education[10] suggest that adults returning to the classroom want mutual planning with the teacher regarding learning needs, course content and sequencing, and means of evaluation; however, the Southern Regional Education Board,[11] in a project report regarding RNs returning to the classroom, found that the traditional lecture mode, instructor-oriented class was preferred by most older students. The reason appears to be that this approach is familiar, more comfortable, and reduces anxiety about returning to the classroom. The implication for the educator is that a variety of teaching methods must be used. The adult learner values the teacher's expertise but does not want to be treated as if any prior experience is useless. For example, the RN returning for a BS degree who has to validate bedmaking and IM injections may resent the remainder of the program. The nursing program with positive instructors has the opportunity to make lifelong learners of RNs returning for advanced degrees.

Transfer of learning from one situation to another occurs when the new situation is related to an earlier learning experience.

Similarities between situations are recognized so that application to new circumstances can occur. Positive transfer is facilitated by assuring the appropriate difficulty level of the learning task and by emphasizing principles and problem-solving methods rather than specific situations.

Nursing educators strive to organize courses and course content so that principles and skills are reinforced and increased. For example, a basic nursing course teaches assessment skills with emphasis on normal findings. Content in the next course includes chronic obstructive pulmonary disease advancing to include abnormal findings. Learning from one situation will be related and transferred to the new situation.

Diagnostic skill and content can be reinforced throughout the program. Specific diagnoses can be emphasized in certain courses. Basic students with few of the skills needed to make diagnoses should concentrate on the less complex diagnoses. The complexity of the diagnoses should increase from course to course as well as the learner's skill in use of the diagnostic process. Adults learn best when new information can be applied to current situations. Adults want immediacy of application. Nurses who are returning for degrees or in hospital inservice education programs want pertinent information that will help them solve practical problems in clinical situations.

The nursing educator should encourage the experienced learner to contribute information and experiences during educational activities and, thereby, relate the diagnostic material in a meaningful way. Clinical situations emphasizing a problem-solving format representative of those encountered in the practice arena are well-suited for this learner. The educator must be highly skilled in making diagnoses and well-informed regarding the professional issues surrounding nursing diagnosis.

The motivation of the learner influences learning.

A learner usually learns best when there is interest or desire. Motives play a role in learning and may be intrinsic, such as the individual's desire for achievement or recognition, or extrinsic, such as money or promotions.

Exactly what motivates a learner is highly individual and difficult to measure or specify. Some learners are highly motivated by a desire to succeed and want to learn everything there is to know. Many nurses seek continuing education out of the desire to learn the "latest thing" in nursing.

Learning to use nursing diagnosis is more complex than learning to use a new chest tube drainage system. Nursing diagnosis often seems new and unfamiliar. Staff nurses may need some convincing about the value of nursing diagnosis; in fact, they may perceive that the actual motive for learning comes from an external source—administration.

The professional significance of nursing diagnosis implies that nurses need to accept and believe in the importance of the process rather than merely follow the policy because it has been mandated. Examination of the process by which individuals accept new ideas provides guidance for the educator. There are four stages of this innovation-decision process model:

Stage One: Knowledge function—becomes aware and gains information
Stage Two: Persuasion function—forms favorable or unfavorable impression
Stage Three: Decision function—tries idea temporarily
Stage Four: Confirmation function—seeks reinforcement of decision[12]

Educators tend to focus on the knowledge function through classroom activities and clinical application. Learners are told what nursing diagnosis is and what they are expected to use. Few educators address the persuasion function in the process of accepting new innovations.

At the persuasion stage, the educator wants the learner to become psychologically involved with the idea and develop an affective "feeling" about it. The learner may seek information about the idea from others and mentally apply the new idea to the present situation. It is at the persuasion stage that the learner's general perception of the idea is developed.

For the learner to obtain a positive attitude about nursing diagnosis, the educator must allow the learner to be persuaded about the new idea. The educator must be positive, well-informed, and enthusiastic about nursing diagnosis. When implementing nursing diagnosis, it is helpful to be as compatible as possible with existing beliefs and attempt change that has a high likelihood of success.

For example, one should not acclaim nursing diagnosis so highly that the clinical expertise of the staff is threatened. The ability to monitor the responses of patient's to medical problems is a highly-valued and necessary function of nursing and should be recognized as such. It is also important to try to make the change a manageable one—avoid changing the entire documentation system, kardex, admission assessment form, *and* implement nursing diagnosis at once.

It may be useful to provide nursing staff with literature about nursing diagnosis and examples of where it has been implemented in other similar settings. If possible, expose the staff to others with positive attitudes about nursing diagnosis. This can be accomplished with one of the videotaped programs currently available that feature nurse leaders discussing the implications of nursing diagnosis.

Finally, allow time for the persuasion stage. Staff will not become involved personally with the idea in a one hour inservice program. Time is needed to seek more information from the literature and others and to contemplate what the change will mean in actual practice.

Staff motivated by money or fear of an unfavorable evaluation will not be enthusiastic practitioners of nursing diagnosis. Particular attention to the persuasion stage of the innovation-decision process model can increase acceptance of new ideas and enhance the development of diagnostic skill.

Organization of the material provides the means by which new information is related to that which is already known.[13]

Brunner[14] describes four advantages of teaching the structure of a discipline. Comprehension is increased because knowledge of structure provides a framework to relate facts and information that otherwise would be isolated and unrelated. Structure promotes memory because details are organized within principles that increase the chances of recall in that the memory of one segment within the pattern may quickly lead to recall of other related elements. Structure appears to promote the transfer of learning. Finally, the advantage of learning the structure of the material is that it will be kept up to date.

Theories describing the organization of knowledge in the long-term memory suggest that biomedical and nursing knowledge is composed of a network of associated concepts stored in a hierarchical manner. Abstract concepts are linked with less abstract concepts and proceeds from the highest most abstract level to the lowest most specific concept.[15]

This principle guides the educator in the organization of material, and it suggests that the taxonomy of nursing diagnosis can be used as an organizing framework. As stated before, not every unit of study must be organized as a nursing diagnosis, but the greater the overall organization into a unifying framework, the greater the student's comprehension and retention of the material.

There are three basic issues related to teaching the process and task of diagnosing that are common regardless of the setting: (1) factors affecting the diagnostician, (2) characteristics of the novice and expert diagnostician, and (3) the diagnostic process. Examination of these issues from the educator's viewpoint will reveal strategies for teaching nursing diagnosis to both novice and experienced nurses.

FACTORS AFFECTING THE DIAGNOSTICIAN

The effectiveness of the individual's diagnostic ability is determined by three factors: (1) the extent of the individual's information and memory, (2) the complex characteristics of the diagnostic task, and (3) the individual's perception of the situation. Differences in the long- and short-term memories of novices and experts were discussed earlier, but there are several additional points pertinent for educators.

Information and Memory

Information in the short-term memory will last only about 30 seconds unless it is rehearsed. This means that facts given to learners will not be remembered unless the learner is given the opportunity to repeat them again and again. Another characteristic of the short-term memory is its very small capacity for numbers or symbols.

The capacity of the short-term memory can be increased immensely by categorizing like pieces of information into similar patterns. In other words, information entering the short-term memory must be categorized and organized so that it is not immediately forgotten. The labels used to define the categories are then stored in the long-term memory for retrieval.[16]

This means that isolated bits of information given to the learner will not be remembered. Information must be connected, labeled, or categorized in some way so that it can be stored in the long-term memory and thus be available for recall. For example, nursing students learn in anatomy and physiology that shallow respirations can result in atelectasis, hypercarbia, and pulmonary infection. The study of chemistry adds to their knowledge of acid/base and the results of hypercarbia. Microbiology contributes to the understanding of infectious processes.

These pieces of information relate directly to clinical nursing practice, but it is when the instructor organizes the information as Impaired Gas Exchange that the information becomes meaningful in a variety of situations. And as the instructor relates the etiologies that can result in Impaired Gas Exchange, such as pain from surgical incision, morbid obesity, muscle weakness, fear of harming incision, or immobility, the student can recognize the need to assess many patients for evidence of Impaired Gas Exchange.

Complex Characteristics of the Diagnostic Task

The diagnostic process is a complex one because of certain characteristics of the task. The relationship between the cues and the actual patient problem is not perfect. That is, the cues assessed from the patient do not lead to one particular diagnosis every time. Therefore, there is a probabilistic relationship between the cue and the diagnosis that changes with the collection of additional data.

Consider a case where a nurse states, "This patient will throw an embolus before she gets out of the hospital." What cues were assessed to trigger such a remark?

1. The patient is 68 years old.
2. The patient is obese.
3. The patient's mobility is decreased because of arthritis.
4. The patient is scheduled for an abdominal hysterectomy.

No one of these cues, alone, would lead the nurse to predict the occurrence of a pulmonary embolus. As additional data are collected, however, the likelihood of this complication increases. The probability is high for an elderly, obese individual with decreased mobility scheduled for surgery, necessitating even more immobility, developing a pulmonary embolus.

The use of probability statements in medicine and nursing is common, especially informal predictions. Some probability predictions are based on systematic observations from large groups of patients, but many nursing probability statements are not based on formal research. Yet, practitioners assign probabilities to data, and later change those probabilities as additional data are collected and validated. Errors in diagnosis are made when the diagnostician fails to recognize the probabilistic relationship between cues and client states.[17] The complexity of the diagnostic task is increased further when one considers that the data necessary to make a nursing diagnosis are not the objective, exact data used in the medical domain. Nurses must rely on their own insight and perception about sometimes vague, imprecise information.

Presented with a patient with the following findings: fidgety, restless, sighs frequently, doesn't complete sentences, and decreased eye contact, the physician can rule out any medical diagnoses with normal results of arterial blood gases, serum electrolytes, EKG, and chest X-ray. The nursing diagnosis, however, could be Anxiety, Alteration in Comfort, Sleep Pattern Disturbance, or others, depending on the result of additional data collection. None of the possible nursing diagnoses can be ruled in or out with a lab finding or even normal vital signs. Nurses must rely almost entirely on their own perceptual ability.[18]

Data collected from a patient or the cues presented by the patient contribute to the complexity of the diagnostic task. For example, more cues often make the diagnostic task more complex. Some cues are infallible indicators of a certain condition; others are not. If a patient exhibits two cues that always occur together, then the redundancy increases and ensures the certainty of the diagnosis. Cues that overlap in different diagnoses increase the complexity of the diagnostic task. Finally, there is some degree of uncertainty in the best circumstances. Expert diagnosticians recognize the uncertainties, the redundancies, and fallibilities of the cues collected.[19]

The Individual's Perception of the Task

The biases of the diagnostician form one of the most important influences in the diagnostic process. These biases can influence the assignment of diagnostic categories that may be drawn primarily from episodic memory—the portion of memory that stores information about the most significant events in one's life.[20]

The first bias is the number of times the event has occurred in the diagnostician's experience. If the nurse has observed many patients develop shortness of breath, who are later diagnosed with pulmonary emboli, then that becomes the most probable diagnosis to that nurse. Indeed, it may be the only diagnosis considered. The novice nurse with limited experiences and knowledge must overcome the tendency to consider only diagnoses previously encountered.

The second bias is the recency of the past experience. The diagnostician may tend to assign a greater probability to experiences more recently experienced and less likelihood to experiences encountered less recently. Tanner[21] studied nursing students, where the students were presented with a patient situation in which the most likely diagnosis was sensory alteration. Students who had just studied diabetes were convinced that the patient was experiencing an insulin reaction, and those students who had just studied neurological problems were as convinced that the patient had increased intracranial pressure.[22]

These biases of the diagnostician have tremendous relevance for the educator. The clinical instructor or preceptor must be aware of content currently discussed in class, and then attempt to assign learners to patients with those problems whenever possible. If that is not possible, the instructor must guide the student to additional diagnostic possibilities and anticipate the student's tendency to diagnose problems most recently discussed. If the didactic material is organized around nursing models, the clinical assignment problem is easier to solve. It usually is possible to find patients with Alterations in Nutrition or Alteration in Comfort, as opposed to finding diabetic patients for forty students who studied diabetes the previous week.

The experienced nurse in the practice setting may also be likely to diagnose problems encountered recently. For example, the nurse who has cared for three patients with unstable angina and who also lack an understanding of the proper use of nitroglycerine for chest pain, very likely will consider the nursing diagnosis of Knowledge Deficit related to use of nitroglycerine for the next angina patient encountered. This nursing diagnosis will be considered initially, even before data collection is begun.

The third bias of the diagnostician is the intensity of the event. Individuals tend to remember dramatic or unusual events. This tendency may bias the probability assigned to a particular diagnosis toward an unlikely one, based on some dramatic event encounter in the past. The novice nurse who cared for lethargic adolescent patient whose CAT scan revealed a bleeding arterio-venous malformation, may associate lethargy in the next patient with an intracerebral bleed. An intracerebral bleed is not as probable as other possible causes of lethargy; but because of the dramatic quality of the events associated with a bleeding AVM, the nurse recalls the situation vividly and frequently.

The use of past clinical experiences as a resource in making diagnoses can be a powerful asset to the nurse. Clinical expertise and judgment is gained and refined over time. Recognition of the potential biases by the learner and the educator can increase the nurse's diagnostic accuracy and help avoid diagnostic errors.

DIFFERENCES BETWEEN THE NOVICE AND THE EXPERT

The novice and expert differ in their use of the diagnostic process and the factors influencing the diagnosis. The most significant difference is the extent of knowledge stored in the long-term memory.[23] Lack of knowledge and experience greatly influence the novice's ability to attend and to attach significance to cues. Benner[24] maintains that this is entirely a function of experience. Furthermore, she[25] has described the use of vague hunches and "gut feelings" by the expert that bypass the classical decision-making process. Experts do not make decisions in elemental, procedural ways and cannot give detailed step-by-step accounts of their decision-making process.[26] The enormous experience repertoire of the expert results in an intuitive approach to clinical situations.[27]

Novices, however, can still derive a likely diagnosis if they are taught to carefully analyze data and avoid common pitfalls and errors.[28] The educator must be aware of the differences between the novice and expert because of the influence education has on the organization of the learner's long-term memory and analytical skills. Many teaching situations involve both novices and experts; therefore, the teaching strategies must be geared to the differing needs of the learners. For example, the insistence of the use of rules and analytical tools for the expert will result in frustration, while rules are appropriate and probably essential for the novice.[29] Differences between novice and expert in which the educator can have maximum influence will be discussed.

The Expert Recognizes the Relationship Between Cues and Between Cues and Diagnosis

While the novice may assume that there is a perfect relationship between the presence of a cue and a given nursing diagnosis, the expert recognizes the tentativeness of cues. The expert is also able to attend to subtle cues and to recognize the probability of one nursing diagnosis over another. The novice has difficulty clustering cues into meaningful patterns, while the expert recognizes relationships between cues and is able to use cue patterns to generate possible nursing diagnoses.

The novice is at that stage of development where no background understanding of the situation exists. The novice must be taught about the situation in terms of objective elements, such as temperature, pulse, and weight, that can be recognized without situational experiences. Novices are taught rigid rules to guide their behavior, rules that may not be within the context of theory or explanation.[30]

Consider a man admitted to the hospital for exacerbation of heart failure. He has 4+ pedal edema and gained 10 pounds in the week prior to this admission. He is accompanied by his wife, who prepares the prescribed low-sodium diet and administers his medications at home. The novice quickly zeroes in on the edema and weight gain with a diagnosis of Fluid Volume Excess related to 4+ pedal edema and begins interventions to decrease the edema such as elevating the patient's feet.

In this example, the novice assumes there is a perfect relationship between the edema, weight gain, and the diagnosis. "Edema means excess fluid" is the rule used. The novice is unable to put the rule into the context of the situation. Other cues such as diet and medication patterns are not considered; therefore, other possible diagnoses are not considered.

Consider the action of the expert in evaluating this patient. The expert recognizes the importance of sodium intake and compliance with prescribed medications and continues data collection to generate other possible diagnoses. These additional cues and possible nursing diagnoses are presented in Table 10–1.

The expert does not assume a one and only relationship between a cue and a diagnosis and, so, continues to collect data. Several nursing diagnostic possibilities were generated on the basis of relationships between cues discovered with additional assessment. The novice uses a rule that limits data collection and is unable to recognize cue patterns in order to generate additional possible diagnoses.

Experts Have a Wide Range and Depth of Experience

The novice's ability to generate likely or probable diagnoses is limited because of a lack of experience with patients. A novice, caring for a patient on the first post-operative day, might make a nursing diagnosis of Impaired Physical Mobility related to refusal to move. When questioned about this nursing diagnosis, the novice responds, "Well, she won't move around—I can hardly get her to help turn herself; and she sleeps all the time and won't do anything for herself." This patient had an extensive exploratory laparotomy with bowel resection and colostomy the previous day. She was hesitant to move for fear of dislodging drains and dressings; she also was having a great deal of pain. Limited experience with surgical patients prevents the novice from knowing what to expect in terms of activity for post-operative patients.

TABLE 10–1. ALTERNATIVE NURSING DIAGNOSES FOR A PATIENT WITH HEART FAILURE, WEIGHT GAIN, AND EDEMA

Knowledge Deficit Related to Insufficient Understanding of Low Sodium Diet
Cues assessed:
- *Usual daily diet*
- *Use of salt shaker*
- *Foods particularly liked or disliked by patient*

Activity Intolerance related to fatigue and shortness of breath
Cues assessed:
- *Changes in ability to perform usual activities*
- *Vital signs at rest*
- *Vital signs with activity*
- *Lung sounds*
- *Use of accessory muscles*
- *Patient's subjective complaint of fatigue and dyspnea*

Potential for alteration in nutrition less than body requirements related to lack of appetite and increased intra-abdominal pressure
Cues assessed:
- *Abdominal girth*
- *Presence of ascites*
- *Bowel sounds*
- *Baseline weight*
- *Thorough assessment of edema*
- *Patient's description of appetite and desire for food*

The novice's lack of experience also may be seen in interviewing and obtaining information from patients. A novice may believe that the patient does not need a nursing diagnosis or have any problem at all. The patient is ambulatory and anticipating discharge. During a brief interview by the instructor, however, the patient indicates that he did not understand "exactly what diverticulitis was and just what foods" he ought to avoid. The student had not been able to elicit this information from the patient. Perhaps the student's interview skills and ability to establish rapport are not yet adequate to obtain the necessary data to formulate a nursing diagnosis. Perhaps because the patient appeared to be doing well and no obvious problems were observed, the student allowed closure to occur prematurely.

The expert knows that even patients who appear well usually have questions or problems requiring nursing intervention and, therefore, require a nursing diagnosis. The interview continues until the expert is satisfied that, indeed, a problem is present and identified as well as supported with adequate data. This leads to the nursing diagnosis Knowledge Deficit related to lack of information about low-residue diet for diverticulitis. The expert's background and experience with patients in clinical practice enables the instructor to continue the data search until a nursing diagnosis is validated.

Experts Have an Extensive Knowledge Base in Their Long-Term Memory

A complex network of categories, subcategories, and concepts of knowledge, as well as special categories developed from experience, characterize the expert's long-term memory. The expert nurse does not rely on rules to guide nursing decisions. The extensive background of knowledge enables the expert to identify pertinent points of the problem without wasting time on alternative diagnoses.[31]

Multiple other categories come to the expert's mind. The retrieval characteristics of the novice might be in the form of memorized lists that are triggered by a diagnostic label. For example, the novice cannot generate all the possibilities but can list signs and symptoms of pulmonary edema once the list has been triggered by the proper name.

The expert nurse's ability to recognize relationships between cues, the background of theoretical knowledge, and experience means that clinical decision making involves an intuitive element. Because of the novice's lack of ability to recognize relationships and the background of knowledge and experience, the novice must rely on rules to guide nursing actions. These differences have relevance for the nurse educator teaching nursing diagnosis. Clinical experience is essential to the development of nursing diagnostic skill, but diagnostic accuracy can be improved and refined with appropriate teaching and learning opportunities.

DIAGNOSTIC REASONING PROCESS

Understanding the elements in the diagnostic reasoning process increases the educator's ability to teach diagnosing and to intervene with students when they have difficulty diagnosing. Collecting, sorting, and identifying the importance of data is a difficult task for the novice with limited theoretical background and clinical experience. Learning the diagnostic process can also be difficult for experienced nurses who do not have extensive theoretical background and for whom the clinical situation is not linked with scientific knowledge. The diagnostic options may be narrowed dramatically to those relating to memorable experience and relevant data are therefore missed.[32] The educator must be able to assist the learner with any element of the process where difficulty is encountered. The steps of the diagnostic reasoning process[33] will be used as a framework for a discussion of specific teaching strategies.

Pre-Encounter Data

Pre-encounter data are information about the client that the diagnostician knows before formally beginning data collection. This information plays an important role in influencing the data-collection process, and it can increase or decrease the likelihood that a nurse will make certain nursing diagnoses. Age and sex are common examples of pre-encounter data that are useful because certain conditions are more common to particular ages and by sex.

Knowledge of certain information about the patient may result in conclusions, opinions, or expectations about the patient. For example, information as basic as "this patient had surgery yesterday" leads the nurse to expect that the patient's activity level might need to be increased. But the nurse, particularly the novice practitioner, must be cautioned about making generalizations based on pre-encounter data. There are patients who resist getting out of bed four days after surgery and others who are ambulating immediately while carrying their urinary drainage system.

Pre-encounter data might have a negative effect on nurse expectations about the patient. For example, it was reported during shift change that a patient complained all night, and that she "was on the light begging for her pain shot every hour." This negative perception may then influence a nurse at the beginning of the shift, before any interaction with the patient, and interfere with any further assessment, diagnosis, and treatment.

Some pre-encounter data may be irrelevant to the client's health status at the moment. Novices can obtain large amounts of pre-encounter data from the medical record and textbooks used in preparation for the clinical experience. Novice nurses will require guidance from a nurse educator or preceptor to be able to differentiate, with accuracy, relevant from irrelevant data, and relate the information to previous experiences. It is noteworthy that experienced nurses in a new and unfamiliar clinical situation can be novices in that clinical situation. Differentiating relevant from irrelevant data can be a difficult task for those nurses.

For example, a novice nurse obtains the following information about the complaining female patient:

1. Frequent expressions of pain, requesting IM medication
2. Had wedge resection of the left lung 4 days ago
3. Has osteoarthritis of lumbar spine
4. Is on Digoxin 0.25 mg daily
5. Husband died last year
6. No bowel movement since surgery

Consider the volume of possible information that can be collected about pain, thoracotomy, arthritis, digoxin, death and dying, and constipation. The educator must be available to assist the novice in deciding which data are most pertinent initially, which situations are appropriate for the application of rules, and if there is a principle in this situation that has been encountered previously.

The expert nurse/novice diagnostician has the ability to differentiate between relevant and irrelevant data and has progressed from the use of noncontextual rules. The expert nurse must be cautioned about biases from other experiences. For example, the negative information received during shift report about the complaining patient is likely to influence the expert nurse who has indeed experienced difficult patients.

Entry to the Data Research Field and Shaping Direction of Data Gathering

The novice diagnostician enters the data search field armed with a tool to guide the assessment process: to learn *what* information to assess and to actually *ask* the questions. It provides the rules, so necessary for the novice, to organize data.

The expert nurse/novice diagnostician will also require a nursing framework, such as Gordon's Functional Health Patterns,[34] to promote organization of data that will lead to a nursing diagnosis. The nursing framework assists in organizing familiar information such as findings on assessment into unfamiliar patterns, the nursing diagnosis terminology.

It may also be helpful to review with the expert nurse/novice diagnostician differences among the independent-dependent-interdependent functions of the nurse. The dependent-interdependent functions of the nurse, such as assessing lab work, vital signs, and the response to medications and treatments, are familiar to the expert nurse. When nursing diagnosis is separated from other familiar, the expert nurse can focus on the collection of data not directly related to the medical diagnosis, data that will lead to a nursing diagnosis.

The diagnostician needs skills for physical assessment as the direction of the data search may be influenced by findings obtained from a quick assessment to determine priorities. The novice has learned rules for physical assessment but may not have palpated or ascultated actual patients. The novice needs time and experience to perfect physical assessment skills, to determine abnormalities, and to know the significance of findings; therefore, the instructor or preceptor needs to validate findings with the novice so that urgent priorities are not overlooked.

Look at the expert's data collection on the previous patient:

1. Frequent expressions of pain, requesting IM medication
2. Had wedge resection of the left lung 4 days ago

This data is relevant; acute pain four days after surgery may indicate the development of complications. Some additional nursing observations based on these data would be: check vital signs, breath sounds, incision, and last chest X-ray.

3. Has osteoarthritis of lumbar spine

This data is relevant; the arthritis could be causing generalized discomfort. Additional nursing observations would be: assess pain thoroughly, ask patient if she takes an analgesic routinely for arthritis pain, Check on ambulation as moving about may decrease stiffness and discomfort.

4. Is on Digoxin 0.25 mg. daily

This data is not relevant to patient's complaints of generalized pain.

5. Husband died last year

This data is not relevant to patient's complaints of pain. Will get more information after pain issue is resolved: check on other family, friends, and visitors since surgery.

6. No bowel movement since surgery

This data is relevant; abdominal discomfort can contribute to generalized discomfort. Additional nursing observations would be: assess abdomen, diet, and work on increasing activity level; offer oral analgesic if possible; consider the possibility that current pain medication is having a constipating effect.

Here, the expert has established directions for the collection of additional data. Early in the diagnostic process, data have been prioritized and several possibilities have been identified to establish the source of discomfort. In contrast, the novice is probably stymied about the patient's pain and the resulting lack of relief from the ordered medication. The novice requires the assistance of an instructor or preceptor to identify priorities and determine the need for additional information.

Coalescing of Cues Into Clusters or Chunks

In this step, the data that have been collected are clustered in short-term memory. Knowledge must be acquired and stored so that when particular cases are encountered, the appropriate knowledge is retrieved. The short-term memory holds limited quantities of data that can trigger long-term memory for more information, associate information with diagnostic labels, and direct the diagnostician in the collection of additional data. A "chunk" of information is any stimulus that has become familiar through previous experience that is recognizable as a unit.[35,36]

The novice nurse's "chunk" contains fewer elements, and recognition of the "chunk" is slower than for the expert. Experts have more items in the unit, and the "chunk" is recognized faster. This concept of memory and its organization has particular relevance to the nurse educator. The novice does not have the facts or experience to put cues together to signal a problem or to sort relevant cues from irrelevant cues. Nor does the novice have the ability to prioritize data, questions, or the probability of the most likely diagnostic label.[37]

The expert nurse collected the following data during the assessment of the previous patient:

1. Surgical incision is clean and dry. Breath sounds are clear bilaterally. Chest X-ray yesterday was WNL. Vital signs are WNL.
2. Pain is 4 on 1–10 intensity scale. Cannot point to a location of severe pain. States "I haven't slept at all. I've just tossed and turned." Takes Motrin at home for arthritis. Usually takes 2 warm showers a day for stiffness. Has not been out of bed except once since surgery. Walks a mile a day when at home.
3. Abdomen is soft with audible bowel sounds in all quadrants. Expresses concern over lack of BM. Oral intake has been primarily liquids since surgery. Does not require laxative at home.

The expert nurse clusters the data in the following manner:

1. Surgical incision, X-ray, vital signs, breath sounds, abdomen all OK. Cannot localize pain. Has not slept well since surgery.
2. Has not had usual analgesic for arthritis. Has not had usual activity level. Has not slept.
3. Concerned about lack of BM. Possibly has been too drowsy from IM medications to eat. Activity level down.

The novice would have difficulty with clustering the data. First, there are a great deal of data to consider. Secondly, it takes a complex organization of the nurse's memory to connect the possibilities of the patient's discomfort: incision, arthritis, abdomen, lack of mobility, and lack of usual arthritis medication. Third, the novice has a rule—relieve pain first—to follow. Additional pain medication would have skewed or prohibited further data collection and any opportunity to cluster pertinent data.

The educator's role is to provide the novice with guidance and support in the activity of clustering cues. This can and must occur in the clinical setting. The post-conference time is an ideal setting to obtain input from the entire group. Change of shift report and patient care influences can provide similar opportunities for exploring cue clusters and appropriate nursing diagnoses. Cluster of cues also occurs in didactic presentations. The nurse educator/preceptor groups cues together to support the nursing diagnosis being discussed.

The defining characteristics of nursing diagnosis, found in handbooks or other references, can assist the novice in cue clustering and formulating a nursing diagnosis. Mallick[38] maintains that most written instructions for making a nursing diagnosis are too advanced for the novice. The novices' lack of experience means they need to be taught in terms of concrete characteristics and rules.[39] Instructions to the novice should include: (1) collect data, (2) compare data to defining characteristics, and (3) choose the diagnosis that best fits the data.[40] The nurse educator/preceptor needs to assist the novice in clustering the data before the data can be compared to the defining characteristics.

Activating Possible Diagnostic Explanations (Diagnostic Hypotheses)

This element of the diagnostic process has been described as tentative, early labels of possible diagnoses.[41] These early labels serve to bring the realm of diagnostic possibilities down to manageable size, and they also guide further data search. After the diagnostician has clustered the cues and compared them to the defining characteristics of the diagnostic categories, the diagnosis that best fits the data is chosen as the nursing diagnosis.[42]

The above description of generating a hypothesis sounds too easy. There are those who argue against the use of such simple rules for the novice diagnostician.[43] Benner[44] has suggested that such simple rules could give the novice a false sense of security, which then disappears when the use of the rule in the clinical situation is not clear.

The clinical instructor or preceptor becomes even more important at this step. Guidance from an expert is vital to determine which clinical situations are appropriate for the use of rules and which are not. Novices, also must be taught that actual patient data will not match exactly with the diagnostic criteria; it is the nursing diagnosis that corresponds most closely with the diagnostic criteria.[45]

While novices are taught to collect data systematically, experienced clinicians do not use this approach. Studies have indicated that experts begin to generate a possible diagnosis very early in the interview from very few cues.[46,47] The cues obtained during the assessment process lead experts to retrieve knowledge associated with those cues, which is a result of theoretical knowledge and experience in the clinical field. The knowledge may be organized according to diagnostic classification, risk factors, or signs and symptoms.[48] The novice, without the well-developed, long-term memory of the expert, is unable to relate cues assessed from the patient with information in the memory.

Guiding the novice to plausible nursing diagnoses is a critical responsibility of the nurse educator, both in the classroom and in the clinical setting. Relationships must be drawn between principles studied in classes or workshops and the actual clinical situations encountered. Often the instructor or preceptor, upon acknowledging that the situation looks similar to one that a learner has encountered before, can provide direction for further data collection. Pertinent questions, additional data, or meanings of data assist the student generate the correct diagnosis. This process assists the novice with clustering cues, assigning meaning to the cues, and associating them with diagnostic labels.

Based on the data collected and clustered by the expert on the previous patient, diagnostic possibilities include:

1. Alteration in Comfort related to generalized arthritis pain and stiffness
2. Alteration in Bowel Elimination: Constipation, related change in diet and mobility since surgery four days ago
3. Physical Mobility: Impaired, related to incisional pain and general discomfort since surgery

The novice would probably miss cue patterns, failing to identify the relationships between patient complaints and possible nursing diagnoses. Furthermore, the problem of pain and recent surgery would probably cause the novice to prematurely close the search for further diagnoses.

The other possibility is that the novice would choose every possible nursing diagnostic category that possibly relates to the cues from the patient; for example:

1. Potential Alteration in Skin Integrity related to prolonged bedrest
2. Oral Mucous Membrane Impairment related to decreased intake of oral fluids
3. Potential Alteration in Nutrition: Less than Body Requirements related to decreased oral food and fluid intake
4. Potential for Injury related to IM narcotic analgesics and chance of falling
5. Anxiety related to hospitalization and surgery

While these nursing diagnoses have some supporting data, they reflect the tendency of novice diagnosticians to identify simplistic patterns in the data and to make every possible nursing diagnosis that might apply.

The clinical instructor or preceptor's primary responsibility, in this step of the diagnostic process, is to assist the novice in identifying the data that substantiate the proposed nursing diagnosis. The process of putting specific data with a particular nursing diagnosis, starts the novice prioritizing diagnostic possibilities. Identifying which nursing diagnosis is supported by the most pertinent data leads into the next step of the diagnostic process.

Directed Search of the Data Field

This stage involves revising and narrowing the diagnostic possibilities generated thus far. The information stored in the diagnostician's long-term memory provides characteristics compatible with the tentative nursing diagnoses. The characteristics considered include risk factors, prevalence of the problem patterns associated with the development of the problem, and signs and symptoms.[49] This step may be familiar to expert nurses as the "differential diagnosis" step often used by physicians. "Sepsis vs. pneumonia" is often seen on medical records as the physician weighs the possibility of each diagnosis while additional confirming data is collected.

The nurse wants to limit the number of diagnostic possibilities to the most likely and to identify the hypothesis that explains most of the findings. In the previous example, Sleep Pattern Disturbance related to inability to rest adequately since surgery is a plausible diagnosis. But the expert realizes that if this patient's discomfort is relieved, sleep would most likely occur without difficulty. Therefore, the most descriptive nursing diagnosis is Alteration in Comfort related to generalized arthritis pain and stiffness.

The novice diagnostician often formulates a list of possible—and plausible—diagnoses, but is then unable to decide which diagnosis is more appropriate or pertinent for the patient. Novices have major disadvantages with "firming up" the diagnosis. Their long-term memory lacks information regarding classic descriptions of diagnoses as well as past clinical experiences with patients. Again, the clinical instructor or preceptor must be the guide as the novice continues to analyze and evaluate the data to narrow the diagnostic possibilities.

Testing Diagnostic Hypothesis for Congruence

Each tentative diagnosis is compared to determine congruence. The diagnostician matches the cues associated with the patient's problem with the profiles or characteristics of the problem according to textbooks and past clinical experiences. The diagnosis with the closest fit is confirmed as the diagnosis.

The instructor or preceptor must help the novice diagnostician match the profiles. For example, the patient does need to move about. Defining characteristics of Impaired Physical

Mobility include the presence of arthritis and surgery as a reason for impaired mobility. The defining characteristics of Alteration of Comfort—the patient's expressions, guarded position—confirm the diagnosis. The instructor or preceptor in the clinical arenas is the resource and guide for the novice diagnostician to confirm the diagnosis and to prioritize the importance of each diagnosis. Testing the diagnosis is based on textbook descriptions as well as past clinical experience. This patient's comfort is the priority and once comfort is improved, other problems may resolve accordingly. Experience is vital for prioritizing diagnoses.

COMPUTER-ASSISTED INSTRUCTION

A variety of instructional techniques necessary to teach nursing diagnosis have been discussed. Some techniques are more appropriate at particular points in the diagnostic process or during didactic presentations. Other techniques may be more effective in the clinical practice area. Certain approaches are selected by the nurse educator based on the experiential background of the learner.

The versatility and possibilities of computers make computer-assisted instruction (CAI) useful for teaching nursing diagnosis to both novice and expert nurses. The use of CAI, as a teaching and learning tool, is increasing in educational programs in nursing schools and practice settings. The computer offers many advantages to the learner such as working at individual speeds, reinforcing and repeating information, giving examples of principles, and working outside formal class time. A major advantage is that the learner can interact with the computer more than once to master difficult content.

Educational software is available for nursing programs and inservice education departments on a variety of subjects, including nursing diagnosis. Some programs are related to the nursing process with emphasis on collecting, clustering, and prioritizing data after the presentation of a clinical situation. Other software programs include NANDA labels as problem statements. There are programs that go through the steps of the diagnostic process. These software packages can be used as an adjunct to the didactic presentation or alone to introduce new or similar content. The learner can review material that was not clear from the lecture presentation or practice clustering data and making diagnoses. The actual practice of selecting data and deciding their relevance can increase the novice diagnostician's skill and confidence in the clinical practice setting.

The use of CAI to teach nursing diagnosis to novice diagnosticians in undergraduate and graduate nursing programs was the basis of a study by Yoder and Heilman.[50] The tutorial program used by the investigators included definition of a nursing diagnosis, the nursing process, common errors in writing a nursing diagnosis, and a practice session for assembling a nursing diagnosis. CAI was used in place of didactic presentation. Although there was no implication that the computer program was a better teaching technique than the lecture format, pretest/posttest results indicated that students were able to make a nursing diagnosis after completing the CAI.

Authoring systems are also available so that nurse educators can write instructional modules that are very specific to the needs of the learner or the content. These authoring systems do not require previous programming experience by the user. For example, the nurse educator introduces the nursing diagnosis Fluid Volume Deficit related to inadequate intake by mouth. Physiology about dehydration and electrolyte changes is reviewed. The example associated with the nursing diagnosis is an elderly patient who forgets to drink and has difficulty swallowing.

As an adjunct to the presentation, a CAI module might include physical assessment data for the learner to cluster and lab data to differentiate. A clinical example could be the identical diagnosis with a different etiology, such as Fluid Volume Deficit related to vomiting and diarrhea. The previously known information about dehydration is transferred and applied to a different clinical situation.

The versatility of authoring systems CAI modules allows the nurse educator to create modules that emphasize rules for the novice diagnostician as well as simulation for practicing and applying those rules. In addition, case studies and clinical situations can be created for experienced nurses to provide practice using new nursing diagnosis terminology. A CAI learning module directed toward differentiating between a medical and nursing diagnosis would be very appropriate for the expert nurse/novice diagnostician.

The use of computers in nursing education is increasing and characteristics of nursing diagnosis lend themselves to computerized learning. CAI programs are invaluable in situations with learners of different experience backgrounds. Of course, the cost factor of the hardware, software, and educator time to learn to use authoring systems will need to be considered by the organization.

CONCLUSION

Acceptance of nursing diagnosis is increasing rapidly in nursing schools and practice settings. Nursing diagnosis is an important professional issue that nurse educators must become prepared to teach. The nurse educator is a vital element in the endeavor for diagnosis-based clinical practice because of the influence the educator has on the neophytes in the profession. As students of nursing become indoctrinated in nursing diagnosis as the basis for nursing clinical practice, nursing diagnosis will emerge in hospitals and other clinical practice settings.

Meanwhile, nurse educators in hospitals must teach nursing diagnosis to practicing nurses. Teaching these experienced nurses requires different techniques because of the distinct clinical decision-making method of experienced nurses. The acceptance of experiential knowledge and intuition for clinical decision making is a major change from the classical problem-solving process traditionally used by educators. Careful attention to the steps of the diagnostic process will assist the nurse educator in making nursing diagnosis meaningful to novice diagnosticians regardless of the background of the diagnostician or the setting of the learning activity.

REFERENCES

1. Reilly, D. & Oermann, M. *The clinical field: Its use in nursing education.* Norwalk, CT: Appleton-Century-Crofts, 1985, p. 156
2. Aspinall, M.J. Nursing diagnosis—the weak link. *Nursing Outlook,* 1976, *24,* 7, 433
3. Matthews, C. & Gaul, A. L. Nursing diagnosis from the perspective of concept attainment and critical thinking. *Advances in Nursing Science,* 2:17–26, October 1977.
4. Frederickson, K. & Mayer, G. Problem solving skills: What effect does education have? *American Journal of Nursing,* 1977, *77,* 7, 1167
5. Lee, H. & Strong, K. Using nursing diagnosis to describe the clinical competence of baccalaureate

and associate degree graduating students: A comparative study. *Image: The Journal of Nursing Scholarship,* 1985, *27,* 3, 82
6. Benner, P. *From novice to expert: Excellence and power in clinical nursing practice.* Menlo Park, CA: Addison-Wesley, 1984
7. *Ibid*
8. Conley, V. *Curriculum and instruction in nursing.* Boston: Little Brown, 1973
9. *Ibid*
10. Knowles, M. *The adult learner: A neglected species* (2nd Ed.). Houston: Gulf, 1978, p. 110
11. Southern Regional Education Board. Understanding the adult student. In *Project report: Faculty*

development in nursing education. Atlanta: Southern Regional Educational Board, USDHEW PHS2D10NU0202904R, 1981

12. Rogers, E.M. & Shoemaker, F.F. Communication of innovations: A cross-cultural approach (2nd ed.). New York: The Free Press, 1971, p. 102–111
13. Brunner, J.S. *The process of education.* New York: Vintage, 1960, p. 17
14. *Ibid*
15. Tanner, C. Factors influencing the diagnostic process, In D. Carnevali, P. Mitchell, N. Woods, & C. Tanner (Eds.), *Diagnostic reasoning in nursing.* Philadelphia: J. B. Lippincott, 1984, p. 71
16. *Ibid.,* p. 69–70
17. *Ibid*
18. *Ibid*
19. *Ibid.,* p. 71
20. *Ibid*
21. Tanner, C. The effect of hypothesis generation as an instructional method on the diagnostic processes of senior baccalaureate nursing students. Unpublished doctoral dissertation, University of Colorado, 1977
22. *Ibid*
23. Tanner. Factors influencing the diagnostic process
24. Benner, P. Characteristics of novice and expert performance: Implications for teaching the experienced nurse. In K.L. Jako (Ed.), *Researching second step nursing education.* Rohnert Park, CA: Sonoma State University, 1981
25. Benner. *From novice to expert*
26. *Ibid*
27. *Ibid*
28. Tanner. Factors influencing the diagnostic process
29. Benner. *From novice to expert*
30. *Ibid*
31. *Ibid*
32. Tanner. Factors influencing the diagnostic process
33. Carnevali, D.L. The Diagnostic reasoning process. In D. Carnevali, P. Mitchell, N. Woods, & C. Tanner (Eds.), *Diagnostic reasoning in nursing.* Philadelphia: J.B. Lippincott, 1984, p. 25–56.
34. Gordon, M. Predictive strategies in diagnostic tasks. *Nursing Research,* 1980, *29,* 39
35. Larken, J. et al. Expert and novice performance in solving physics problems. *Science,* 1980, *208,* 1335
36. Simon, H. How big is a chunk? *Science,* 1974, *183,* 482
37. Tanner. Factors influencing the diagnostic process
38. Mallick, J.M. Nursing diagnosis and the novice student. *Nursing and Health Care,* 1983, *4,* 8, 455
39. Benner. Characteristics of novice and expert performance
40. Mallick
41. Carnevali
42. Tanner. Factors influencing the diagnostic process
43. Mallick
44. Benner. Characteristics of novice and expert performance
45. Mallick
46. Elstein, A., Shulman, L., & Sprafka, S. Medical problem solving: An analysis of clinical reasoning. Cambridge, MA: Harvard University Presses, 1978
47. Gordon
48. Tanner. Factors influencing the diagnostic process
49. *Ibid*
50. Yoder, M. & Heilman, T. The use of computer assisted instruction to teach nursing diagnosis. *Computers in Nursing,* 1985, *3,* 6, 262

CHAPTER 11

Nursing Diagnosis:
The Legal Foundations

Judith Rocchiccioli and Carolyn C. Lavecchia

Nursing care is changing. High technology, decreasing lengths of stay in acute-care hospitals, increasing patient complexity, and prospective payment have dictated new arenas of nursing practice. Early discharge of patients from acute-care institutions has created intensely sophisticated nursing care needs in the community. Home intravenous therapy, enteral feeding, ventilator maintenance, wound care, and oxygen therapy are becoming routine aspects of home care. Nurses working in nursing homes are also seeing a group of patients with more complex needs and in need of more skilled care than ever before. In order to meet these increasingly demanding needs, both in the hospital setting and in newer arenas, nursing must organize itself systematically with a common language. Nursing diagnosis is that language.

In Chapter 2, the historical development of nursing diagnosis was discussed. The efforts to identify nursing care issues, and to separate these from the medical care of the patient, have been taking place for the last 50 years. The Nursing Problems Classifications[1] and the Basic Human Needs Classification[2] were early attempts to categorize the problems nurses treat. Many terms have been used to avoid the word diagnosis, which was perceived during that time to belong only to the physicians. These terms included nursing problem, patient need, clinical judgment, and the ambitious, multisyllabic trophicognosis[3].

The term diagnosis was first used in the nursing literature in 1950.[4] Concern that nurses would be making medical diagnoses, outside the legal scope of nursing practice, had an inhibiting effect on the evolution of a system for identifying and naming nursing problems; however, as the practice of nursing has defined nursing diagnosis, it is clear that nursing diagnoses and medical diagnoses are distinctly different.

Consider a widely accepted definition of nursing diagnosis. Gordon states:

> Nursing diagnoses, or clinical diagnoses made by professional nurses, describe actual or potential health problems which nurses by virtue of their education and experience are capable and licensed to treat.[5]

This definition focuses on the patient's health problems that can be addressed through nursing care.

Medical diagnosis, on the other hand, has a very different focus. It has been defined as:

> the determination of which disease the patient is actually suffering from, especially the art of distinguishing between several possibilities.[6]

An examination of these two definitions demonstrates several important differences between nursing and medical diagnoses.

Disease is the primary concern of the physician. This includes identifying the disease as well as determining which treatments are indicated. Medical diagnoses, then, are the names of specific diseases, disorders, or syndromes. Examples of medical diagnoses might be congestive heart failure, diabetes mellitus, malignant melanoma, and multiple sclerosis.

Nursing diagnoses are concerned with health problems and the patient's responses to these. The naming of disease is not the focus of nursing diagnosis. Nursing diagnoses are labels that describe the patient's response and prescribe the appropriate nursing treatment. Examples of nursing diagnoses are Self-Care Deficit related to left hemiparesis, Ineffective Airway Clearance related to weakness and fatigue, and Impaired Physical Mobility related to pain. It is clear from these examples that nursing diagnoses and medical diagnoses, although drawing on recognized medical terminology, describe different patient conditions and reflect different professional concerns.

THE SCOPE OF NURSING PRACTICE: ISSUES RAISED BY NURSING DIAGNOSIS

According to the American Nurses' Association (ANA) Social Policy Statement, "Nursing is the diagnosis and treatment of human responses to actual or potential health problems."[7] Again, this definition identifies a realm of practice for nursing that is distinctly different from the practice of medicine. The definition of nursing and the definitions of nursing and medical diagnoses are important because physicians, lawyers, legislators, and even nurses themselves may be unsure of exactly what the practice of nursing is.

The practice of nursing is becoming a more distinct science, grounded in nursing theory and research. Nurses are forced to respond more and more to professional and social demands. The profession has developed standards of nursing practice, has formed numerous specialty organizations within the practice of nursing, is working on standards for advanced and specialty nursing practice including credentialing, and has a Code of Ethics and a Social Policy Statement. These nursing standards must then be incorporated into the clinical practice of the individual nurse within the context of the health care organization.

The nursing profession has always been committed to caring for the sick and well, either individually or in a group. This has not changed. The phenomena of concern to nurses are human responses to actual or potential health problems. Any observable manifestation, need, condition, concern, event, dilemma, difficulty, occurrence, or fact that can be described or scientifically explained and is within the target area of nursing practice is of interest to nurses.[8] The question then, is what is different about nurses treating these actual or potential health problems. Why are so many nurses, physicians, and other professionals worried about the term "nursing diagnosis."

Many physicians question the concept and idea of nurses making diagnoses about patients. There are several possible reasons for their concern. One is territoriality, where physicians are fearful that nurses will infringe upon and erode their professional arena. Since it has been shown that nurses are highly effective providers of low cost, comprehensive, quality health care,[9] it is no wonder that physicians are concerned about nurses encroaching upon their well-founded and very solid economic base. If a nurse can diagnose, many physicians might view this as a threat to their economic well being.

Another possible concern of physicians is that they will be held liable and accountable for the nurse's diagnosis. Many physicians do not realize that nursing is an entirely separate and distinct profession from medicine, founded on its own theory and grounded by its own research.

A more understandable reason for physician non-support of nursing diagnosis is the lack of knowledge and understanding about the concept, its use, and current practice of nursing. Educating physicians about nursing diagnosis will be integral to the success of its implementation.

It is not unusual to find nurses that are nonsupportive of the concept and use of nursing diagnosis. Many nurses are concerned about the legal implications and feel diagnosing is outside the arena of acceptable, safe nursing practice. This is certainly true if the nurse attempts to diagnose diseases or syndromes, or to apply medical therapies for these.

The use of nursing diagnosis does not abrogate the nurse's responsibility to monitor the patient's condition for critical changes, significant symptoms, progress of the medical condition, and responses to medical treatment. These activities are an important part of nursing practice; however, they are a part of the delegated responsibility from the physician and distinctly different from the practice of medicine.

Nursing interventions based on judgments made by the nurse about the patient's disease-related condition fall into one of several categories: notify the physician, record the information in the patient's record, carry out or withhold treatments designated by the existing physician's orders, carry out palliative treatments based on nursing judgment, or a combination of these.[10] A critical distinction is that these nursing interventions are directed toward disease rather than dealing with the patient's human response.

Nursing activities have traditionally been viewed in three categories: dependent, independent, and interdependent. Dependent nursing activities or interventions are those which are carried out under medical order, without judgment or discretion by the nurse playing a significant role in their execution. An example of this type of nursing intervention might be: Gentamicin 80 mg. IV q8h. This situation does not remove the nurse's responsibility to question inappropriate medical orders; rather, it describes those situations where the orders are correct and the nurse carries them out as ordered.

At the other end of the continuum are independent nursing interventions. These are decided and implemented based upon the professional knowledge and judgment of the nurse, without consultation from the physician or other health care professionals. Examples of this type of nursing intervention include patient education and daily living activities.

The third category, interdependent nursing interventions, falls in between the dependent, delegated activities and independent nursing interventions. In this situation, an activity ordered by the physician requires a high degree of judgment by the nurse for its accomplishment. Consider the post-operative patient, who has an order for Demerol for pain. The nurse makes a nursing diagnosis of Impaired Physical Mobility related to pain, and a care plan is identified to alleviate the patient's pain with the goal of preventing the complications of immobility.

The nurse decides that a useful nursing intervention for this patient is to administer the Demerol about 45 minutes prior to assisting the patient to ambulate. In this situation, the medication has been ordered by the physician; however, the nurse is using independent clinical judgment as to the timing of the medication in an effort to accomplish specific nursing goals for the patient. This example demonstrates the professional decision-making that can make nursing practice both challenging for the nurse and effective for the patient.

In diagnosis-based nursing practice, assessment of the patient focuses on the responses of the patient to the medical condition for purposes of delegated monitoring functions and identification of nursing diagnoses. Some nurses criticize nursing diagnosis because they believe it "labels" or "stereotypes" patients by giving them all the same diagnosis. This is not the case. While nursing diagnosis does employ consistent, standardized language, it does allow for individualized nursing care based on problem identification. (See Chapter 2 for a detailed discussion of nursing diagnosis) The concept is the same in medical diagnosis. We know that all patients with a diagnosis of peptic ulcer will not follow the identical medical treatment regime, nor will patients diagnosed with Activity Intolerance related to imbalance between oxygen supply and demand follow the same nursing care plan. Nursing diagnosis encourages individualized problem identification based on sound nursing assessment.

Nursing diagnosis only seems new or different. It merely puts a new name or label on what nurses have been doing for years. With the increasing complexity of nursing practice, it is becoming more and more evident that we must have a way to organize and direct nursing care delivery. Nursing diagnosis does not change the nurse's legal or professional accountability. Nurses are still accountable for patient care and the quality of patient care delivery. Indeed, the actual formulating and documenting of nursing diagnosis can help nurses and institutions avoid malpractice actions.

Nurse Practice Acts and Nursing Diagnosis

Although reviewing the statutory language of Nurse Practice Acts may be considered less than exciting, the acts are invaluable reading because of their importance in defining and regulating nursing practice.[11] Also of great importance in defining nursing practice are State Board of Nursing rulings, which aid in determining the scope of nursing practice in a given state. Before embarking upon a "grey" area of practice, a nurse may do well to check with that state's board to determine rules, regulations, board rulings, and advisory opinions. It may also be useful to check with professional nursing organizations, particularly if the nursing practice issue is a specialized one.

The definition and regulation of nursing practice are issues of growing national interest. A variety of factors are responsible for this, including rising health care costs, increased consumer awareness, and cost constraints. In a climate of changing professional and economic competition, state legislatures, state boards of nursing, courts, and professional nursing organizations are in the process of changing, adapting, or interpreting existing Nurse Practice Acts to meet the needs of the changing health care system.[12]

In response to these needs, the ANA surveyed the Statutory Definitions of Nurse Practice and their Conformity to Certain ANA Principles.[13] The ANA principles were set forth in the Nurse Practice Act: Suggested State Legislation.[14] The ANA recommends that nurse practice should be broadly defined. Furthermore, the definition should be stated in terms that permit flexibility of nursing personnel with accountability vested in the registered nurse. Additionally, the ANA recommended that the definition should recognize the breadth and depth of educational preparation that justify entrusting overall responsibility for nursing services to the judgment of the registered nurse.[15] (See Table 11–1.)

It is interesting to note that the Nurse Practice Acts of only 33 states make any reference to the nursing process while 32 states do not refer to the traditional five-step nursing process in their definitions of nursing. No reference to a nursing process of any description is made in 17 states. A different approach from the traditional nursing process is used in 15 states to delineate the services performed by nurses. For this chapter, we will be looking specifically at application of the nursing process to nursing functions that includes assessment, diagnosis, planning, intervention, and evaluation.

TABLE 11–1. THE AMERICAN NURSES' ASSOCIATION MODEL NURSE PRACTICE ACT, 1981

The practice of nursing means the performance for compensation of professional services requiring substantial specialized knowledge of the biological, physical, psychological, and sociological sciences and of nursing theory as the basis for assessment, diagnosis, planning, intervention, and evaluation in the promotion and maintenance of health; the casefinding and management of illness, injury, or infirmity; the restoration of optimum function; or the achievement of a dignified death. Nursing practice includes but is not limited to administration, teaching, counseling, supervision, delegation, and evaluation of practice and execution of the medical regimen, including the administration of medications and treatments prescribed by any person authorized by state law to prescribe. Each registered nurse is directly accountable and responsible to the consumer for the quality of nursing care rendered.

Nursing diagnosis directs patient care. It is the second step of nursing process and is based on the assessment data gathered by the professional nurse. Nursing diagnosis allows for the development of specific, individualized nursing care plans to meet the requirements of state agencies, institutions and the Joint Commission on Accreditation of Health Care Organizations. The addition of nursing diagnosis to the practice of nursing does not alter the legal responsibilities of nurses; rather, it adds a mechanism for clearly identifying the patient conditions that require nursing care; From a legal perspective, however, the implications of a standardized language for nursing problems remain to be seen. Nurses have always been liable and accountable for their judgments and decisions about patient problems and nursing interventions, and this responsibility is not increased by the use of nursing diagnosis.

THE LAW AND NURSING DIAGNOSIS

Two areas of the law that primarily affect the practice of nursing are state Nurse Practice Acts, which define the legal scope of the practice of nursing in a given state, and tort law. The practice of nursing in a given state is usually regulated by the State Board of Nursing.

The State Board generally has the authority to promulgate rules and regulations that have the force of law. All nurses are legally accountable to their state regulatory board and may be subject to criminal prosecution or revocation of their license if board compliance is not met. Nursing misconduct that can result in an action by the regulatory board would include unauthorized practice of nursing, as in the case of medication being prescribed for a patient by the nurse who is not permitted to do so.

Tort law is the area of law that has the greatest impact on nursing diagnosis. Torts are civil wrongs that are either intentional or negligent. Slander, libel, assault, and battery are examples of torts that are found in the general practice of law. In nursing practice, negligence or malpractice is by far the most common tort affecting the practice of nursing.

Nursing malpractice or negligence is an act or a failure to act by the nurse that causes a patient harm. In order to prove nursing malpractice, a patient or plaintiff must establish that (1) the nurse had a duty to the plaintiff (2) that was breached (3) causing (4) damage to the plaintiff. All four of these elements must exist to establish nursing malpractice. Not every adverse patient outcome is due to malpractice. Nurses, physicians, and other health care providers cannot guarantee or insure the outcomes of health care. They do, however, have a duty to use reasonable care.

If the nurse is found negligent, the nurse's employer is also held liable for nursing negligence even though the employer may not be at fault. The employer is held liable for the employee's negligent acts if the employee is acting within the scope of employment. This is the legal doctrine of *respondeat superior.*

The most significant implication for nursing diagnosis in alleged nursing malpractice is in the area of breach of the duty of care. Generally, the duty of care owed to the patient is that of the reasonable, prudent nurse. All health care providers including nurses have a duty to exercise reasonable, ordinary care, skill, and diligence in their practice. The measuring tool for this duty is called the standard of care. For the purposes of nursing neglience, the law will adopt the definition of standards used by the profession. For example, because the ANA has incorporated nursing diagnosis into the ANA standards, this represents a standard of care recognized and accepted by the nursing profession. Accordingly, the ANA standards can be admissible in court to establish the standard of care. The nurse's failure to comply with this standard may result in liability for the nurse.

Traditionally, acts of nursing liability for negligence were focused on the role of the nurse in carrying out physician orders and caring for the physical needs of the patient. Common acts of nursing negligence were:

1. Carrying out physician orders inappropriately
2. Improper administration of medications and solutions, that is, medication orders
3. Improper use of nursing skills, that is, burns, injection injuries
4. Foreign objects left inside a patient, that is, incorrect sponge count

The fourth act, listed above, presents an interesting point of view: even though it is the physician who actually left the object inside the patient, it is the nurse who is held legally accountable. This is because the nurse is considered to have a duty to count sponges accurately.

The developing professionalism of nursing has shifted the focus of malpractice concern to include those areas where the nurse has independent, professional responsibilities. The emergence of nursing diagnosis as a responsibility of the professional nurse identifies clear responsibilities for nursing practice. Although there are no reported cases involving nursing diagnosis, courts are beginning to recognize the nurses's duty to make appropriate patient assessments and to act upon these.

At this point the use of nursing diagnosis in clinical nursing practice is new, and the diagnostic labels are still being identified. Although the term diagnosis is included in many state Nurse Practice Acts, what this actually means is unclear from both a clinical practice and a legal standpoint; however, as more and more nurses use nursing diagnosis in their clinical practice and more health care organizations include nursing diagnosis in their documentation standards, this situation will change.

As nursing diagnosis becomes the standard of nursing practice, it will become the standard of care or duty that the nurse owes the patient. Thus, failure to make an appropriate nursing diagnosis and carry out an appropriate plan of nursing care may meet several of the requisite elements of nursing malpractice. This failure alone will not constitute malpractice unless damage or harm to the patient results.

In some situations physicians may forbid nurses to make nursing assessments or nursing diagnoses. Such a directive by a physician does not relieve the nurse of legal accountability for making an assessment or diagnosis if the nurse has a duty or responsibility to do so. Indeed, if nursing diagnosis is the standard of care, the nurse's failure to diagnose may result in professional negligence if this omission causes harm to the patient.

LEGAL PITFALLS IN THE USE OF NURSING DIAGNOSIS

Incorrect nursing diagnoses may result in nursing malpractice and negligence. Although there have been no reported nursing malpractice cases for incorrect nursing diagnoses, as nursing diagnosis becomes more widely used in clinical practice, the expectations of nurses making these diagnoses will change. Court decisions in nursing malpractice cases will reflect these changes, as the law will adjust the definitions and standards used by the nursing profession.

Incorrect nursing diagnoses arise out of three situations: lack of diagnostic skill and experience, diagnostic errors, and incorrectly written nursing diagnoses. These situations are discussed below. It is essential to recognize that these situations are most likely to be present during the implementation of nursing diagnosis. During the implementation process, a fine balance must be struck between assisting nurses in identifying accurate and appropriate phraseology for nursing diagnoses without frightening them unnecessarily with legal implications.

The ability to make clinically accurate nursing diagnoses is a skill, and experience and practice are critical factors in the development of diagnostic skill. In order to accomplish this, the nurse must be able to interview and examine patients effectively. The next step is to organize the assessment data within the framework of nursing diagnosis. The nurse must be familiar with the defining characteristics of nursing diagnoses as well as the diagnostic labels themselves. An important aspect is the determination of when a nursing diagnosis is required and when the clinical situation must be referred to the physician or other health care provider. (See Chapter 4 for a detailed discussion of clinical thinking and nursing diagnosis.)

Another source of incorrect nursing diagnoses are diagnostic errors. Diagnostic errors may result from faulty data collection, where either too much or too little information is used in formulating the nursing diagnosis. Another type of diagnostic error occurs when the relationships between data are misinterpreted or not recognized. Assessment data that is inaccurate or unsubstantiated may also contribute to erroneous diagnoses.

Consider the patient who is found crying in his room. The nurse observes the crying and knows that the surgeon saw the patient today to inform him that the results of the biopsy showed malignancy. It would be easy and reasonable to assume that these two events are related, and the nurse might then formulate a nursing diagnosis of Anxiety related to poor prognosis. This, however, might not be the case.

It might be that the patient is in pain, that he is worried about his family, or that some other event has distressed him. Perhaps the surgeon indicated that the prognosis was good, but only if the patient has disfiguring surgery. If the nurse stays with the initial diagnostic conclusion and fails to validate the data with the patient, then a significant diagnostic error may occur.

The third situation where incorrect nursing diagnoses are found is in the writing of nursing diagnoses. If the diagnostic conclusion is in error, then the written diagnosis will be in error as well; however, it may also be the diagnostic thinking is accurate, but the transition to the written word may be faulty. Some examples of poorly written diagnoses follow.

Potential for Injury related to leaving foreign object in wound[16] was a nursing diagnosis recommended for use in a hospital operating room. This diagnosis has significant legal implications. It implies negligence by the hospital for not removing all foreign objects, such as sponges or instruments, from the surgical wound before closure. Furthermore, this nursing diagnosis is incorrect because it does not meet the necessary criteria for a useful and precise nursing diagnosis. (See Chapter 2.) First of all, there is nothing within the realm of nursing practice that a nurse can do to correct or "treat" this situation. There are no nursing actions or interventions that can result in an improvement of the condition; an exploratory laparotomy would be necessary to retrieve the foreign object. Since nursing diagnoses are problems that nurses can "treat" based on their experience and education, this would be a meaningless diagnosis.

Another concern reflects simple common sense. Even the average lay person knows that foreign objects are not supposed to be left in the body following a surgical procedure. It is an important responsibility for nurses in the operating room to perform and record correct needle, instrument, and sponge counts; however, describing this responsibility as the patient's problem in the form of a nursing diagnosis is confusing at best and may be misleading at worst.

Another error in writing nursing diagnoses is the use of the phrases, "caused by," "secondary to," and "due to," that imply causation. These phrases indicate a cause-and-effect relationship between the nursing diagnosis and the etiology statement. For example, the nursing diagnostic statement Potential for Injury secondary to improperly maintained skin traction suggests that the nurse has failed to manage the skin traction correctly, and the patient has been harmed as a result. Another example might be Altered Mental Status due to multiple brain surgeries. This diagnostic label attributes causation of the problem to the surgical treatment provided by the physician. No wonder that physicians are apprehensive about nursing diagnosis! Furthermore, this nursing diagnosis also identifies an etiology statement that cannot be used to direct the nursing care plan because it is not a problem that nurses treat.

It is recommended that the terminology "related to" be used when writing nursing diagnoses.[17-19] While "related to" indicates an association between factors, it does not necessarily mean there is a direct cause and effect between the two parts of the diagnostic statement. When phrases as "caused by," "secondary to," and "due to" are used, the second part of the diagnostic statement could be interpreted as the specific cause of the problem.[20]

Errors in Nursing Care Planning

Another pitfall in the use of nursing diagnosis occurs when there are discrepancies in the care plan. Nursing care plans are central to nursing practice. The nursing diagnosis, the expected outcomes, and the nursing interventions are contained in the written plan of care. The addition of nursing diagnosis provides a focus for the care planning process. Patient problems are clearly identified through the use of nursing diagnosis; therefore, there should be a clear and discernible linkage between the identified problem and the activities in the care plan for the treatment of the problem. (See Chapter 2 for a discussion of nursing diagnosis and the nursing care plan.)

Nursing care plans are the written manifestation of the nursing process. For this reason, only professional nurses should develop and contribute to the nursing plan of care. The nursing process is based on the scientific method of problem solving. Nursing care plans promote the quality of care by determining (1) individualized care, (2) continuity of care, (3) communication, and (4) evaluation.[21] Nursing interventions are the actions that nurses take in order to accomplish the expected outcomes for the problem identified in the nursing diagnosis.

In order for the nursing care plan to provide useful guidance for nursing activity, the nursing diagnosis must be correctly identified. It must also be accompanied by appropriate outcome statement against which the patient's progress can be judged. Finally, the plan must include nursing interventions that will be effective in dealing with the problem.

Since the professional nurse is accountable for the nursing care plan that is directing the patient's care, it is of the utmost importance that any staff member who reads the plan is able to comprehend necessary nursing actions and tasks. The deliberate omission of a nursing action necessary to patient care is an act of negligence and can be a basis for action against nursing personnel. Consequently, if another staff member did not understand the care plan, this too can cause significant problems. Clarity of the nursing care plan also enhances interdisciplinary teamwork because the responsibilities and contributions of nurses are identified clearly.

In order to achieve this clarity, the nursing care plan must include a correct nursing diagnosis, realistic and measurable statements of patient outcomes, and clinically appropriate nursing interventions. Once the nursing diagnosis is identified, the next step is the determination of outcome statements based on the clinical situation and a realistic understanding of nursing practice.

It is the purpose of outcome statements to identify specific patient behaviors or clinical findings that are observable and measurable. Vague statements or abstract concepts, such as improved nutritional state or optimal ventilation, are not helpful in evaluating the patient's condition and response to nursing care. Avoidance of statements that are too narrow or too global in the description of the patient's progress is important from a clinical and a legal perspective.

Consider the example of a patient with multiple trauma in the intensive care unit. This patient's injuries included open, contaminated wounds as well as internal injuries. Three surgical procedures were done within the first 24 hours of hospitalization. Multiple invasive lines have been placed for monitoring blood pressure, pulmonary artery pressure, and intracranial pressure. There are also two IV lines, a foley catheter, and an endotracheal tube in place to permit mechanical ventilation.

The nursing diagnosis Potential for Infection related to invasive lines and procedures could certainly be considered for this patient; however, what possible outcome statements are appropriate for this situation? The outcome statement of infection will not occur is a goal that nurses will endeavor to accomplish. In view of the multiple insults that this patient has experienced, is this statement a realistic one?

From a clinical perspective, the outcome statement infection will not occur does offer a standard against which the patient's progress can be monitored. There are many observable and measurable criteria for determining whether or not an infectious process is present. From a nursing perspective, however, this outcome statement is problematic for several reasons.

The first problem is that this outcome is affected by many variables other than nursing care. The initial contamination of the wounds at the time of injury, the operative techniques, and the nutritional state of the patient are just a few of the factors that can influence the development of an infection.

Another problem with this statement is that it gives no specific parameters for evaluating the patient's progress. Infection will not occur is a fairly global statement. What are the areas of concern for this patient? Should individual wounds be evaluated for signs of infection, or is laboratory data more important? A useful outcome statement will provide specific criteria against which the patient may be judged.

In the event that this patient does not develop an infection, then the outcome has been successfully accomplished. From a clinical point of view, however, it is likely that this patient will become infected. In that situation, failure to accomplish this outcome could have legal repercussions if the nursing care necessary to avoid infection was not documented, or if changes in the patient's condition were not monitored and addressed. While failure to document is not negligence, the absence of documentation of appropriate nursing care activities to prevent infection and the existence of an outcome statement that infection will not occur might raise questions about the duty owed this patient by the nurse to prevent infection.

The use of realistic, clinically appropriate outcome statements can help avoid this type of confusion. An accurate nursing diagnosis, amenable to nursing intervention, is an essential foundation for determining appropriate outcome statements; furthermore, identification of a patient condition with a nursing diagnosis indicates that the nurse has assumed treatment responsibility for that problem. Oftentimes, clinical situations require treatment from several health care providers and the responsibility for treatment outcomes is shared. In this type of situation, the use of shared terminology is appropriate. Rather than making a nursing diagnosis of Potential for Infection, the nurse could carry out and document the appropriate activities as part of the medically delegated or protocol-directed aspects of nursing care. This does not mean, however, that the patient does not have any conditions that could be named with nursing diagnosis and treated with nursing intervention.

In this example, the patient is unconscious, intubated, and receiving mechanical ventilation. An appropriate nursing diagnosis for which the nurse can assume a major aspect of treatment responsibility would be Ineffective Airway Clearance related to decreased level of consciousness and thick, tenacious secretions. For this nursing diagnosis, realistic and appropriate outcome statements would be:

- Breath sounds will be present and clear bilaterally
- Breath sounds will clear after suctioning

Here the nurse can use objective clinical findings to determine the effectiveness of the nursing interventions.

Once the appropriate outcome statements have been identified, the next step is selecting nursing interventions. A key factor in the selection of nursing interventions is the predicted effectiveness of the intervention. For many nursing diagnoses there are a wide range of available nursing interventions. The predicted effectiveness of nursing interventions will depend upon the unique characteristics of the patient, the patient's perception of the problem and treatment options, the degree to which the patient already has begun to compensate for the condition, the magnitude and urgency of the situation, and the cost-benefit considerations.[22] (See Chapter 4 for a detailed discussion of nursing treatment options.)

From a legal perspective, the area of nursing interventions can be another source of concern. Errors in selecting, carrying out, and documenting nursing interventions may create legal problems in a number of situations. These include the identification of appropriate interventions on the care plan that are not carried out, the absence of clinically indicated nursing interventions on the care plan, and clinically inappropriate nursing interventions.

In the first situation, there are appropriate nursing interventions on the nursing plan of care; however, the implementation of these interventions is not apparent in the patient's record. This situation is commonly seen in the use of standardized nursing care plans. These plans may be in manual format or in a computerized information system. It is not unique, however, to the use of standardized care plans; failure to carry out and document nursing interventions can and does occur in many nursing situations.

Of importance here is whether or not the plan is actually implemented. If an entire standardized plan of care is chosen, it is important that the plan of care be followed. If only specific interventions in the care plan are appropriate, only those interventions should be selected as necessary. If interventions have been chosen that are not appropriate for the patient, then the nurse's practice may be questioned. Additionally, if interventions have been selected and not implemented that affect the patient's well being, then the nurse could possibly be judged negligent.

A case to illustrate this point may be helpful. An 84-year-old white female patient was admitted to a medical unit with a primary admission diagnosis of CVA. Additional history revealed weakness, Parkinson's disease, anemia, and the inability to walk. The admitting nurse found the patient to be at high risk for falling and developed the nursing diagnosis: Potential for Injury related to weakness and inability to walk.

The interventions for this nursing diagnosis were directed towards keeping the side rails up on the bed, placing the call bell within reach, and keeping a night light on in the patient's room. Unfortunately the patient fell, broke her hip, and it was determined that all side rails were not up on the bed. Consequently, an action was brought against the hospital alleging that the nurse was negligent. Here a problem and an approach were identified; however, failure to carry out the identified nursing interventions was considered to be a breach in the standard of care.[23]

It is mandatory that the nursing care plan is implemented as it is written. When standardized nursing care plans are used, inappropriate nursing interventions must be deleted and appropriate nursing interventions must be carried out and documented. It is also important to note that the nurse is also legally accountable for actions and interventions that should have been part of the nursing care plan but were omitted. Acts of omission as well as acts of commission may be grounds for nursing negligence. The completeness, clarity, timeliness, and appropriateness of the nursing interventions are all factors that influence the quality of care and increase patient satisfaction, thereby serving as a safeguard should legal action arise.

The case of *Darling vs. Charleston Community Hospital*[24] demonstrates this point. In this case, a patient was admitted with a leg fracture that was casted in the emergency room. The hospital was found liable for failure of the nursing staff to assess the circulatory status of the patient's toes and to recognize that the cast was too tight. This omission led to the amputation of the patient's leg. In this case, the nursing interventions were related to the responsibility of nurses to monitor medical therapy and the patient's responses. Oftentimes, these assessments may not be included on the nursing care plan as they are considered standard practice for the medical condition in question, and the execution of routine assessments or nursing care activities must be documented even though there is no specific order.

The clinical appropriateness of nursing interventions is another area that can have legal ramifications. If a nursing diagnosis is identified, the interventions on the nursing care plan should be clinically appropriate. They also should reflect the approach that the reasonable, prudent nurse would use for this nursing diagnosis. When the nursing interventions are clinically inappropriate, or if certain standard nursing interventions are not included, this situation could be problematic in the event that the patient comes to harm.

When nursing interventions are not adequate for successful treatment of the patient, then referral to another health care professional must be considered. Referral may be necessary if the nurse does not have the authority or expertise to order certain treatment options or if those options fall outside the realm or scope of nursing practice. Another situation that requires referral is a critical change in the patient's condition.

Consider the patient recovering from a myocardial infarction. The patient has been highly upset about his illness and its effects on his life. A nursing diagnosis of Anxiety related to situational crisis has been made. Nursing interventions include an educational program, supportive listening, and reassurance.

Later that evening the patient becomes increasingly apprehensive, his respiratory rate increases to 28, accompanied by diaphoresis and slight dyspnea. Although he denies chest pain, he does describe a vague "twinge" in his epigastric area. These symptoms could very well be the result of myocardial ischemia or a pulmonary embolus. Continuing with the nursing interventions for Anxiety will be ineffective and could delay appropriate medical treatment. Failure to refer this situation to the physician could result in significant harm to the patient.

In clinical nursing practice, the selection and implementation of nursing interventions is a critical step in the nursing process. The use of nursing interventions that are ineffective, inappropriate, or inconsistent with the standard of care certainly have an effect on the patient's progress; however, grounds for a malpractice action exist only if there is harm or damage to the patient as a result of the nursing interventions. There also must be proof that the nursing interventions in question were below the standard of care and that this is the cause of harm to the patient.

Failure to Evaluate Nursing Diagnoses and Interventions

Evaluating the effectiveness of nursing care is essential, because it provides information for the nurse about the accuracy of the nursing diagnosis and the effectiveness of the nursing interventions. Failure to evaluate the nursing diagnoses and interventions may result in attempts to treat a nonexistent problem or ineffective treatment of an actual problem that could prolong or worsen the patient's condition. This could contribute to a breach of the standard of care and may have legal implications if harm to the patient occurs.

Evaluation is not a static process. The condition of the patient should be assessed on a frequent and regular basis. This ongoing assessment must evaluate the effectiveness of the current nursing plan of care, as well as detect changes in the patient's condition that indicate the plan of care should be modified.

There are two situations when failure to evaluate the nursing care plan may present legal pitfalls. The first situation is when the correct nursing diagnosis and nursing interventions have been identified; however, a subsequent change in the patient's condition is not incorporated into the plan, thereby making the plan inaccurate and ineffective.

An appropriate nursing diagnosis for a patient who is unconscious, immobilized, and malnourished might be Potential for Impaired Skin Integrity related to immobility. Nursing interventions would focus on turning, skin care, and hygiene. A related concern would be to provide adequate nutritional support.

This patient develops a sacral decubitus despite implementation of the nursing interventions on the care plan. At this point, failure to evaluate the plan and modify the nursing interventions could lead to further skin breakdown and possibly sepsis. This harm to the patient could result from the nurse's failure to evaluate the care plan and to make modifications based upon changes in the patient's condition.

A second situation when failure to evaluate the plan of care may have legal implications is when the plan is not effective. In this instance the nursing interventions are unsuccessful in achieving the desired patient outcomes. Failure to evaluate the effectiveness results in continuation of nursing interventions that are not working, and the patient's condition may worsen.

Consider the patient with chronic obstructive pulmonary disease, who has thick secretions and becomes fatigued very easily. A nursing diagnosis is made of Ineffective Airway Clearance related to weakness and fatigue, and nursing interventions consist of instructing the patient in pursed lip breathing, use of the incentive inspirometer, and encouraging the patient to cough. Despite the implementation of the interventions, the patient continues to have rhonchi bilaterally and is too tired to participate in any self-care activities.

At this point, evaluation of the plan shows that the selected interventions are not successful in moving the patient toward the desired outcomes of clear breath sounds and sufficient energy to participate in self-care activities. In the absence of evaluation, and a substantial change in the nursing interventions employed in the care plan, the patient probably will be unable to make any progress toward those outcomes. The retained secretion might even develop into a pneumonia. Harm to the patient could result from both the selection of ineffective nursing interventions and failure to evaluate and modify the situation.

The legal pitfalls of nursing diagnosis fall into three categories: incorrect nursing diagnoses, inappropriate or ineffective nursing interventions, and failure to evaluate the success of the plan of nursing care. These are also pitfalls of clinical nursing practice. In the next section, some guidelines for avoiding these problem areas will be presented.

GUIDELINES FOR PRUDENT PRACTICE USING NURSING DIAGNOSIS

The ability to make appropriate nursing diagnoses is an evolutionary process. While basic nursing diagnosis theory is taught in nursing schools along with a limited clinical application, the true ability to diagnose comes with practice and experience. In this way nursing diagnosis is not unlike medical diagnosis. The ability of the practitioner to diagnose correctly and appropriately, in both medicine and nursing, is enhanced over the years with experience and the refining of skills.

As indicated earlier, however, a nurse is legally accountable for her nursing diagnoses. Here are some guidelines that a nurse should use to avoid legal pitfalls when developing nursing diagnoses and writing nursing care plans:

1. Stay within the scope of nursing practice. If a diagnosis is made outside the scope of accepted nursing practice for your state, legal problems could result. The use of the medical diagnosis as an etiology statement could be construed as the nurse making a medical diagnosis.

2. The nursing care plan must be easily understood by all levels of nursing personnel. Take care that the plan does not become too "nursy" to be professionally interpreted by other disciplines, or too sophisticated to be understood by nursing aides, assistants, and students.

3. Avoid the use of terms in outcome standards that are either too global or too narrow. Since outcome standards are used to determine the success of the nursing care plan as well as to direct the evaluation or the re-evaluation of care, they should be patient-specific with a definite timeframe identified in which change should occur.

4. A mechanism for referral is an essential action in any nursing care plan. The referral can be to a physician, a clinical nurse specialist, or any member of the health care team. A referral can in essence "get the staff nurse off the hook" if a patient problem is beyond the nurse's area of expertise. This could protect the staff nurse, who is beginning to work with nursing diagnosis, against liability by demonstrating that resources were used or more expert opinions were solicited.

5. Since only registered nurses can diagnose, it is essential that their physical assessment skills be at the level necessary to allow for a comprehensive evaluation of the patient's condition. The initial nursing assessment upon admission sets the tone for the plan of care. Emphasis on a comprehensive assessment, using a nursing framework such as functional health patterns[25] or Unitary Persons[26] in conjunction with a physical examination, is essential.

6. The documentation guidelines for nursing care planning must be consistent with prudent, clinical practice and the standards for the respective professional organization. Reasonable timeframes should be set for completing the nursing assessments and updating care plans.

7. Be sure that there are data in the initial assessment or in the patient record to support the nursing diagnosis. The presence of a nursing diagnosis and the absence of defining characteristics is a discrepancy that can have legal ramifications. The opposite situation also holds true; if defining characteristics of a nursing diagnosis are documented, but a nursing diagnosis and care plan were not formulated, then this lack of treatment might possibly be considered negligent if harm occurs to the patient.

8. Evaluation of the nursing care plans, including the clinical relevance of the nursing diagnoses and nursing interventions, is essential. This evaluation should be conducted at both the unit and department of nursing levels. Information from this process can be used for guidance and feedback for individual nurses and as a part of the quality assurance process.

Following these guidelines makes the implementation of nursing diagnosis a smoother process and results in prudent nursing practice as well.

CONCLUSION

Nursing diagnosis is here to stay. As more and more individual nurses and health care organizations begin to use it, nursing diagnosis will become the standard of nursing practice. Indeed, this is reflected already in a number of state Nurse Practice Acts that identify nursing diagnosis as a foundation of professional nursing practice.

The role of diagnostician for the professional nurse demonstrates the changes occurring in nursing practice. O'Neil states, "The role of professional nursing, for at least the past decade, has been the subject of extensive political, social, and legal change."[27] Nowhere are these changes more exciting and challenging than in the area of nursing diagnosis.

Avoiding the pitfalls and anxieties about the legal issues related to nursing diagnosis can be accomplished by an understanding of a number of factors. Of first and foremost importance is the understanding of what a nursing diagnosis is and is not. The clinical expertise necessary to apply nursing diagnosis in clinical practice must accompany this knowledge.

Awareness of the scope of both nursing and medical practice, and a knowledge of the state Nurse Practice Act with its related rules and regulations is another critical factor. All of this knowledge and understanding can be used in order to adhere to the standard of nursing practice and prudent use of nursing diagnosis.

REFERENCES

1. Abdellah, F., Beland, L., Martin, A., & Matheny, R. *Patient centered approaches to nursing.* New York: Macmillan, 1960
2. Henderson, V. *The nature of nursing.* New York: Macmillan, 1966
3. Levine, M. *Introduction to clinical nursing,* 2nd ed. Philadelphia: F.A. Davis Company, 1969
4. McManus, R.F. Assumptions of the functions of nursing. In *Regional planning for nursing and nursing education.* New York: Bureau of Publications, Teacher's College, Columbia University, 1950
5. Gordon, M. Nursing diagnoses and the diagnostic process. *American Journal of Nursing,* 1976, *76,* 8, 1299
6. Schmidt, J. E. *The attorney's dictionary of medicine and word finder.* Albany, NY: M. Bender, Publishers, 1962
7. American Nurses' Association. *Nursing: A social policy statement.* Kansas City: American Nurses' Association, 1980, p. 9
8. *Ibid*
9. Greenlaw, J. Definition and regulation of nursing practice: An historical survey. *Law, Medicine, & Health Care,* 1985, 117
10. Gordon, M. *Nursing diagnosis: Process and application* New York: McGraw-Hill, 1982, p. 248
11. Cushing, M. Expanding the meaning of accountability. *American Journal of Nursing,* 1983, *83,* 10, 1472
12. Greenlaw
13. LaBar, C. Legal regulation of nursing practice. Unpublished paper presented at American Nurses' As-

sociation credentialing meeting, San Antonio, Texas, March 1982
14. American Nurses' Association. *The nursing practice act: Suggested state legislation.* Kansas City: American Nurses' Association, 1981
15. *Ibid*
16. Yoder, M.E. Nursing diagnosis: Applications in perioperative practice. *AORN Journal,* 1984, *40,* 2 185
17. Carpenito, L.J. *Nursing diagnosis: Application to clinical practice.* Philadelphia: J. B. Lippincott, 1983
18. Kelly, M.A. *Nursing diagnosis source book: Guidelines for clinical application.* Norwalk, CT: Appleton-Century-Crofts, 1985
19. Mundinger, M. & Jauron, G. Developing a nursing diagnosis. *Nursing Outlook 23,* 94
20. Iyer, B. W., Taptich, B. J., & Bernocchi-Losey, D. *Nursing process and nursing diagnosis.* Philadelphia: W.B. Saunders, 1986
21. Bower, F.L. *The process of planning nursing care,* 3rd ed. St. Louis: C. V. Mosby, 1982
22. Gordon. *Nursing diagnosis: Process and application*
23. *Bosemen v. Medical Center Hospitals,* Circuit Court of the City of Norfolk, Virginia, 1987
24. *Darling v. Charleston Community Memorial Hospital,* 33 Ill. 326, 211 N.E. 2d 253, 1965
25. Gordon. *Nursing diagnosis: Process and application*
26. Guzzetta, C.E., Bunton, S.D., Prinkley, L.A., et al. *Clinical assessment tools for use with nursing diagnosis.* St. Louis: C.V. Mosby, 1989
27. O'Neil, E.A. A gavel falls for nursing: *Sermchief v. Gonzales. Nursing Economics,* 1984, *2,* 102

Implementing Diagnosis-based Nursing Practice: Specialty Issues and Clinical Applications

Implementation Strategies for Diagnosis-based Nursing Practice in Psychiatric Nursing

Katherine Norfleet Berry

Diagnostic thinking is not new to the psychiatric nurse; nursing diagnosis is. Many questions remain to be answered about nursing diagnosis, but the time to begin working with it is now. Implementation of nursing diagnosis in psychiatric settings offers significant rewards even in this early stage of development.

Psychiatry is a specialty area where professional roles are often blurred. The acceptance and integration of nursing diagnosis within the nursing process for psychiatric patients will lead to a more solid nursing identity and the delineation of a unique nursing role with patients. When patient problems are more clearly identified, psychiatric nurses will be able to define the most effective interventions they have to offer.

Most psychiatric nurses are familiar with diagnostic thinking in relation to psychiatric patient problems due to their exposure and involvement with *The Diagnostic and Statistical Manual of Mental Disorders* (DMSIII). Some nurses even propose the DSMIII for their own diagnostic nomenclature.[1]

Expert nurse clinicians have long been contributing their assessments of psychiatric patients for the formulation of DSMIII diagnoses. In this approach, signs and symptoms have been examined and clustered using a medical model approach. Nurses have been rewarded for these assessment skills by their physician colleagues.

Psychiatrists have often relied on nurses in psychiatric settings to collect the data they need to make medical or DSMIII diagnoses. For example, nurses routinely monitor target symptoms associated with the medical diagnosis of depression, such as changes in sleep patterns, appetite, weight, mood, and activities of daily living. Physicians value and give recognition to nurses for this sort of data seeking and communication. Many psychiatric nurses, because of this powerful reward system, have adopted a sort of quasi-medical model for their own thought processes about patient problems.

In 1980 the American Nurses' Association (ANA) challenged this medical-model way of thinking by defining nursing as "the diagnosis and treatment of human responses to actual or potential health problems."[2] Soon thereafter, the term nursing diagnosis was included in the

Standards of Psychiatric and Mental Health Nursing Practice. Gordon defines nursing diagnosis in this way:

> Nursing diagnoses' or clinical diagnoses, made by professional nurses describe actual or potential health problems that nurses, by virtue of their education and experience are capable and licensed to treat.[3]

Since 1973, the National Conference Groups on Nursing Diagnosis have been working to identify and classify the human responses that nurses treat. To date, 98 nursing diagnoses have been accepted and classified within the North American Nursing Diagnosis Association's (NANDA) Taxonomy I. These human responses to actual or potential health problems are phenomena of unique concern to the profession of nursing. Work is continuing to identify new diagnoses for use in clinical practice that will be incorporated into Taxonomy I. The taxonomy serves as a classification system for the human responses that all professional nurses treat and is organized around nine human response patterns. The intent is for the taxonomy to classify phenomena of concern for all nursing specialty areas.

Some psychiatric nurses have noted gaps in Taxonomy I for the responses they treat. Two particular problems have been identified with the use of nursing diagnosis for psychiatric patients: The insufficient number of diagnoses for phenomena of concern to psychiatric nurses, and the lack of specificity of many of the diagnoses.[4] Many nurses have found diagnoses such as Ineffective Individual Coping and Altered Thought Processes to be too broad or abstract to be clinically useful to direct the care of individual patients.

A review of the literature reveals little clinical application of nursing diagnosis in the psychiatric setting. Only one study[5] of nursing diagnoses for patients with the medical diagnosis of depression appears in the literature. Twelve nursing diagnoses were identified for six depressed patients. Only three were noted to be similar to the NANDA-approved diagnoses. These were Fear of Loss of Control of Feelings, similar to Fear and to Grieving, and Potential for Self-harm similar to Potential for Violence: Self-directed. The other nine are not included in NANDA's Taxonomy I. These include Emancipation, Emancipation of Child, Emotional Detachment, Lack of External Resources, Neediness in Interpersonal Relationships, Passivity, Post-overdose Syndrome, Somatization, and Uncertainty about Life Direction. None of the nursing diagnoses identified in the study included etiology statements.

It has been clearly stated that Taxonomy I is an incomplete classification of the problems nurses treat.[6] Efforts are underway to fill gaps for phenomena of concern to psychiatric nurses. Diagnostic labels such as Inappropriate Aggression, Depressive behavior, and Suspiciousness[7] are offered in the literature for use in psychiatric settings.

The ANA Council of Psychiatric Mental Health Nurses has even begun work on a separate Taxonomy of Phenomenon of Concern to Psychiatric Mental Health Nurses.[8] This classification system lists diagnoses at a highly specific level of abstraction such as Blocking of Ideas, Circumstantial Thinking, Flight of Ideas, and Indecisiveness. These are only four of 13 subcategories of Alterations in Judgment.

The recommendation here is for psychiatric nurses to unite their efforts on nursing diagnosis and work with only one classification system—Taxonomy I. The clinical application of nursing diagnosis holds the key to further development and refinement of Taxonomy I. The answers to nurses' questions lie with actual patients in actual practice settings.

Obviously, to change the way a psychiatric nurse defines the nursing role to "the diagnosis and treatment of human responses to actual or potential health problems"[9] is a major undertaking. Without a deliberate, well-organized plan for implementing nursing diagnosis at the unit or organizational level, efforts will be useless. Learned behavioral patterns will be maintained and the existing practice culture (see Chapter 1) will likely impede progress toward the desired change.

The purpose of this chapter is to demonstrate how to integrate nursing diagnosis into nursing practice in the inpatient psychiatric setting. Implementation strategies are presented according to Lewin's planned change model.[10] The unique aspects of psychiatric nursing in relation to nursing diagnosis are discussed.

UNIQUE ASPECTS OF PSYCHIATRIC NURSING PRACTICE

Certain aspects of the psychiatric milieu must be considered before discussing how to implement nursing diagnosis in this specialty area. The psychiatric inpatient setting presents significant challenges and distinct advantages in terms of the integration of nursing diagnosis into the psychiatric nursing process. The abstract nature of most psychiatric patient problems often overwhelms nurses in initial attempts to make nursing diagnoses. Once nurses acquire more advanced diagnostic thinking skills, though, they realize how nursing diagnosis enables them to label problems with greater specificity unique to individual patients.

Mental health problems are often not observable in the concrete sense as, for example, a fractured tibia in orthopedics, a left hemiparesis in neurology, or an infected wound in general surgery. Psychiatric patients are hospitalized for health problems more complex and abstract in nature. A suicidal teenager who has just been rejected by her boyfriend may present the concrete symptom of a slashed wrist, but the core problem precipitating the suicidal attempt are more difficult to define.

Other examples might be a man with the medical diagnosis of schizophrenia who is admitted to the hospital with fixed delusional thoughts that his workplace has been bugged and his food is being poisoned, or a recent widow admitted to a psychiatric facility for evaluation and treatment of depression evidenced by difficulty sleeping, lack of appetite, and severe feelings of guilt and self-worthlessness. An elderly gentleman may be hospitalized when his family no longer feels able to care for him due to his intermittent wandering and physically aggressive behavior. These health problems certainly are more abstract than the those examples treated in other health specialty areas.

Psychiatric illness by its very nature often affects many human response patterns. Consider the elderly man in the preceding example. This individual could be experiencing responses in virtually all of the nine human response patterns. The usefulness of nursing diagnosis is in breaking this abstract, complex patient experience down into observable responses. Any of the nursing diagnoses in Table 12–1 might apply to this patient. (See Table 12–1.)

Thus, the use of nursing diagnosis enables the professional nurse to identify a particular patient's individual response to dementia amenable to nursing intervention. Patients respond in unique ways to illness. Quality nursing care plans can be developed and implemented when individual patient problems are effectively described.

The Role of the Psychiatric Nurse

What is the role of the nurse within the psychiatric setting? How does nursing define its unique role with these patients with such abstract health problems?

TABLE 12–1. POSSIBLE NURSING DIAGNOSES FOR AN ELDERLY, DELUSIONAL PATIENT

Potential for Injury: Falls related to disorientation to place at night

Self-Care Deficit: Feeding, Toileting, Grooming related to short-term memory impairment and decreased concentration

Potential for Impaired Skin Integrity related to urinary and bowel incontinence

Potential for Violence: Other-Directed related to suspiciousness of others

Powerlessness related to progressive loss of memory and functional abilities

Alteration in Family Process related to ambivalence over nursing home placement

Noncompliance: Medications related to memory impairment and suspiciousness

Grieving related to loss of previous family role

Mereness and Taylor define psychiatric nursing as:

> The process whereby the nurse assists persons, as individuals or in groups, in developing a more positive self concept, a more harmonious pattern of interpersonal relationships, and a more productive role in society. The achievement of these goals results in the establishing of patterns of behavior that are more satisfactory to others and more satisfying to the individual. Helping persons to accept themselves, to improve their relationships with other people, and to function independently are the most fundamental goals in psychiatric nursing.[11]

The role of the psychiatric nurse in the inpatient setting, therefore, is the therapeutic use of self with individuals, groups, and families within the milieu to achieve these fundamental goals. The nurse manipulates the environment and interactions within the milieu to deliver effective interventions for individual patients according to their unique responses to their health problems.

For example, for a man diagnosed with Powerlessness related to progressive loss of memory and functional abilities, the nurse can structure the milieu in such a way as to promote this man's sense of control and autonomy despite his limitations. Numerous visual cues such as: a calendar clock, a large print name, or a photograph on his hospital room door could be used to provide frequent reminders as to time, place, and date so that he can reorient himself as needed. Clear, step-by-step directions can be given this gentleman so he could participate in routine activities of daily living. The nurse would allow this patient to make as many of his own decisions about his care as possible to maintain his sense of control, but intervene when necessary to assure successful completion of activities of daily living.

Another intervention for the nurse can be to spend time with this patient to explore his thoughts and feelings about his loss of memory and functional abilities. Positive feedback regarding his unique strengths and contributions to the milieu would also be indicated. A familiar and successful life role such as "mailman" might be employed within the milieu to achieve a sense of accomplishment.

The Nursing Domain with Psychiatric Patients

Psychiatry is an area where professional roles are especially blurred. Interdisciplinary care plans often are developed without clear delineation of professional roles with the patient. The DSMIII has been used by various professions, including medicine, social work, and psychology as well as nursing. The tendency has been for nurses to view patient problems according to this medical diagnosis classification system. In other words, nurses often planned their nursing care according to the diagnosis of depression or schizophrenia rather than the patient's individual response to these illnesses.

A major advantage from the implementation of nursing diagnosis is delineation of the unique role of the nurse with psychiatric patients. This delineation is not only helpful for colleagues in the other disciplines but for nurses themselves. The focus that nursing diagnosis places on the human responses to health problems versus the health problems or diseases themselves serves to define nursing's unique role with patients. Medicine focuses on identification and treatment of disease; nursing focuses on the identification and treatment of the human responses to disease.

Psychiatric nurses in an inpatient setting most often diagnose and treat patient responses to the mental disorders listed in the DMSIII and the diseases listed in the International Classification of Diseases-9. Before the advent of nursing diagnosis, this distinction was less evident. It was more difficult to carve out a distinct role for the nurse in the often complex abstract problems of psychiatric patients.

Psychiatric illness often affects all aspects of health presenting significant problems of living for the individual. Nursing diagnosis enables the nurse to break down the individual experience into measurable responses amenable to nursing therapy. One model of the nursing discipline's distinctive domain in health care that is particularly applicable to psychiatric nursing practice is illustrated in Figure 12–1.

Carnevali maintains that nursing is concerned with the interaction between daily living and its environment and functional health status.[12] The model is two-directional. Alterations in activities or demands of daily living and the nature of the environment affect functional health status. In turn, functional health status affects daily living and relationships to the daily living environment.

The key to the implementation and integration of nursing diagnosis into nursing practice is the clear understanding of this unique domain of the nursing profession. When nurses have a firm grasp on what they have to offer patients, the desire for accountability for that autonomous role with patients can be both the most important motivating factor for change as well as the most significant and rewarding outcome of the change to a diagnosis-based psychiatric nursing practice.

IMPLEMENTATION OF NURSING DIAGNOSIS AS A PLANNED CHANGE PROCESS

Organizational change to a diagnosis-based psychiatric nursing practice involves four levels of change: knowledge, attitude, individual behavior, and group or organizational behavior.[13] Diagnosis-based practice involves more than just individual nurses using nursing diagnosis to name their patients' problems. (See Chapter 1.)

Change to a diagnosis-based practice implies change in the nursing culture itself. The way

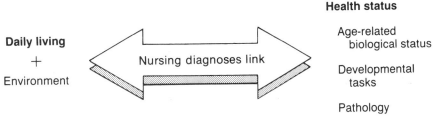

Figure 12–1. Nursing discipline's distinctive domain in health care. *(From Carnevali, D. Nursing Care Planning: Diagnosis and Management (3rd ed.). Philadelphia: J.B. Lippincott, © 1983, p. 12. Reprinted with permission.)*

nurses think, behave, and value their roles must change to integrate nursing diagnosis success-fully into practice. Change of such magnitude clearly requires thorough planning.

Lewin's framework for the three phases of planned change: unfreezing, change, and refreezing[14] is used to organize the recommended implementation strategies. Ideas presented have been generated from the author's experience as a change agent in the nursing diagnosis process at the psychiatric-unit level and the hospital-wide level.

ASSESSMENT OF UNIT FOR READINESS TO CHANGE

Before a decision to implement nursing diagnosis is made, it is important to evaluate the nursing climate for certain factors that signal readiness for change. If present, these factors will greatly influence the change process to proceed in a positive manner. If overlooked, the absence of any one of these factors could block the change to nursing diagnosis.

Professional Identity

The nurse's professional identity is the key to nursing diagnosis. A major benefit of using nursing diagnosis is to define the nurse's role in patient care. Some nurses may be satisfied solely with their medically-dependent role. Some nurses are enmeshed in the medical-model approach to nursing practice. Nursing diagnosis concepts will be difficult to grasp for these nurses.

If the nursing staff is able to conceptualize both their independent and collaborative functions, then the likelihood of a successful transition is greater. The absence of this profes-sional identity factor need not prevent implementation, however. Nursing diagnosis can, in fact, provide the necessary direction for nurses to assume a stronger professional identity.

Model of Nursing Practice

The model of nursing practice used is an important factor. (See Chapter 6.) Does the model effectively support the nursing process? Are individual patients linked with individual nurses? Primary, team, and case management models of nursing practice can provide this link effec-tively. Furthermore, a practice model will support nursing diagnosis only if the role of the registered nurse is clearly defined to make the nurse truly accountable for the diagnosis and treatment of specified patients.

Administrative Support

Effective administrative support consists of much more than an organizational decision to implement nursing diagnosis. Nurse managers at the unit level must possess significant investment and skill, or at least be willing to develop skills in nursing diagnosis for the process to work. Resources of people, time, and money must be allocated for effective change.

A nurse manager who demonstrates effective diagnostic skills can influence the success of nursing diagnosis through role modeling, teaching, and the development of unit systems that promote effective use of nursing diagnosis. The influence of a nurse manager who values nursing diagnosis is critical for successful implementation. Conversely, if the frontline nurse managers are not invested in nursing diagnosis, do not consider implementation. Change is often slow but without the support of the key unit leaders, change is difficult if not impossible!

Clinical Resources

At least one expert clinician within the unit system must be available to provide clinical leadership and role modeling during the change process. This nurse expert must be skilled in psychiatric nursing, and ideally should already be skilled in diagnostic thinking and successful in applying nursing diagnosis in actual practice. Familiarity with the work of NANDA and Taxonomy I is essential.

The leader must be the first to communicate diagnostic language and clinical thinking to others. This resource person will need to be the first to use nursing diagnosis terminology in clinical practice as well as with other disciplines or in interdisciplinary care plans. Staff nurses may not feel comfortable taking this risk without a role model. When the other disciplines begin to see the benefits of nursing diagnosis and form a clearer perspective on the nurse's unique role in patient care, their positive comments will serve as strong motivators and reinforcers of change.

The initiator of the change to nursing diagnosis must be in close communication with the administrative staff throughout the implementation process. The initiator and administrators must hold similar values related to nursing practice and be in agreement about goals, processes, and outcomes of the change process. The staff must see mutual support and hear consistent messages from the initiator and the administrative staff.

A psychiatric clinical nurse specialist is ideal for this resource role due to the direct patient-care focus of the role as well as the level of expertise already established in the specialty area. The clinical specialist could serve as a consultant, educator, and role model during the change process; however, nurses in other roles may assume this function. The major requirements are expertise in psychiatric nursing, sound assessment skills, teaching skills, knowledge of change theory, and *time* to devote to the project.

Satisfaction with Current Care Plans

An important question is "How do the staff nurses view their current care plans?" Readiness to change to nursing diagnosis implies that nurses see the need to alter their current care planning practices.[15] Prior to the implementation of nursing diagnosis, many staff nurses view care plans negatively, and the major motivating force for plan development is external audit procedures.

If the nurses do not value the current care plans, then use that dissatisfaction to an advantage. The transformation of nursing care plans from cumbersome, generic exercises to practical, useful tools should help to sell the concept of nursing diagnosis.

Nursing diagnosis assists nurses to develop practical, functional care plans. Nursing care plans have not always served this intended purpose. Unfortunately, nurses providing direct care to patients have overlooked valuable information in care plans because the plans were often too long, impractical, or idealistically worded in textbook fashion. On the other hand, a care plan directed toward the following specific nursing diagnoses for a depressed patient pinpoints the patient's individual responses to the depression and thus provides helpful direction.

Self-care Deficit: Grooming related to decreased motivation
Potential for Intentional Self-harm related to low self-esteem

Assessment

A necessary implementation step for nursing units and organizations is to institute the use of a nursing assessment framework that supports the use of nursing diagnosis. Assessment tools that are organized according to a nursing framework such as Gordon's Functional Health Patterns[16] or the nine human response patterns of NANDA's Taxonomy I are particularly useful. The use of such a form for the initial nursing assessment cues the nurse to assess patient conditions in all areas of health.

One area of assessment of particular concern to psychiatric nursing practice is the mental status examination. Guidelines for mental status examination[17,18] are available in the literature. These guidelines may be used to supplement the nursing assessment form, or selected items may be included in the assessment questions for the "Perceiving" and "Knowing" patterns if the NANDA Taxonomy I framework is used. Different specialty areas may choose to specify certain assessment questions. For example, nurses working in an eating disorder unit might add items to evaluate body image, while nurses in a geriatric setting might add questions to assess memory function.

In summary, if the factors described in Table 12–2 are in place, proceed in the change process. Any work done to strengthen these influencing factors before change begins will be well worth the time and effort.

UNFREEZING

The unfreezing phase in the implementation process is critical in terms of setting the stage for staff nurses to redefine their role with human responses to actual or potential health problems. The time prior to actual implementation of nursing diagnosis should be a testing or practice period. Nurses should be given the freedom to try out diagnostic thinking in safe situations. Staff nurses need, however, a resource person to help them learn and test new diagnostic skills.

The first step in implementing nursing diagnosis on the unit or organizational level is to identify a resource person or the individual who will initiate efforts to implement nursing diagnosis. Field describes three major roles of this change agent: leader, resource person, and role model.[19] This individual should have recognized clinical expertise as well as a firm grasp of how to apply nursing diagnosis concepts to clinical practice.

The staff needs a readily available resource person, involved in direct day-to-day patient care, who can offer assistance, support, and validation in the identification of nursing diagnoses for specific patients.[20] In most organizations, this role function is particularly well suited for a clinical nurse specialist; however, other nursing roles such as head nurse, staff educator, or "expert"[21] staff nurse could function effectively as the resource person if given adequate time for the project.

Desensitizing Efforts

Next, certain desensitizing efforts can begin. The resource person can begin to use nursing diagnosis in all aspects of actual practice: documentation, patient-care conferences, rounds, individual consultations. Field points out that a change agent's decision to take the initiative in practice both reinforces the value assigned to the process and lessens the stress and risk for less proficient nurses.[22]

The resource person or designated change agent in any practice setting implementing

---

TABLE 12–2.   FACTORS INFLUENCING READINESS FOR CHANGE TO NURSING DIAGNOSIS

- *Strong professional nursing identity*
- *Team, primary, or case management nursing models*
- *Administrative support*
- *Clinical resources/experts*
- *Dissatisfaction with current care plans*
- *Human response-based assessment tool*

nursing diagnosis must be willing to serve this role-model function. In patient-care conferences and unit inservices, the resource person must begin to expose the nursing staff to the ANA's definition for nursing: "the diagnosis and treatment of human responses to actual or potential health problems."[23] For nurses who are comfortable with a medical model of practice, this focus on the patient's response to illness can help to distinguish nursing's unique and autonomous role in patient care.

The initiator might facilitate discussions during patient-care conferences regarding the unique role of the nurse in specific patient-care situations. Again, reinforcing the nurse's role in treating the patient's individual response should be helpful. Be aware of the tendency for novice diagnosticians to search for one comprehensive diagnosis to name the patient's problem, rather than focusing on particular patient conditions.

For instance, with complex patient presentations within the psychiatric setting, such as borderline personality disorder, clear direction for nursing treatment is often difficult to determine. Focus on the nine human response patterns helps nurses identify the patient's individual problems amenable to nursing intervention such as potential for Intentional Self-harm related to rejection from boyfriends, Potential for Violence related to lack of impulse control, self-concept Disturbance: Low Self-esteem related to sexual abuse as child, and Impaired Social Interaction related to intense anger/rage.

The next step is learning the language. This can begin with exposure to NANDA's 88 accepted diagnoses, their definitions, and defining characteristics. The initiator should carry a nursing diagnosis handbook[24] at all times to use for impromptu diagnostic thinking with staff nurses. Handbooks should be located on the unit so nurses have quick access to the diagnoses and defining characteristics.

Difficult patient presentations during patient-care conference may be used to illustrate how nursing diagnoses can clearly define the nurse's role in an otherwise overwhelming and complicated situation. Nurses can learn the diagnostic process by using Gordon's "problem/etiology/signs and symptoms" format[25] to identify the nursing diagnoses. Exercises such as listing all the available data about the patient help staff nurses learn the diagnostic process. Data from the initial nursing assessment, physical assessment data, behavioral observations, historical data from patient and family may then be clustered into logical groups according to some pattern or recognition or organization of the diagnostician.[26] Table 12–3 illustrates this method of data clustering.

The nursing staff may be more comfortable naming symptoms that point to a DSMIII diagnosis such as depression rather than the response to the depression. If this is the case, use the familiarity with DSMIII diagnostic thinking as a strength. Build on these diagnostic skills and have the nurses cluster data according to nursing diagnoses. It is helpful to view the DSMIII diagnosis as the health problem itself; then the nurse can define the patient's individual human responses amenable to nursing treatment.

Overcoming Resistance

Be prepared for some experienced psychiatric nurses to show signs of resistance to the change. These expert practitioners may have gathered many rewards from physicians over the years for their assessments and judgments regarding medical problems and treatments.[27] These skills certainly are valued and continue to be part of the collaborative nursing role. One way to encourage these nurses to begin to label patient problems in terms of nursing diagnoses is to demonstrate the effectiveness and practicality of this kind of diagnostic thinking. By comparing medical diagnoses to possible co-occurrent nursing diagnoses, a number of benefits can be seen.

Table 12–4 compares medical and nursing diagnoses for two patient problems. These

TABLE 12–3. CLUSTERING OF THE DATA FOR A DEPRESSED PATIENT

Patient Data	Nursing Diagnoses
56-year-old woman	*Potential for Intentional Self-Harm related to command hallucinations*
School teacher	
Diagnosis of depression	
Overdose, lethal amount of elavil	
Flat affect, no eye contact	
Emanciated	*Alteration in Nutrition: Less than Body Requirements related to lack of initiative and suspiciousness*
Appears older than stated age	
10 pounds weight loss in last 2 weeks	
Admission weight: 95 pounds, height: 5'6"	
Scheduled for ECT to begin in 2 days	
Husband asking every staff member questions regarding ECT	
Husband threatened to sign wife out AMA	
Seclusive in her own room	
Will miss meals if left to own initiative to eat	
Appears preoccupied at times	
Reports hearing voices telling her to kill herself	*Fear related to upcoming ECT treatments*
Occasionally seen peering out of her room	

examples illustrate how nursing diagnoses clarify the specific role of the nurse with individual psychiatric patients. Most experienced psychiatric nurses are familiar with the generic standards of care for certain groups of patients such as the hallucinating patient or the manic patient. The goal of nursing diagnosis and care plans is for the professional psychiatric nurse to use this knowledge to outline a realistic plan for the nursing treatment of individual patients with individual human responses. In this way, nursing interventions may be developed to treat more concrete patient-specific responses versus abstract and complex patient experiences.

A change strategy that builds upon this advantage of nursing diagnosis is to begin with the highest priority diagnoses, or the diagnoses that are most meaningful to nurses in day-to-day practice. These diagnoses can be those that describe life-threatening patient states such as Potential for Intentional Self-harm or Potential for Violence, or those that describe patient states requiring a large amount of nursing time and intervention such as Self-care Deficit. Initial focus on these frequently occuring diagnoses helps the staff nurses describe the nursing role with patients more clearly and in more concrete terms. This focus increases the ease of staff in dealing with these problems because they are identified clearly and consistently. Most importantly, when problems are identified in care plans, interventions are planned and higher standards of patient care can be achieved.

Using only a few diagnoses in the beginning implementation stages facilitates familiarity with associated defining characteristics and risk factors. The resource person and others skilled in nursing diagnosis should assist work groups and individual nurses to develop care plans for the identified diagnoses. To promote maximal acceptance of the new care-planning approach, the patient outcomes should be achievable and the nursing interventions practical and patient-specific.

TABLE 12–4. CO-OCCURRENT MEDICAL AND NURSING DIAGNOSES

Medical Diagnosis	Nursing Diagnosis
Schizophrenia	*Social Isolation related to suspiciousness of others*
	Self-Concept Disturbance: Low Self-Esteem related to poor work tolerance
	Potential for Violence related to command hallucinations
	Sleep Pattern Disturbance related to anxiety
	Noncompliance: Medications related to denial of (mental) illness
	Potential for Intentional Self-Harm related to command hallucinations
	Self-Care Deficit: Grooming related to decreased motivation
	Impaired Mobility related to catatonic rigidity
	Fluid Volume Deficit related to suspiciousness of fluids
Bypolar Disorder: Mania	*Sleep Pattern Disturbance related to psychomotor agitation*
	Impaired Social Interaction related to intrusive behavior
	Alteration in Nutrition: Less than Body Requirements related to distractibility
	Impaired Verbal Communication related to flight of ideas
	Impaired Social Interaction related to grandiose delusions
	Potential for Injury: Head Banging related to psychomotor agitation

A conscious and spoken effort to get away from the flowery, impractical, "school book" approach to care plans should be employed at this stage. "Less is best!" is a welcome phrase to staff nurses that describes this new approach to care planning. A move towards a more qualitative versus quantitative approach to auditing care plans can be an effective change strategy. Nurses feel rewarded to know that their efforts to identify accurate, descriptive, and directive nursing diagnoses are valued. Loosening auditing standards during the change process is helpful to promote acceptance of nursing diagnoses.

Introduce NANDA's Diagnoses

As nurses begin to express interest in naming the phenomena of nursing concern, familiarize them with the 98 diagnoses accepted by NANDA's membership. Some frustration and resistance may surface, evidenced by comments like "there are not enough psychiatric nursing diagnoses" or "this might work for medical/surgical patients but not psychiatric patients." Reassurance that all the diagnoses have not yet been identified may help; freedom to practice without being "wrong" and encouragement to give the diagnoses a try can also lessen resistance.

Structured time should be provided for nurses to review patient data, cluster the data, and make diagnostic decisions about the problems they treat. Nurses need time to practice diagnostic thinking and experiment with different diagnostic labels and etiologies. At first, nurses may become frustrated to find there are not always clear-cut answers to their diagnostic questions. They may want the answers provided them rather than appreciating that the answers will emerge from their practice.

A certain tolerance for the yet imperfect nature of the classification system must develop so that nurses do not become too frustrated. Nurses may become impatient when the diagnostic decision is difficult to reach. Other nurses may be stimulated by lively discussion regarding diagnostic dilemmas such as the differentiation among the diagnoses Powerlessness, Self-concept Disturbance, Hopelessness, and Grief. When a tolerance for such differential diagnostic discussions is evident, the climate is ripe for change.

Etiology Statements

At first glance many of the diagnoses and even some of the response patterns seem of limited value for the psychiatric patients. An excellent example is Activity Intolerance. Most nurses think of patients with some sort of energy depletion or oxygen depletion for this diagnostic label; however, the label can be effectively applied for patients within the psychiatric milieu who lack tolerance for activity because of misperception of their abilities. The diagnosis Activity Intolerance related to perceived helplessness describes the phenomenon effectively and provides direction for nursing interventions. Through the use of etiology, all of the diagnostic categories become applicable to psychiatric nursing practice.

At this point in the implementation process, the creative use of etiology should be explored so that diagnostic statements may name, in the most effective manner, the problems psychiatric nurses treat. Some questions regarding the use of etiology have emerged in the literature in recent years. (For a complete discussion of the concept of etiology refer to Chapter 3.)

This author strongly supports the naming of etiology, or contributing factors, for patients' responses. In fact, the use of etiology is crucial to the diagnostic process for naming phenomena that psychiatric nurses treat.

Consider the difference in these diagnostic statements:

Self-care Deficit: Bathing related to left hemiparesis
Self-care Deficit: Bathing related to decreased motivation

Alteration in Nutrition: Less and Body Requirements related to lack of appetite
Alteration in Nutrition: Less than Body Requirements related to suspiciousness of food

Clearly, the nursing interventions indicated for these diagnoses are quite different. The etiology statement directs patient specific interventions.

Common Problems

A significant and somewhat surprising problem encountered during the implementation of nursing diagnosis in the psychiatric setting has been the difficulties associated with the nursing diagnoses, Altered Thought Process and Sensory-Perceptual Alterations. Since patients in psychiatric settings frequently respond to health problems with altered thoughts and perceptions, nurses in these settings must develop the skill to apply clinically useful nursing diagnoses for these patients. Even though experienced psychiatric nurses are quite familiar with disordered thinking and perceiving patterns, nursing diagnoses that are descriptive of the patient and prescriptive of nursing intervention are often very difficult to formulate for these patient groups.

The problem with the two diagnostic labels, Altered Thought Process and Sensory-Perceptual Alterations, is not theoretical but a practical one. These two broad diagnostic labels name phenomena of concern to the nursing profession. They have been described as categories with exhaustive lists of defining characteristics, naming various cognitive and perceptual deficits. (See Table 12–5.)

Many defining characteristics of these two nursing diagnoses overlap, such as inaccurate interpretation of stimuli, hallucinations, distractibility, and disorientation. The critical indicators, nonreality-based thinking processes and reality distortion as judged against some set of normative criteria, respectively, are quite similar.[28] Carpenito discusses the differential diag-

TABLE 12–5. ALTERED THOUGHT PROCESS AND SENSORY-PERCEPTUAL ALTERATIONS DEFINING CHARACTERISTICS NOTED BY VARIOUS AUTHORS

Altered Thought Process		
Kim McFarland McLane	*McFarland Wasli*	*Carpenito*
Inaccurate interpretation of environment	Inaccurate interpretation of environment	Disoriented in time, place, or person
Cognitive dissonance	Cognitive dissonance	Altered abstraction
Distractibility	Distractibility	Distractibility
Memory deficit or problems	Memory deficit or problems	Memory deficits
Egocentricity	Egocentricity	Inaccurate interpretation of stimuli
Hyper/hypovigilance	Hyper/hypovigilance	
Decreased ability to grasp ideas	Inability to follow directions	
Impaired ability to make decisions	Delusions, flight of ideas, disorganization	
Impaired ability to problem solve	Word salad, neologisms, echolalia, condensations	
Impaired ability to reason	Perservation	
Impaired ability to abstract or conceptualize	Circumstantiality	
Impaired ability to calculate	Difficulty in interacting with others, withdrawal, unpredictability	
Altered attention span, distractibility	Obsessions	
Commands; obsessions	Decreased ability to grasp ideas	
Inability to follow	Impaired ability to make decisions	
Disorientation to time, place, person, circumstances, and events	Impaired ability to problem solve	
Changes in remote, recent, immediate memory	Impaired ability to reason	
Delusions	Impaired ability to abstract or conceptualize	
Ideas of reference	Impaired ability to calculate	
Hallucinations	Disorientation to time, place, person, circumstances, and events	
Confabulation	Ideas of reference	
Inappropriate social behavior	Hallucinations	
Altered sleep patterns	Confabulation	
Inappropriate affect	Altered sleep patterns	
Other possible defining characteristic	Inappropriate affect	
Inappropriate/nonreality-based thinking		

(continued)

TABLE 12–5. (Continued)

Sensory-Perceptual Alterations		
Kim McFarland McLane	McFarland Wasli	Carpenito
Disoriented in time, place, or with persons	Disoriented in time, place, or with persons	Disoriented in time or place
Altered abstractions	Altered abstractions	Disoriented about people
Altered conceptualization	Altered conceptualization	Altered ability to problem solve
Change in problem-solving abilities	Change in problem-solving abilities	Altered behavior or communication pattern
Reported or measured change in sensory acuity	Reported or measured change in sensory acuity	Sleep pattern disturbances
Change in behavior pattern	Change in behavior pattern	Restlessness
Anxiety	Anxiety	Reports auditory or visual hallucinations
Apathy	Apathy	Fear
Change in usual response to stimuli	Change in usual response to stimuli	Anxiety
Indication of body-image alterations	Indication of body-image alteration	Apathy
Restlessness	Restlessness	
Irritability	Irritability	
Altered communication patterns	Altered communication patterns	
Disorientation	Unpredictability	
Lack of concentration	Mumbling to self	
Daydreaming	Talking about unseen objects	
Hallucinations	Looking about in a frightened, guarded manner	
Noncompliance	Unusual interest in television or radio	
Fear	Complaints of headache	
Depression	Withdrawal	
Rapid mood swings		
Anger		
Exaggerated emotional responses		
Poor concentration		
Disordered thought sequencing		
Bizarre thinking		
Visual and auditory distortions		
Motor incoordination		
Complaints of fatigue		
Alteration in posture		
Change in muscular tension		
Inappropriate responses		

Kim, M. J., McFarland, G., & McLane, A. *Pocket Guide to Nursing Diagnosis* (2nd ed.). St. Louis: C.V. Mosby, 1987
McFarland, G. & Wasli, E. *Nursing Diagnosis and Process in Psychiatric Mental Health Nursing*. Philadelphia: J. B. Lippincott, 1984
Carpenito, L. *Handbook of Nursing Diagnosis*. Philadelphia: J. B. Lippincott, 1984

nosis of Altered Thought Process and Sensory-Perceptual Alterations and uses etiological factors to distinguish between the two categories.[29]

Another way to distinguish between these two nursing diagnoses might be to view altered thoughts as faulty interpretation of *internal* stimuli, while altered perceptions are seen as faulty interpretation of *external* stimuli; however, even the experienced clinician, who is skilled at recognizing signs and symptoms associated with delirium, dementia, or functional psychosis, may have difficulty deciding how to group patient data to determine which of these two nursing diagnoses to make. Furthermore, the broad, abstract nature of these nursing diagnostic categories does not offer much, if any, patient specific direction for nursing intervention than do the medical diagnoses of schizophrenia or organic mental disorder, for example.

In addition to choosing which of these two nursing diagnoses to use, another significant problem that nurses face in the clinical application of Altered Thought Process and Sensory-Perceptual Alterations is the determination of the etiology component for specific patients. Few of the suggested etiology statements for these nursing diagnoses provide direction for nursing intervention. (See Table 12–6.) A useful nursing diagnosis must name human responses amenable to nursing treatment. Many of the etiology statements listed, such as biochemical changes, genetic predisposition, and chemical alterations, lie more in the realm of medical practice than nursing practice. Academically or theoretically speaking, these etiological labels do name causes or contributing factors of altered thought and perceptions. In terms of clinical application for nursing practice, however, etiology determination for Altered Thought Process or Sensory-Perceptual Alterations is quite complex and of limited value.

An example is helpful at this point. Consider a young woman with a medical diagnosis of schizophrenia and a history of physically abusive behavior when threatened. She appears withdrawn, seclusive, frightened, and is talking to someone not in the room. During a patient group, she runs out of the room yelling, "They are all talking about me!" She refuses all liquids, stating, "That drink is poison." Her skin is dry, and her urine is concentrated. Orthostatic hypotension is observed, and her serum sodium is elevated. When approached by staff or other patients, she steps backwards and shouts, "Get away from me! Don't come any closer!"

What should the nursing diagnoses for this patient be? Clearly, Altered Thought Process can be considered, but what etiology statement could be identified? Altered Thought Process related to schizophrenia? Altered Thought Process related to neurochemical imbalance? Altered Thought Process related to ineffective coping? How can the nurse determine the cause of the altered thinking pattern? Why even try? These nursing diagnostic statements would give very few clues as to appropriate nursing interventions for this particular patient. A useful nursing diagnosis in this situation should direct the nurse to assist this patient with her individual responses to the health problem of schizophrenia.

The nursing diagnosis Altered Thought Process seems too broad and abstract to be helpful to the nurse who must care for this patient in day-to-day clinical practice. Finding an etiology or contributing factor for the altered thought process further complicates the diagnostic decision and lies more in the realm of medical practice. When nurses in clinical practice settings do make a diagnosis of altered thoughts and perceptions, often a defining characteristic is listed as the etiology. For example, Altered Thought Process related to auditory hallucinations, is used frequently in practice. This diagnostic statement, although more patient-specific, does not provide direction for individualized nursing interventions for the patient.

This scenario points out the need to identify and classify more discrete subcategories within this nursing diagnostic category of Taxonomy I. Although there is value in naming more specific subsets of these two nursing diagnoses in terms of naming the specific phenomena of

TABLE 12–6. ALTERED THOUGHT PROCESS AND SENSORY-PERCEPTUAL ALTERATIONS ETIOLOGIES NOTED BY VARIOUS AUTHORS

Altered Thought Process		
Kim McFarland McLane	McFarland Wasli	Carpenito

Physiological changes
Psychologic conflicts
Loss of memory
Impaired judgment
Sleep deprivation
	Genetic factor
	Neurotransmitter dysfunction
	Developmental stage fixation
	Anxiety
	Crisis,maturational or situational
	Central nervous system dysfunction
	Chemical alteration
	Aging process
	Trauma
	Sleep deprivation
	Negative thought patternings
		Pathophysiological
		  Personality and mental disorders related to alteration in biochemical compounds
		  Genetic disorder
		Situational
		  Depression or anxiety
		  Substance abuse (alcohol, drugs)
		  Fear of the unknown
		  Actual loss (of control, routine, income, significant others, familiar object, or surroundings)
		  Emotional trauma
		  Rejection or negative appraisal by others
		  Negative response from others
		  Isolation
		Maturation
		  Adolescent: peer pressure, conflict
		  Elderly: Isolation

Sensory-Perceptual Alterations		
Kim McFarland McLane	McFarland Wasli	Carpenito

Environmental factors
  Therapeutically restricted environments (isolation, intensive care, bedrest, traction, confining illnesses, incubator)
  Socially restricted environment (institutionalization, home-bound, aging, chronic illness, dying, infant deprivation); stigmatized (mentally ill, mentally retarded, mentally handicapped); bereaved
Altered sensory reception, transmission, and/or integration
  Neurologic disease, trauma, or deficit
	Altered stimuli, excessive or insufficient
	Altered sensory reception, transmission, and/or integration (i.e., pain, sleep deprivation, diseases affecting neurological system, problems in communication such as language differences, normal aging processes)
	Chemical alterations (i.e., electrolyte imbalances, lack of oxygen in blood and other alterations blood composition, CNS stimulants, depressants, hallucinogens)
	Psychological stress
	Brain dysfunction
		Pathophysiological
		  Sensory organ alterations (visual, gustatory, hearing, olfactory, and tactile deficits)
		  Neurologic-alterations
		  Cerebrovascular accident (CVA)
		  Neuropathies
		  Encephalities meningitis
		  Metabolic alteration
		  Fluid and electrolyte imbalance
		  Elevated blood area nitrogen (BUN)
		  Acidosis
		  Alkalosis
		  Impaired oxygen transport

(continued)

TABLE 12—6. (Continued)

Sensory-Perceptual Alterations

Kim McFarland McLane	McFarland Wasli	Carpenito
Altered status of sense organs Inability to communicate, understand, speak, or respond Sleep deprivation Pain Chemical alteration Endogenous (electrolyte imbalance, elevated BUN, elevated ammonia or hypoxia) Exogenous (central nervous system stimulants or depressants, mind-altering drugs) Psychologic stress (narrowed perceptual fields caused by anxiety)		Cerebral, cardiac Respiratory, Anemia Musculoskeletal changes Paraplegia Quadriplegia Amputation Situational Medications (sedatives, tranquilizers) Surgery (glaucoma, cataract, detached retina) Social isolation (terminal, or infectious patient) Physical isolation (reverse isolation, communicable disease, prison) Radiation therapy Immobility Pain Stress Environment (noise pollution) Mobility restrictions (bedrest, traction, casts, Stryker flame, Circoelectric bed) Biorythm alterations (travel, shift-work, hospitalization, special care units [cardiac, trauma, burn]) Substance abuse (alcohol, drugs) Different culture or language Maturational Infant/child: Maternal deprivation, excessive stimulation Elderly: Hearing or vision loss, gustatory/olfactory deficits, decreased potential for tactile stimulation, isolation, custodial care

Kim, M. J., McFarland, G., & McLane, A. *Pocket Guide to Nursing Diagnosis* (2nd ed.). St. Louis: C.V. Mosby, 1987
McFarland, G. & Wasli, E. *Nursing Diagnosis and Process in Psychiatric Mental Health Nursing*. Philadelphia: J. B. Lippincott, 1984
Carpenito, L. *Handbook of Nursing Diagnosis*. Philadelphia: J. B. Lippincott, 1984

concern to nursing, problems with practical application would remain. Again, the issues lie with etiology determination.

For example, "auditory hallucinations" describes a specific, more concrete altered thought pattern. But how would the nurse identify the causative or contributing factors for the individual patient's auditory hallucinations? At times, this kind of diagnostic process may be possible. When such data exist, the altered thoughts and perceptions diagnoses can be made effectively. For example, the nursing diagnosis Sensory-Perceptual Alterations related to sensory overload has been suggested by Carpenito,[30] and this nursing diagnosis clearly identifies a problem within the realm of nursing practice. In many situations, however, the nurse may be unable to identify a contributing factor for the thought or perception that is amenable to nursing intervention. In these instances, using these two nursing diagnoses may not be the most effective approach.

A more concrete nursing diagnosis of Sensory-Perceptual Overload[31] has been proposed. This label, when combined with the suggested etiology statements such as bombardment with tasks, persistent auditory stimulation, and decisional overload, may provide clear and useful direction for nursing intervention for certain patients.

A proposed solution for the difficulties found in using the nursing diagnoses Altered Thought Process and Sensory-Perceptual Alterations takes the diagnostic thinking process one step beyond the alterations to identify the specific human responses to the thought or perceptual problem. In this approach, nursing diagnostic labels are chosen according to the data that represent the patient's unique response to the altered thoughts and perceptions, such as Potential for Injury, Impaired Social Interaction, Fear, Fluid Volume Deficit, Potential for Violence, or Potential for Intentional Self-Harm. Furthermore, labels such as Suspiciousness or Visual Hallucinations, which refer to more discrete categories within the altered thought process and sensory-perceptual alterations, may be used more effectively to name contributing factors rather than the nursing diagnostic label, unless there are other etiological factors that can be identified and treated with nursing intervention.

Returning to the young woman with schizophrenia, described earlier, instead of making a nursing diagnosis of Altered Thought Process or Sensory-Perceptual Alterations, the data might be clustered in a different fashion (see Table 12–7) to reach nursing diagnoses that are clinically descriptive and prescriptive. These nursing diagnoses provide the nurse with clear

TABLE 12–7. ALTERNATIVE NURSING DIAGNOSES FOR A PATIENT WITH SCHIZOPHRENIA

Clustering of the Data	Alternative Nursing Diagnosis
History of physically aggressive behavior when threatened *"You are trying to poison me!"* *Upon approach, yells: "Get away from me . . ."*	*Potential for Violence: Other-Directed related to suspiciousness*
Dry skin, orthostatic hypotension, concentrated urine, elevated serum sodium *Refuses all liquids* *"You are trying to poison me!"*	*Fluid Volume Deficit related to suspiciousness of p.o. fluids*
Runs out of patient group screaming that: "They are all talking about me!" *Talks to someone not in room* *Withdrawn, seclusive*	*Impaired Social Interaction related to auditory hallucinations and suspiciousness*

direction to develop a practical and effective plan of nursing care. The nurse is able to identify priorities quickly and to communicate these to all health care providers involved with this patient. Several human response patterns are addressed by using the disordered thought as an etiology rather than the problem component of the nursing diagnostic label. In this approach, the nursing diagnosis directs the nursing staff to focus on various aspects of daily living that, for this particular patient, are affected by the thought disorder.

Consider another example of a patient in an intensive care unit experiencing multiple metabolic disturbances that have resulted in delirium. This patient is a 68-year-old man recovering from abdominal surgery. He misperceives objects and persons in the environment, and he is disoriented to time and place. Sometimes he is lethargic, while at other times he becomes very restless. Both blood pressure and heart rate are elevated. He frequently calls out for protection against "strange men" in his room. Despite the nurses' attempts to reorient him to his surroundings and their constant reminders not to pull out his tubes, he frequently tries to pull out his IV and remove his nasogastric tube.

For this patient, nursing diagnoses of Sensory-Perceptual Alterations: Visual or Acute Reversible Confusion[32] could be considered in the differential diagnostic process. But what etiologies could be identified? A specific electrolyte imbalance? Hypoxia? Drug toxicity? If these are, indeed, the etiological factors, does not this diagnostic question fall more correctly within the realm of medical practice? A more useful approach, consistent with the goals of nursing diagnosis, is to cluster this patient's data in the manner presented in Table 12–8.

The nursing diagnoses Fear related to misperception of the environment and Potential for Injury related to short-term memory impairment alert the nurse to this patient's specific responses that require nursing intervention. Nursing intervention aimed at decreasing the fear by providing clear explanations of the external stimuli and minimizing the stimuli whenever possible are helpful. Reality orientation, using both verbal and visual cues can augment the patient's memory and assist him in interpreting the environment around him. The nurse is also guided by the second nursing diagnosis to institute special precautions to prevent injury such as wrist restraints and frequent observations of the patient.

These two patient examples demonstrate how the more discrete nursing diagnostic labels provide more direction for the practicing nurse in the acute-care setting. The diagnostic process is useful only when it leads to the clear description of patient conditions and appropri-

TABLE 12–8. ALTERNATIVE NURSING DIAGNOSES FOR A DELIRIOUS PATIENT

Clustering of the Data	Alternative Nursing Diagnoses
Restless	Fear related to misperception of the environment
Increased BP, heart rate	
Frequent calls for help	
"Strange men"	
Misperceives objects, people	
Disoriented to time, place	Potential for Injury related to short-term memory impairment
Attempts to pull tube, IVs despite frequent reminders	
Unable to follow directions	
Lethargic at times	

ate prescription of nursing interventions to treat the identified conditions. Furthermore, the approach presented here to the diagnosis of altered thoughts and perceptions can do much to assist novice diagnosticians in making clinically accurate and useful nursing diagnoses for this patient population, and that can be a very effective implementation strategy in the psychiatric setting.

Problems with the determination of appropriate, useful nursing diagnoses for patients with altered thoughts and perceptions should be anticipated during the implementation of nursing diagnosis in the psychiatric setting. Two other issues that may require specific implementation strategies are the reliance on protocols or standard plans for this group of patients and the time required for the development of diagnostic skill in a specialty area.

Some nurses may experience a hesitancy to give up reliance on standard care plans or textbook guidelines for the care of certain groups of patients. Guidelines for care of the hallucinating patient, the delusional patient, or the manic patient are valuable resources and serve as foundations for psychiatric nursing practice; but, they direct care for groups of patients not individual patients. A nursing diagnosis is formulated to direct care for an individual patient. A strategy for this situation is to focus on how those guidelines can be made specific for a particular patient.

Finally, a definite time for nurses to develop diagnostic thinking skills should be provided. During implementation it is important to recognize that diagnostic decisions regarding the responses of psychiatric patients are quite complex for the novice as well as the expert nurse. Much of the expert nurse's planning and thinking about patients is often embedded in the nurse's learned intuition about patients.[33] Since many psychiatric nurses have experience with large numbers of patients with some sort of altered mental status or psychosis, they may intuitively or automatically evaluate a suspicious patient's social interaction, nutritional state, fluid balance, and the potential risk the patient poses to self or to others. New graduates or advanced beginners,[34] on the other hand, do not have this experiential knowledge-base to use in clinical thinking. As a result of their recent educational experience, however, nursing diagnosis terminology and concepts may be more familiar.

Freedom to practice and experiment with nursing diagnosis prior to formal expectations should minimize the fear often associated with change. Change to nursing diagnosis will be more successful if individual nurses support the change and feel comfortable with their skills before implementation is mandated. Table 12–9 summarizes the implementation strategies suggested for the unfreezing phase of the change process.

CHANGE

Once nurses begin to show interest and some beginning skill in diagnostic thinking, an official implementation date can be set. A formal educational activity should be provided at this point

TABLE 12–9. UNFREEZING IMPLEMENTATION STRATEGIES

1. *Identify a change agent who is a clinical expert with diagnostic skills and who is familiar with work of NANDA.*
2. *Desensitize staff to idea of new definitions of nursing and nursing diagnosis.*
3. *Saturate environment with nursing diagnostic terminology.*
4. *Begin with highest priority nursing diagnoses.*
5. *Creatively explore etiology for use with psychiatric patients.*
6. *Allow structured time for nurses to develop diagnostic thinking skills prior to administrative expectations for implementation.*

TABLE 12–10. OBJECTIVES FOR INTRODUCTORY PROGRAM ON NURSING DIAGNOSIS FOR PSYCHIATRIC NURSES

The learner will:

1. *Define nursing in the psychiatric setting as the diagnosis and treatment of human responses to actual or potential health problems*
2. *List the nine human response patterns in Taxonomy I*
3. *Explain the concept of nursing diagnosis/DMSIII diagnosis*
   - *Define nursing diagnosis with attention to the differentiation between nursing diagnosis and medical diagnosis/DSMIII diagnosis*
   - *Describe the relationship of nursing diagnosis to the nursing process*
   - *Describe the nursing diagnostic format of problem, etiology, and defining characteristics*
   - *Discuss common pitfalls of using nursing diagnosis in the psychiatric setting*
4. *Discuss the historical development of nursing diagnosis*
5. *Identify the uses and value of nursing diagnosis in the nursing care of psychiatric patients*
6. *Demonstrate beginning level skills in the recognition and formulation of nursing diagnoses*
7. *Demonstrate beginning level skills in the clinical application of NANDA's Taxonomy I nursing diagnoses for the psychiatric patient*
8. *Use nursing diagnosis to articulate the unique role of the nurse in the psychiatric setting*

to develop a consistent knowledge-base for nursing diagnosis. A set of objectives for such an educational program has been presented by Field.[35] Educational objectives for nurses working in the psychiatric setting are presented in Table 12–10.

Diagnostic Consultation and Decision Making

Following the formal instruction, the resource person should continue to be available on the unit for consultation regarding diagnostic decisions. Immediate reinforcement of the content with actual patients on the unit is essential and enhances learning while demonstrating clinical value.

Frequent patient-care conferences to enhance diagnostic-thinking skills should be held. The resource person may facilitate the group process by stimulating the group to list and cluster patient data in order to make diagnostic decisions. Tolerance for diagnostic dilemmas may be enhanced by reiterating that there are no absolutes at this stage of nursing diagnosis development.

Nurses can feel frustrated when they realize that their diagnostic questions do not always have clear-cut answers or that labels have not yet been identified to name some of their patients' problems. It is important to allow flexibility and assist nurses to try out different diagnostic labels and etiologies without the fear of being "wrong."

Nurses will need help naming phenomena they are familiar with in nursing diagnostic language. The strategy of confronting head-on the issues related to diagnosing altered thoughts and perceptions plays a critical role at this point. If confusion is present about the approach to making nursing diagnoses for this aspect of psychiatric nursing, major problems with the implementation process can result.

Sometimes nurses may identify phenomena of concern that they elect not to treat. At times, problems such as suspiciousness or short-term memory impairment may be observed in a patient, but this finding cannot be clustered with other relevant data. The identified phenomenon may be an important clinical finding that requires continued assessment, observation, documentation, or referral. In the event that this finding has an effect on the patient's functional ability, then it would be useful to formulate a nursing diagnosis to describe the patient's response. An example might be Self Care Deficit: Feeding related to short-term memory impairment.

Administrative Support

Change to a diagnosed-based psychiatric nursing practice model requires significant administrative support. Crucial to such an organizational change are certain administrative actions that facilitate professional nursing practice. This aspect of implementation *must not* be overlooked.

Administrative expectations regarding the role of the registered nurse within the nursing process must be clearly defined. Significant changes in assignment patterns may need to be made in order to allow the registered nurse the time for effective nursing diagnosis and treatment planning. Managers may need to redefine the roles of all members of the nursing staff in order to facilitate nursing diagnosis activities. The message must be clear that nursing diagnosis and treatment planning are highly valued and that unit systems and staff functions will be organized in order to achieve their successful completion. (See Chapter 6 for a complete discussion of practice models in relation to nursing diagnosis.)

Diagnosis should be incorporated into all clinical systems such as patient-care conferences, reports, rounds, and team meetings during this phase. The resource person needs to initiate and maintain these new diagnosis-based practice systems through role-modeling behaviors and lots of positive feedback for individual nurse participation. Formal evaluation criteria also may include development of nursing diagnosis skills and participation in the change process. Table 12–11 summarizes the necessary steps in the actual change phase to nursing diagnosis.

REFREEZING

The refreezing phase, in the planned change to nursing diagnosis, involves strategies designed to maintain or solidify the use of nursing diagnoses in daily care-planning activities and to proceed towards a truly diagnosis-based practice model. Nurses must perceive that their care-planning time is both valued and rewarded for the desired change in behavior to take hold. "The pattern of using nurses as interchangeable bodies on a shift in order to get work done does not foster nurses valuing nursing diagnosis."[36]

Purposeful linkage of nurses to patients must be maintained and rewarded for the kind of accountability inherent in the diagnostic process to develop. As mentioned earlier, primary nursing, team nursing, and case-management models of nursing practice with direct linking of RNs to specific patients supports adequate accountability.

Lack of continued reinforcement for the use of nursing diagnosis often interferes with the refreezing phase. Young and Lucas describe how continuous and intermittent reinforcement schedules in combination may result in nurses both learning the nursing diagnostic process more quickly and the change lasting longer.[37] Nurse managers should not only consistently reward staff nurses for their diagnostic efforts during the initial implementation period, but

---

TABLE 12–11. CHANGING PHASE IMPLEMENTATION STRATEGIES

1. *Present a formal education program.*
2. *Assure the availability of a resource person/role model in day-to-day practice to help facilitate the diagnostic process.*
3. *Work in groups to improve diagnostic thinking skills and to identify diagnostic labels and etiologies for psychiatric patients.*
4. *Build nursing diagnosis into all unit clinical systems.*
5. *Demonstrate administrative support for the change to nursing diagnosis by establishing systems in which diagnostic thinking may occur.*

also should provide intermittent rewards on an ongoing basis. The power of a simple comment from a head nurse like, "What nursing diagnoses are you working on today?" should not be overlooked.

The unit systems adopted in the changing phase to promote nursing diagnoses must be developed further. Clear guidelines for the use of nursing diagnosis in report, patient-care conferences, and team meetings could be written and implemented to help solidify the new diagnosis-based practice model. Job descriptions and performance evaluation criteria should be modified to reflect the value placed on professional nurses' diagnostic skills. Indeed, Gordon suggests:

> if the central focus of professional practice is nursing diagnosis and treatment, the major factor in a primary nurse's hiring, retention, and performance-review and merit salary increases should be the level of competency in diagnosis and treatment.[38]

While this quotation is framed within the context of primary nursing, the sentiment holds true for any model of nursing practice when diagnosis-based nursing practice is used. (See Chapter 5 for further discussion of job description criteria and related issues in diagnosis-based nursing practice.)

Taxonomy I

The introduction of NANDA's Taxonomy I is recommended during the refreezing phase in the change process. After nurses have gained a certain level of competence with diagnostic decision making, exposure to the classification system serves to clarify the importance and scope of nursing diagnosis for the nursing profession. The sense that nurses who use nursing diagnosis in actual practice are involved in developing the future knowledge-base for the profession serves as a strong motivator and reinforcer of change.

Time for structured group work to determine solutions to diagnostic dilemmas is imperative at all stages of the change process. Nurses in practice need time to experiment with newly accepted diagnoses as well as to develop labels not yet identified and classified. Psychiatric nurses who focus on a specific groups of patients, such as adolescents, geriatric patients, and those with personality disorders, should join efforts to answer remaining questions.

The resource person should be available to assist nurses to expand to other less concrete nursing diagnoses such as Self-concept Disturbance, Grieving, Powerlessness. As nurses begin to make diagnoses in all the human response patterns, the benefit to the patients should become more evident through successful care-planning activities and serve to reinforce their efforts. Staff nurses may need help applying newly accepted nursing diagnoses as they are approved by NANDA.

Educate Other Nursing Staff Members and Other Disciplines

Also during the refreezing phase, efforts should continue to explain the development of the nursing diagnosis classification system to other nursing staff members and other disciplines. It might be wise to assume that other disciplines may be thinking nursing diagnosis means "nurses making medical diagnoses." Simple terms should explain the difference: "Doctors treat disease. Nurses treat the response to disease." It is, however, not that simple.

Psychiatric nurses play an important role on the psychiatric treatment team. As the size of this team has increased, the boundaries between the professional roles of the team members, including psychiatrists, psychologists, social workers, occupational therapists, and, of course, nurses, have become blurred. The introduction of nursing diagnosis into the care plan can create role confusion and discomfort among team members. For the nurse, the result of

TABLE 12–12. REFREEZING PHASE IMPLEMENTATION STRATEGIES

1. *Set up administrative rewards for nursing diagnosis skills.*
2. *Introduce Taxonomy I.*
3. *Structure time for group diagnostic thinking.*
4. *Expand to nursing diagnoses in all nine human response patterns.*
5. *Educate other disciplines about nursing diagnosis.*
6. *Expect documentation of nursing diagnoses and care plans in the patient record.*

this situation may be feelings of vulnerability when faced with the challenge of defending the nursing role.

The treatment of the patient with anxiety illustrates the role confusion that can occur with the introduction of nursing diagnosis. The diagnostic label of anxiety can be found in both the DSMIII and Taxonomy I. Who has the responsibility for this diagnosis? While there are no easy answers for this question, strategies for dealing with this complex situation include defining clearly the purposes of nursing diagnosis, negotiation of goals and interventions for patient problems with shared accountability, and sensitivity and professional courtesy on all sides.

In addition to the multidisciplinary treatment team, other nursing staff members, such as LPNs, nursing assistants, or psychiatric technicians, require a more in-depth explanation of nursing diagnosis since they are responsible for following through on the care plans developed by the registered nurse. If the RNs have successfully learned to develop plans of care that are patient specific, practical, and achievable, then nursing diagnosis should sell itself. Plans developed to treat nursing diagnoses will provide much more direction for these care givers than previous plans that were less patient specific.

Documentation

A very effective refreezing strategy is the administrative expectation that registered nurses document their nursing diagnoses in their patients' records. Certain formats have been suggested in the literature and are described in Chapter 7.

When nurses must document against their own diagnoses in the progress notes, incentives to identify accurate, useful, and practical nursing diagnoses develop. In other words, the nursing diagnoses and care plans must effectively direct the nursing care of the patient, which is after all the whole idea!

The use of nursing diagnoses in documentation of nursing care is one more step to a diagnosis-based nursing practice model, but this involves certain theoretical problems that must not be overlooked. Young and Lucas[39] point out how the nurse risks being perceived by others as "wrong" when documentation of nursing diagnoses occurs. Again, the resource person is an invaluable consultant to provide validation and support for novice diagnosticians. Table 12–12 summarizes the steps in the refreezing phase of nursing diagnoses implementation in the psychiatric setting.

CONCLUSION

Implementation of diagnosis-based nursing practice involves considerable change in the way nurses think, view their roles, and organize nursing care delivery. Fortunately, psychiatric nurses have experience in diagnostic thinking. The beauty of nursing diagnosis is that it enables the psychiatric nurse to move from the medical model approach to diagnosis to a nursing model of naming the individual human responses to health problems. Experience with the DSMIII should ease the transition to the diagnosis of the phenomena of unique concern to nursing.

Strategies for the implementation of nursing diagnosis in the psychiatric setting are presented and organized according to Lewin's framework for planned change. Suggestions for how to change knowledge, attitudes, individual behavior, and organizational behavior in order to effect a significant organizational change are noted throughout the chapter.

Patient examples demonstrate how to effectively apply the nursing diagnoses currently classified within NANDA's Taxonomy I to psychiatric patient problems. Nursing diagnosis offers psychiatric nurses a way to communicate unique aspects of their roles in a specialty area where professional roles are often blurred. With the implementation of nursing diagnosis, too, comes patient-specific, nurse-directive care plans. The overwhelmingly complex and often quite abstract problems that psychiatric patients frequently present can be clearly defined.

Nursing diagnosis is still relatively new and more work is needed to identify the phenomena of concern for psychiatric nurses, but this early stage of nursing diagnosis development should not impede implementation. In fact, implementation is the very path through which more effective nursing diagnoses for all specialty areas will emerge. The time to implement a diagnosis-based psychiatric nursing practice model is now. Nursing diagnosis is not merely a new way for psychiatric nurses to think about patient problems, but an effective way to actualize what has always been nursing.

REFERENCES

1. Williams, J.B.W., & Watson, H.S. A psychiatric nursing perspective on DSM-III. *Journal of Psychosocial Nursing and Mental Health Services,* 1982, 14
2. American Nurses' Association. *Nursing: A social policy statement,* Kansas City: American Nurses' Association, 1980, p.9
3. Gordon, M. Nursing diagnosis and the diagnostic process. *American Journal of Nursing,* 1976, *76,* 8, 1299
4. Thomas, M.D. et al. Nursing diagnosis of depression. *Journal of Psychosocial Nursing and Mental Health Services,* 1986, 6
5. *Ibid*
6. North American Nursing Diagnosis Association. *Nursing Diagnosis Taxonomy I.* 1986
7. McFarland, G., & Wasli, E. *Nursing diagnosis and process in psychiatric mental health nursing.* Philadelphia: J.B. Lippincott, 1986
8. American Nurses' Association Council of Psychiatric Mental Health Nurses. *Taxonomy of phenomenon of concern to psychiatric mental health nurses.* 1986
9. American Nurses' Association. A social policy statement
10. Lewin, K. Frontiers in group dynamics: Concept, method and reality in social sciences; social equilibrium and social change. *Human Relations,* 1947, *1,* 1, 5
11. Mereness, D.A., & Taylor, C.M. *Essentials of psychiatric nursing.* St. Louis: C.V. Mosby, 1978, p.6
12. Carnevali D. *Nursing care planning: Diagnosis and management* (3rd ed.). Philadelphia: Lippincott, 1983,
13. Hersey, P. & Blanchard, K. *Management of organizational behavior* (4th ed.). Englewood Cliffs, N.J.: Prentice-Hall, 1982
14. Lewin
15. Young, M.S., & Lucas, C.M. Nursing diagnosis: Common problems in implementation. *Topics in Clinical Nursing,* 1984, *5,* 4, 70
16. Gordon, M. *Nursing diagnosis: Process and application.* New York: McGraw-Hill, 1982,
17. McFarland & Wasli
18. Folstein, M.F., Folstein, S.E., & McHugh, P.R. Mini-mental state, a practical method for grading the cognitive state of patients for the clinician. *Journal of Psychiatric Research,* 1975, *12,* 189
19. Field, L. The implementation of nursing diagnosis in clinical practice. *Nursing Clinics of North America,* 1979, *14,* 3, 498
20. *Ibid*
21. Benner, P. *From novice to expert.* Menlo Park, CA: Addison-Wesley, 1984,
22. Field
23. American Nurses' Association. *A social policy statement*
24. Kim, M.J., McFarland, G.K., & McLane, A.M. *Pocket guide to nursing diagnoses* (2nd ed.). St. Louis: C.V. Mosby, 1987
25. Gordon, M. The concept of nursing diagnosis. *American Journal of Nursing,* 1979, *79,* 9, 490

26. Carnevali

27. Field

28. Thompson, J. et al. *Clinical nursing.* St. Louis: C.V. Mosby, 1986

29. Carpenito, L.J. Altered thoughts or altered perceptions? *American Journal of Nursing,* 1985, *85,* 5, 1283

30. *Ibid*

31. Gettrust, K., Ryan, S., & Engelman, D.S. *Applied nursing diagnosis: Guides for comprehensive care planning.* New York: John Wiley and Sons, 1986

32. *Ibid*

33. Benner

34. *Ibid*

35. Field

36. Carnevali, D. Nursing diagnosis: An evolutionary view. *Topics in Clinical Nursing,* 1984, *5,* 4, 16

37. Young & Lucas

38. Gordon, M. Implementation of nursing diagnoses: An overview. *Nursing Clinics of North America,* 1987, *22,* 4, 877

39. Young & Lucas

CHAPTER 13

Implementing Nursing Diagnosis in Critical Care

Sherry Williams Fox

In the critical care unit, the nurse must take responsibility for the unique aspects of nursing practice as well as working collaboratively with the health care team.[1] The interdisciplinary teamwork required in this area demands clarity of roles and responsibilities in order to achieve the best outcome for the patient. Accomplishing this clarity of roles is challenging, however, as the distinctions in roles can be very subtle.

Distinguishing the contributions of the critical care nurse, within the context of the health care team, is a challenge that must be met in order to establish diagnosis-based nursing practice in the critical care area. Additional challenges arise from the characteristics of critical care nurses, the patients for whom they care, and the environment in which critical care nurses function.

Characteristics of the Critical Care Nurse

The essence of critical care nursing is often thought to be a function of the specialized environment and advanced technology. While these factors are important influences on the practice of critical care nursing, they do not explain its unique character. Rather the essence of critical care nursing lies in the decision-making process of the nurse, coupled with a willingness to act upon those decisions.[2]

The critical care nurse must be knowledgeable, motivated, independent, and decisive. These characteristics are necessary for the nurse to work within the rapidly changing critical care area. The decisions made in critical situations require a degree of speed and decisiveness rarely found in other health care settings. The critical care nurse must be adept at integrating information and establishing priorities in order to meet this challenge.[3]

Making nursing diagnostic and treatment decisions in this setting is complicated by three factors: the speed with which these decisions must be made; the data available for making these decisions, often too little or too much; and a lack of awareness of how the data were used to make the decisions. These factors are important considerations in determining the implementation strategies for nursing diagnosis in critical care.

The Critical Care Patient Population

This group is unique as compared to other settings, and this presents a number of challenges in defining nursing problems. The degree of physiologic instability can be astounding. When illness strikes one body system, the other systems rally in an effort to cope with the disequilibrium, and the physiologic state becomes more complex.[4] This physiologic complexity maybe compounded by the existence of significant psychological and even social problems. As biopsychosocial complexity increases, length of stay can increase that may lead to iatrogenic problems.

As a result of the advancing skills of pre-hospital providers and advances in medicine, patients are surviving longer to get to the acute care hospital. They bring complex problems in larger numbers. Along with this, the rising pressure to control health care cost has lead to an emphasis on discharging patients sooner. It has become imperative for nurses to be able to rapidly and correctly identify problems and solve them in order to send patients home in a maximum state of wellness.

The Critical Care Environment

The third and final challenge in delineating the unique role of nursing is the high-tech—high-touch critical care environment. Technology continues to increase at an amazing rate. The nurse must stay abreast of these advances, deal with the data that the technology provides, and in the midst of the instrumentation maintain a focus on the responses of the patient as an individual.[5]

ISSUES IN THE USE OF NURSING DIAGNOSIS IN CRITICAL CARE

Nursing diagnosis is a tool the critical care nurse can use to identify human responses and to provide quality care for individual patients. However, the identification of those human responses that are amenable to nursing intervention in the high-tech—high-touch environment of the Intensive Care Unit (ICU) is complicated by the highly interdependent clinical practice in that setting. It is helpful to examine two issues at this point: the debate about physiologic nursing diagnoses and the interdependent clinical practice in the critical care area.

Physiologic nursing diagnoses pose a number of questions for the critical care nurse. The first aspect to be considered is the naming of a human response, once it has been identified. Use of the names of actual diseases, disorders, or syndromes correctly falls within the practice of medicine. The diagnostic language of nursing is still evolving, and, for those nursing diagnoses that describe physiologic problems, the clarity and descriptiveness of these diagnostic labels is sometimes less than optimal. Furthermore, this issue of physiologic nursing diagnoses is fraught with controversy.

The debate about the use of physiologic nursing diagnoses is organized around two major positions. One states that these problems must be referred to the physician or managed under medical protocol and are not amenable to nursing intervention.[6] The other side of the argument is that physiologic nursing diagnoses are *not* medical diagnoses renamed, but that these nursing diagnoses describe issues which are not the unique domain of medicine.[7] An important consideration is that most nurses are practicing in settings where physiologic alterations are a major focus of nursing care. To exclude these from the nursing diagnostic realm, especially in critical care, would place a significant restriction on the ability of nurses in that environment to make nursing diagnoses.[8,9]

One strategy for dealing with physiologic problems is the collaborative problem approach suggested by Carpenito. Collaborative problems are:

physiologic complications for which nurses use monitoring skills to detect onset or status so that nursing can collaborate with medicine to provide definitive treatment . . . When the nurse diagnoses a collaborative problem, the nurse confers with the physician regarding treatment.[10]

In effect, the focus of nursing activity in regard to collaborative problems is monitoring the disease-related condition of the patient rather than identifying unique human responses. Examples of collaborative problems using this approach are dysrhythmia, allergic reaction, and hemorrhage.[11]

This description of nurse-physician collaboration is a familiar one to nurses, and, indeed, collaboration is an important aspect of all nursing practice, not just critical care. The development of nursing diagnoses, however, as names for human responses requires an analytical and open-minded approach to the patient. By simply labeling physiologic problems in the manner suggested by Carpenito, this critical analysis of patient conditions may be inhibited or restricted. Such an examination of patient conditions is necessary to identify human responses that are relevant to the practice of nursing in general, and critical care nursing in particular. Only when patient conditions are clearly defined can nursing practice issues be defined; there is still much work to be done in this area.

The types of nursing interventions that are frequently found in critical care offer an alternative strategy for considering the issues of physiologic nursing diagnoses. Nursing interventions have traditionally been divided into three categories: dependent, independent, and interdependent. Dependent nursing interventions are those delegated medical functions ordered by the physician and not requiring exercise of nursing judgment in their execution. At the other end of the spectrum are independent interventions that are initiated by the nurse without consultation from other health care professionals including physicians. The last category, interdependent nursing interventions, fall somewhere in between these two positions. Interdependent nursing interventions are therapeutic actions performed by the nurse with reciprocal dependence on a physician or other health professional for the prescription of that action, including nursing judgments when carrying out physicians orders.[12]

While the majority of interventions for the patient in critical care are ordered by the physician, these often fall into the interdependent category in that they require a high degree of judgment by the nurse in their implementation. There are also a number of independent nursing interventions, based on professional nursing knowledge and judgment. It could also be argued that the physician is dependent upon the observations and analysis of data from clinical assessments and invasive monitoring that the ICU nurse provides! This makes carving out the unique contributions of nursing care a true challenge.

It is helpful to discuss an example of independent/interdependent nursing practice. Of concern to every critical care nurse is the physiologic phenomenon of hypoxia that can be a potential problem for any critically ill patient. Some of the diseases frequently associated with hypoxia are acute respiratory distress syndrome, sepsis, and pulmonary contusion.

Fortunately, there are numerous ways to determine the presence and degree of hypoxia in patients. Physical assessment can reveal the presence of hypoxia through changes in color of the skin and mucous membranes. Likewise, arterial blood gas measurements can reveal the presence and the precise degree of hypoxia. Several new methods are being used in critical care to provide continuous monitoring of oxygenation. These methods are pulse oximetry and mixed venous oxygen saturation (SvO_2) monitoring. Both methods can provide continuous data and allow the medical team to see minute-to-minute changes in oxygen saturation.

This continuous monitoring of data is particularly useful to the nurse at the bedside. The nurse can see the effects of activity, procedures, and other care on the patient. Based on these cues, the nurse can diagnose nursing problems and plan interventions.

For example, if the nurse caring for a patient with a left pulmonary contusion notes that O_2 saturation changes when the patient is turned on the left side, then a nursing diagnosis of Impaired Gas Exchange related to left side positioning can be made. Once this nursing diagnosis is made, nursing interventions can be planned to treat the problem, such as position changes from supine to right side only and continued correlation of changes in SvO_2 and patient activity. This demonstrates the independent role of the critical care nurse.

It can also be argued that interdependent nursing practice exists in this example. When the physician has ordered monitoring, drugs, or other therapeutic modalities to improve oxygenation, the nursing interventions are interdependent because the nurse is following an order to provide these therapies; however, the effective use of these treatments still depends on the high-level assessment and decision-making skills of the nurse. For example, narcotic medication may be ordered by the physician to facilitate mechanical ventilation and prevent the patient's resisting the ventilator because of pain. The nurse must exercise judgment and discretion as to the timing of medication administration based on available data from SvO_2 monitoring, assessment of the patient's respiratory function, and pain perception to provide a smooth level of pain control that contributes to effective ventilation and oxygenation.

BENEFITS OF NURSING DIAGNOSIS IN CRITICAL CARE

With so many issues unresolved, it is a challenge to implement nursing diagnosis in critical care. One important benefit that results from taking on this challenge is the contribution that the use of nursing diagnosis makes to the development of a professional nursing model. Indeed, the most important reason for changing from a medical model nursing practice to diagnosis-based nursing practice is to allow nursing to determine its practice.

"Historically, nurses have been held accountable for their actions, but have not had the autonomy to determine those actions."[13] Lack of autonomy is the most frequent reason cited in job satisfaction surveys for nurses leaving their jobs.[14] The concerns about autonomy and job satisfaction in critical care nursing are important factors in the clinical nursing practice environment. Examining ways that these issues affect nurses in critical care, or any nursing area, is an integral part of the implementation of nursing diagnosis and leads to increased professional autonomy.

Job satisfaction is a complex phenomenon. Two aspects have been identified that are relevant to this discussion: task identity and task significance are important components of job satisfaction.[15] The use of nursing diagnosis establishes nursing accountability for clearly identified problems through its focus on patient conditions and their treatment. As nurses use this focus, they are directed toward the most effective solutions for problems. As a result, nurses are able to achieve task identity by participating in a complete process as opposed to performing tasks with no direction or end goal.

Participating in the nursing diagnosis-directed process of naming and solving patient problems can also provide increased satisfaction, allowing the nurse to appreciate the significance of tasks performed. As each step is taken, the nurse can evaluate the effect of the solutions on the patient, thus providing immediate feedback and reward. If the process of planning and evaluating care is appropriately documented, then peers and supervisors can also recognize the contributions of the nurse.[16]

The nurse who makes a nursing diagnosis of Ineffective Airway Clearance related to thick secretions is acting in an autonomous manner. Once the diagnosis is made, there is an explicit accountability for identifying appropriate treatment for the patient and evaluating its effectiveness. When the care plan is carried out, by this nurse and other nurses who care for the patient, its effectiveness can be determined. If this evaluation does not take place, the progress of the patient cannot be determined, and movement toward desired goals will probably not occur.

The nurse who has made an accurate diagnosis and formulated a effective plan can receive the rewards of task identity and significance, improved patient status, and feedback from peers and colleagues. In the absence of a clearly identified nursing diagnosis and care plan, there can be little or no accountability for the improved state of the patient except on a short-term, shift-by-shift basis. Furthermore, without clearly defined accountability to make nursing diagnostic and treatment decisions, the progress of the patient can be difficult if not impossible to determine.

Critical care units cannot afford to ignore the issue of professional nursing practice, autonomy, and job satisfaction. In the face of today's nursing shortage, it is essential to recruit and retain experienced nurses to care for an increasingly complex group of patients. The implementation of nursing diagnosis in critical care shifts clinical thinking from an emphasis on tasks and diseases to the needs of the whole patient. Particularly in the critical care area, where nurses deal with tremendous amounts of data about the patient's condition, nursing diagnoses can provide a focus and a strategy for organizing clinical thinking and clinical practice that contributes both to professional nursing practice and the job satisfaction of nurses in the area.

While there are a number of benefits from implementing nursing diagnosis in critical care, there are other aspects that present serious challenges. One of the most difficult challenges is the familiarity, experience, and expertise that the critical care nurse has using the medical model for clinical thinking. Nurses in the critical care unit gain reinforcement, satisfaction, and support from the physician because they are skilled in assessing for medical problems, carrying out medical interventions, and reporting patient responses to medical therapy.[17] This reinforcement makes it difficult for the nurse to change focus.

The inability of the nurse to change from a disease focus to a nursing diagnosis-based focus may be evidenced in the desire to use medical diagnosis within the context of nursing diagnosis. Many nurses, well-ingrained in the medical model, use medical diagnosis as the etiology component of the nursing diagnosis. This is often an attempt to express their perceptions of nursing activity, limited by the mind-set and language of medicine. This use of the medical diagnosis as the etiology statement for nursing diagnoses has been described as an interim strategy in the implementation of nursing diagnosis. It appears to offer a bridge from medical model-based thinking to nursing diagnosis.[18] This can offer a way to assist critical care nurses in working with nursing diagnosis in the short run. The challenge, however, is moving from this interim strategy to identifying descriptive etiology statements that critical care nurses diagnose and treat.

Another difficulty that may surface as the change in accountability becomes apparent is an increase in concerns about legal issues. Nurses may believe that if the problem is not worded correctly that they could be sued; however, these fears are not supported by the current case law. (See Chapter 11 for a discussion of the legal issues of nursing diagnosis.)

A review of available literature indicates that the majority of legal claims against nurses are not scope of practice but the result of carelessness and poor communication with colleagues, physicians and patients. The best protection against legal claims is sound nursing judgment and adequate documents, two of the areas on which nursing diagnosis can have the most impact.[19]

Nurses have always been accountable for identifying patient problems. The use of nursing diagnoses to name these problems does not relieve the nurse of this responsibility, nor does it increase it. The nurse is still accountable for the accuracy and timeliness of problem identification. In a similar fashion, failure to identify a pertinent problem has legal implications whether or not nursing diagnosis is used.

The ability to use nursing diagnosis in critical care nursing practice is a skill and, like any skill, requires practice. In the initial phases of the implementation of nursing diagnosis, anxiety about these legal concerns will be present along with other issues. The careful selection and execution of strategies for the introduction of nursing diagnosis in critical care can do much to make the implementation of nursing diagnosis easier and more effective.

STRATEGIES FOR IMPLEMENTATION OF NURSING DIAGNOSIS IN CRITICAL CARE

The process for implementing nursing diagnosis in critical care is much like the nursing process used for patient problems. The implementation process is based on a well-defined philosophy and includes careful assessment, a well-developed plan, an implementation and action phase, and an ongoing evaluation of progress. (See Chapter 5 for a detailed discussion of the implementation process.)

Pre-implementation Issues and Assessment:

The first phase of the change process is unfreezing, where the target population and environment are prepared for change.[20] Beginning this process for the implementation of nursing diagnosis in critical care must include a careful assessment of the existing nursing practice systems and staff resources. Assessment is an essential part of the process as planning based on inaccurate information, misperceptions, or fantasy cannot succeed.

In the assessment of nursing practice systems, important aspects will be the behaviors of nurses in the critical care area as well as the results and outcomes of their practice. The model of nursing practice, routines for shift report, and the information networks of the unit are vitally important clinical practice systems. The behavior of nurses within these systems and their effectiveness must be scrutinized for those aspects that support diagnosis-based nursing practice. There are a variety of strategies available in terms of practice models or report routines. The decisions that are made about the clinical practice systems should be consistent with the philosophy and values of the unit.

A Philosophy for Implementation.   Before beginning the assessment phase for the implementation of nursing diagnosis, it is crucial to establish a well-defined philosophy of how nursing diagnosis will be utilized in the critical care area. This must be the first step. A well-defined philosophy is essential because there are many approaches to the use of nursing diagnosis, and a philosophy can be invaluable in guiding the decision-making process. For example, whether nursing diagnosis will be used only as a documentation format or become the foundation of nursing practice is a reflection of the philosophy guiding the implementation process.

Establishing a philosophy begins with a vision of what nursing practice can and should be, based on the values, beliefs, and attitudes toward nursing process and nursing diagnosis. Deciding upon a philosophy gives direction to the overall implementation process, but more importantly, it guides the assessment toward important cues in the environment. From this assessment, specific goals and outcome criteria for the change process can be determined, along with intervention strategies to accomplish them. Often times, the development of a philosophical foundation for the change process, as well as the change plan itself, can be enhanced by the use of a nursing theory or model.

Assessing Readiness for Change. What are the cues that a critical care area is ready or would benefit from the implementation of nursing diagnosis? Readiness for this change might be seen when critical care nurses express frustration with focusing only on diseases or machines, existing documentation formats that do not include nursing assessments and judgments along with the huge amounts of medical data, or the lack of consistency and follow-through on nursing care plans. This frustration may be verbally expressed; however, it may be seen in decreasing scores on documentation audits or high turnover rates if nurses become so frustrated that they leave the unit.

Other indicators that might suggest the readiness for implementation include frequent expressions of job dissatisfaction, blaming colleagues for problems, and distortion of communication networks. These all may be cues that this unit needs guidance in focusing on nursing practice issues. The communication network is an essential feature of an effective critical care unit. The volumes of patient information that must be communicated, and the serious consequences if this information is not accurately conveyed, make the issues of communication and information flow pressing ones for nurses in the critical care area.

An example of cues suggestive of a need for diagnosis-based nursing practice might be shift reports that fail to communicate pertinent patient information because they have become a forum for airing complaints. This might take the form of patient descriptions that are focused on machines and numbers instead of the unique individual. Another cue might be seen when nurses fail to relate to the family members of their patients, hiding during visiting periods or showing inflexibility and rigidity about rules and regulations that actually interfere with meeting patient needs. Requests for a different patient assignment every day, rather than efforts to promote continuity of care, can also indicate that a nursing staff could benefit from shifting the focus of the unit to a nursing model based on nursing diagnosis.

An important part of assessment is comparison of actual nursing practice to the philosophy statement. Consider example of the lack of congruence between the nursing philosophy and actual clinical nursing practice. The belief that all patients should have a complete assessment prior to development of the nursing care plan is a part of the professional philosophy of nursing. If the critical care nurse believes, however, that it is the written care plan document that is important, rather than individualized nursing care, then the nurse may believe that it is efficient to develop a nursing care plan in advance of the patient's arrival from the recovery room rather than waiting to assess the patient and formulate the plan based on that assessment. The driving philosophy, in effect, is efficiency from a time perspective rather than careful patient assessment based on the philosophy of individualized care planning.

Differences in nursing practice and philosophy should be identified. These areas are essential targets of the change process. Defining the philosophy of how nursing diagnosis will be used in critical care is paramount to a smooth implementation. It is the foundation on which the entire process will build.

One area to be clarified is the manner in which individual patient problems will be addressed. Should nurses be allowed to experiment with the wording of nursing diagnosis or should only accepted (NANDA*) diagnoses be used? Depending on the experience level of the staff with nursing diagnosis, it would be helpful to offer the NANDA list as a guideline or

---

*North American Nursing Diagnosis Association

starting point. Encourage nurses to experiment with wording to give them some control over their practice and to enhance the learning process. It must be recognized, however, that the approved NANDA list is in its early stages, and there are many areas where nursing diagnostic labels are lacking. Indeed, it is incumbent upon critical care nurses, who are working with the physiological human responses, to define and refine nursing diagnostic labels for submission to NANDA and ultimately for use in nursing practice.

In addition, it is very important to maintain the perspective that nursing diagnosis is evolving, especially in specialty care areas. Creativity and experimentation should be encouraged; however, this experimentation must be done within the accepted principles of nursing diagnosis (See Chapter 2) and clinical resources should be readily available.

Procedures, Protocols, and Nursing Diagnosis. A second area that must be clearly defined is the use of procedures and protocols or guidelines. The nursing diagnosis and related nursing interventions are designed to meet the unique needs of a particular patient. These must be distinguished from those routine interventions provided to all patients who require certain types of nursing care.

At this point it is helpful to consider an example of the use of procedures, protocols, and nursing diagnosis. (See Chapter 2 for a complete discussion of these directives for nursing care.) The needs of head-injured patients who may be unable to eat and require nasogastric feedings for nutritional support provides such an example. The procedure for giving a nasogastric tube feeding would be consistent from patient to patient. The protocol for providing nutritional support for head-injured patients will be specific for a given institution.

The nursing diagnoses for three different head-injured patients would depend upon the human responses that each of them demonstrated. For example, one might have a Potential for Injury related to confusion, another have a Self-Care Deficit related to left sided weakness, while Ineffective Airway Clearance related to thick secretions is the biggest problem for the third. Yet all three patients are receiving nasogastric feedings as a part of the nutritional support protocol for head-injured patients.

The question must be asked as to whether the nursing diagnosis Alteration in Nutrition should be made for these three patients. If the nasogastric tube feedings are providing adequate nutritional intake, then these patients do not have any alteration in their nutritional status and Alteration in Nutrition is an unnecessary nursing diagnosis. Nursing time is better spent on diagnosing and treating patient problems than in re-naming existing treatments. On the other hand, if the patients were not receiving adequate nutritional support, a nursing diagnosis of Alteration in Nutrition: Less than Body Requirements should be considered. Other nursing diagnoses that should be considered in the differential diagnosis process might include Fluid Volume Deficit, Self-Care Deficit: Feeding, Potential for Aspiration, and Impaired Swallowing.

Attitudes, Education, and Resources. In continuing the pre-implementation analysis, it is important to examine several other areas including staff attitudes toward nursing process, internal/external educational resources, the model of practice in the unit, and the documentation system.

Analysis of staff attitudes and values in relationship to nursing care planning and its effect on nursing practice can be extremely beneficial in planning the implementation of nursing diagnosis. An understanding of the attitudes and values of the staff is very useful in designing the unfreezing phase of the change process, and can be employed to enhance the driving forces for a change to diagnosis-based nursing practice, as well as minimizing any restraining forces. Areas that should be specifically examined include the nursing staff's attitudes and perceptions about the appropriate role of the medical model in directing nursing practice, the values of task accomplishment versus holistic patient care, and the role of the professional nurse.

An assessment of this type can be done using a formal survey or questionnaire or through discussion. A survey has the advantage of confidentiality, which may elicit more honest information than an open discussion, although many useful responses have been obtained through discussion. Furthermore, consideration should be given to repeating either strategy at regular intervals during the implementation process to continue to elicit feedback, ideas, and suggestions about the use of nursing diagnosis.

Another practice system to carefully consider is the educational system within the institution and within the unit. It is important to determine what systems exist for the sharing of new information within the unit. Examples of these might be the orientation for new staff, inservices, and patient care conferences. If these systems do not exist, then consider which ones might reasonably be added. If the systems do exist, then determine how they can be used to promote the implementation of nursing diagnosis.

Let us consider the orientation of new nurses to the critical care unit. A method for progressively incorporating nursing diagnosis into the existing orientation plan might include a number of strategies. An information-giving session to ensure that the orientee has the necessary information about nursing diagnosis might be a useful starting point. The next step would be the application of nursing diagnosis information in case studies and supervised clinical situations. During the first week of patient care experiences, the new nurse should focus on identifying one nursing diagnosis for each patient. This process of supervised, directed diagnostic thinking should continue until the orientee is able to select nursing diagnoses and etiologies and determine nursing interventions that are clinically accurate and relevant.

In addition to the actual educational systems, it is imperative to delineate resource persons. It may be helpful to ask, "Are there individuals on the staff who have had prior experience with nursing diagnosis who could be developed as a unit resource?" "How can clinical specialists be utilized to implement nursing diagnosis?" "How can the hospital or department education system be used to assist in educating staff about nursing diagnosis?"

Do not exclude outside educational resources. It can be very beneficial, if money and time exist, to employ a consultant to assist in beginning the implementation of nursing diagnosis. Valuable information and insight can also be obtained from attending workshops presented on local as well as national level.

Along with human resources, analysis of material resources and supports should not be forgotten. Look at what material support already exists for the implementation and what will need to be obtained. An important area to examine is the existence of written educational materials, such as books on nursing diagnosis, charts, posters, and other instructional materials. A new area for many nurses is computer-assisted instruction, which permits interactive learning between the learner and the automated educational content. The presence of protocols, policies, procedures that guide the use of nursing diagnosis, forms necessary to promote the actual documentation of nursing process, and any additional material supports such as monitors and computers to trend and store data should also be considered in a review of educational materials and systems. (See Chapter 9 for a discussion of nursing diagnosis and information systems).

The Model of Nursing Practice. The model of nursing practice is of extreme importance in the practice system assessment. A model of nursing practice defines the nursing care delivery systems for the unit. Ideally, the model used should reflect the institution's philosophy; furthermore, it should be one that allows the RN to have maximum contact with the patient.

Specific aspects of the model should address nurse-patient assignments, the use of nursing diagnosis and nursing care planning responsibilities, and the coordination of unit activities. Defined nursing practice models that are consistent with these requirements include primary nursing, total patient care, and the case management model.

Some of the professional nursing activities that should be included in a model of nursing practice for critical care include report strategies, patient assignment continuity, and coordination of patient admission and discharge from the unit. The report at the change of shift in the critical care unit should be given from care giver to care giver; this permits the most accurate transmission of information and encourages the communication of subtle data that might get lost if the report were channeled through the charge nurse, as well as providing an opportunity for shared assessment of clinical findings. Providing for continuity of nurse-patient assignments requires active coordination of nurses' schedules as well as daily assignments, and often this will fall to the nurse manager to provide the structure and the administrative support for this. Creating and maintaining the values and beliefs that are necessary to support continuity are also a part of the model of nursing practice. Finally, the admission and discharge of patients from the unit must be included in the model of nursing practice. Specific strategies for pre-admission visits and post-transfer visits can do much to enhance the job satisfaction and task identify of the critical care nurse while providing meaningful clinical follow-up for the patient.

An effective model of nursing practice must be supported by a documentation system that is consistent in philosophy and assists in recording pertinent patient information. The issues of documentation in critical care are complicated by the tremendous volumes of patient data that must be recorded, analyzed, and interpreted. A useful documentation system must be organized to show the relationship between the data and trends in data so that they can be seen and easily accessed by care givers.

Another influence on the documentation process is the interdependence of these data, much of which can be used by nurses, physicians, and other health care professionals to formulate their respective diagnostic and treatment decisions; however, documentation of nursing care must demonstrate the unique, discipline perspective of nursing rather than simply recording data for others to use. The use of nursing diagnosis, within the context of nursing process, can facilitate and enhance the recording of data and information by nurses that reflects professional nursing practice. (See Chapter 7 for a complete discussion of documentation in diagnosis-based nursing practice.)

APPLYING CHANGE THEORY IN CRITICAL CARE IMPLEMENTATION PLANNING

After a complete analysis of practice/support systems has been completed, an implementation plan can be developed. The implementation plan should be comprehensive, goal-directed, and address every phase of implementation. For instance, the plan should begin with goals for preparatory interventions to address needed changes in practice systems, then address the unfreezing, the change, the refreezing, and evaluation phases respectively.

In planning the implementation process several ideas are paramount. (1) Do not begin without a comprehensive plan. This can lead to haphazard decision making and difficulty in evaluating the change process. (2) Allow for evaluation by targeting individuals to examine the progress of the plan at specified times. This will assist in addressing small problems before they become large and unmanageable. (3) Keep in mind that flexibility must be maintained as each step is taken. The pitfalls can be numerous and often unpredictable; however, by maintaining flexibility with clear goals as the guide, it is possible to change successfully to diagnosis-based nursing practice.

Awareness of certain pitfalls unique to critical care is particularly helpful in implementing nursing diagnosis. Particularly challenging to the smooth implementation of nursing diagnosis is the complexity of the critically ill patient. The complex interaction of physiologic and psychologic patient conditions as well as the sophistication of current critical care therapeutics creates a clinical situation where medical and nursing activities overlap. Indeed, it is often hard to distinguish boundaries in responsibilities of the health care team in critical care. This overlap can result in frustration and confusion for the critical care nurse who is attempting to work with nursing diagnosis. When should a patient's condition be described with a nursing diagnosis? Examples of when a nursing diagnosis might not be appropriate are cardiac arrest, tentorial herniation, or when a patient is in multi-system failure. It is imperative that staff be clear that not every situation requires a nursing diagnosis, and guidelines should be developed to assist the staff in making these distinctions.

Another pitfall is to underestimate the time needed for care planning. When nursing diagnosis is first implemented, it takes extra time for nurses to work on care plans. While this is not necessarily unique to critical care, the complexity of the patient problems, the demands of frequent evaluation and intervention activities, and the unpredictable nature of the critical care environment make the time issue especially pressing. Strategies must be explored to provide the extra time needed for care planning. Using group work, such as a patient care conference, to develop care plans is a strategy to assist the nurse with these time constraints. Having extra resources available on the unit during the implementation period to assist staff with questions and skill development should also help decrease the time needed for care planning.

Failure to assess the skill of professional nurses to use nursing diagnoses in clinical practice is another pitfall that can impede implementation. This issue may affect experienced clinicians who are novice diagnosticians, or it might be that there are new nurses who have learned to use nursing diagnosis in their educational programs but lack clinical expertise with the complex, critically ill patient. It is very important that the implementation assessment and plan include strategies to assist staff in the development of diagnostic skills.

One pitfall that units may encounter, if there are varying levels of nursing personnel, is the failure to address the roles of the different classifications of staff in the nursing process. Certainly all staff contribute a great deal to the care of the patient, but only the professional nurse has the skill and educational background to develop nursing diagnoses. A system must be worked out to maximize the data collecting skills of the LPN and the diagnostic skills of the RN, as both are necessary to provide quality care for the patient.

Physician reaction, whether anticipated or actual, can also become a pitfall. In the critical care environment, where the medical model is ingrained and where the physician is dependent on the critical care nurse, a strong reaction should be expected; however, this does not have to be negative. One way to minimize this is to provide educational sessions for physicians and keep them informed as changes occur. Critical care nurse managers should meet with medical directors of units to discuss scheduled changes and any impact on medical staff before implementation begins.

Unfreezing

As the implementation plan is finalized, the unfreezing phase of the planned change can begin. The aim of the unfreezing phase is to motivate and make the individuals or the group ready to change. It is a crucial phase to the successful implementation of nursing diagnosis because failure on the part of the staff to see the value in the proposed change and to commit to the change will severely inhibit progress toward a complete change. (See Chapter 5 for a discussion of general implementation issues and strategies.)

One key step with unfreezing is exposing staff to nursing diagnosis. Exposure can be accomplished by having brief workshops that familiarize staff with nursing diagnosis. The objectives should include a definition of nursing diagnosis, showing how it should be written; a differentiation of nursing diagnosis from medical diagnosis; the relationship of nursing diagnosis to nursing process; and the value of nursing diagnosis to nursing practice. Most importantly, the workshops need to be long enough to present examples relevant to that staff's practice and to allow staff to ask questions. Each participant should be provided a handout with key information and examples that relate to practice in that area.

During this exposure period, a discussion of the controversies can be used to diffuse many of the problematic issues with nursing diagnosis in critical care. A particularly problematic issue is physiologic nursing diagnoses. There are many areas of critical care nursing practice that are not yet adequately described with nursing diagnoses. An up-front acknowledgement of this situation, combined with the challenge of identifying those nursing diagnoses from clinical practice and expertise, can do much to ameliorate the frustrations that can result from lack of nursing diagnostic labels for certain critical care situations. Failure to address this issue can cause tremendous frustration, if nurses feel obligated to "fit" patient problems into imprecise or cumbersome diagnostic labels.

Another way to expose staff to nursing diagnosis is to use visual media to present and reinforce clinical content about nursing diagnoses for the unit's patient population. Bulletin boards, signs, and posters about nursing diagnostic issues can provide continuing exposure and reminders of this new approach to critical care nursing. For example, a unit that frequently cares for patients with myocardial infarctions could display posters, created by interested staff members, that describe assessment and possible nursing diagnoses for the patient with MI.

Presenting articles that contain information about nursing diagnosis for critically ill patients along with a display of a "care plan of the week" is another strategy for exposing staff to nursing diagnoses. The care plan can either be from an article related to critical care nursing or be done by a staff member on the unit who is attempting to work with nursing diagnosis. Place these near areas where nurses work on care plans as reminders and as teaching aids. If money permits, one or two staff members could be sent to out-of-hospital programs on nursing diagnosis. These key people should share the information obtained from these programs with their peers in some type of presentation. Encourage staff to contact critical care staff in other institutions as another excellent strategy to determine how they work with nursing diagnosis.

As unfreezing progresses, it is very important to show and generate enthusiasm for nursing diagnosis, give positive feedback to staff who begin to use nursing diagnosis in their practice, and talk the language whenever possible especially at change of shift report, patient care conferences, and unit educational events. It is also important to provide support to staff if negative feedback comes from other services that function within the unit.

As the activities of the unfreezing phase take place, note the people in the group who are interested and motivated in working with nursing diagnosis. These people may be key people to form a task-force to assist, as supporter change agents, with the implementation plan for nursing diagnosis within the unit or department. If the staff can be participative planners in the change that will occur in their practice, then the actual implementation should be much smoother.

As enthusiasm is generated for nursing diagnosis and more people become exposed to it, it can be useful to hold group discussions. Question the group concerning feelings about the current care planning system and what would improve it. Generate lists of the pros and cons of each system to let the group visualize the differences. For example, a staff nurse may complain that with the current care planning system no one uses the plans despite the time and effort put into them. This provides an opportunity to demonstrate the recording and follow through with interventions that can be accomplished using a nursing diagnosis-based practice. Other nurses might express a lack of sense of accomplishment due to the numerous medical tasks to be done in the critical care unit. This scenario provides the opportunity to challenge the nurse to compare the sense of accomplishment achieved with the nursing diagnosis system and the accomplishment felt with using the old system.

Once staff have had initial exposure, then nursing diagnosis should begin to be included in patient care conferences and other events on the unit so that nursing diagnosis actually relates to the care of the patient. One method to accomplish this is to have staff share information in a group setting about a patient they are caring for. Write all the data on a flip chart or board where it is clearly visible. Have the staff group relate the data together, then encourage brainstorming on a possible nursing diagnosis based on the clustered data. Have the group decide on the diagnosis that best addresses the individual patient's problem. This process allows nurses to see nursing diagnosis as it relates to their patients.

Throughout the unfreezing phase, it is necessary to have strong administrative support as well as role modeling. The problem solving that must occur here is painstaking and crucial. Good problem-solving skills and strong management skills are necessary to help the group move toward change in the most efficient manner.

Implementation and Changing

Four types of strategies for implementing nursing diagnosis were discussed in Chapter 5: educational strategies, clinical strategies, systems strategies, and administrative strategies. While these same general areas are appropriate for the critical care area, the particular strategies used will depend upon the clinical population of the unit, the skill and experience of the nursing staff with nursing diagnosis, and the unique issues of physiological nursing diagnoses and interdependent clinical nursing practice.

Educational Strategies. Educational strategies should focus on the essential clinical knowledge that critical care nurses must possess to make nursing diagnoses. An important aspect of the educational strategies is assisting nurses in applying the existing physiological nursing diagnoses and in identifying when a nursing diagnosis is required or when the patient's condition should be named in medical terminology. (See Chapter 2 for a discussion of this issue.) For those critical care nurses who are experienced with nursing diagnosis and interested in research, educational activities about research methods would be useful and exciting for examining their patient population to identify new physiological nursing diagnoses and for validating existing diagnoses.

Other educational strategies for the critical care area include the availability of specialty reference texts and journals on the unit, presentation of educational programs, and attendance at workshops and conferences on particular clinical issues. The use of educational consultants and guest speakers can also be highly effective.

Clinical Strategies. The clinical strategies chosen for a particular unit must be based in the clinical practice activities and philosophy of the critical care unit. Indeed, there must be synergy between the various aspects of clinical practice and agreement that nursing practice will be directed by nursing diagnosis. Some clinical strategies to accomplish this include the selection of a nursing assessment framework that supports the identification of nursing diagnoses accompanied by deliberate decisions about which patient problems will be described with nursing diagnoses and which diagnostic labels will be used.

A number of assessment frameworks have been proposed to assist nurses in formulating nursing diagnoses. One that has been specifically designed for the critically ill patient is the Unitary Person Assessment Tool; indeed, one of the benefits of using this tool is that the "data collected is so rich that nursing diagnoses appear to 'fall out' following the nursing assessment."[21] In addition to the choice of an appropriate assessment framework, it can be helpful for a critical care unit to identify which nursing diagnoses will be used in certain clinical situations or to target certain nursing diagnoses as a starting point for differential diagnostic decisions.

Another clinical strategy, which is particularly important in critical care, is the determination of which problems can be addressed through nursing care and which problems should be referred to the physician. Many times there is a progression in the patient's condition from a state where nursing intervention is adequate and appropriate to a situation where medical treatment may be required, or vice versa. Identifying exactly where on the clinical continuum this decision for patient management should be made can provide assistance to critical care nurses beginning to work with nursing diagnosis. These decisions can be structured into a clinical protocol, consisting of clinical patient findings and parameters, that would identify when the patient should be referred to the physician for medical therapy.

An example of the decision-making process in regard to nursing and medical diagnoses is helpful at this point. A critical care unit with a respiratory care focus should use the Unitary Person Assessment Tool[22] to assess their patients and to then make nursing diagnoses of Ineffective Airway Clearance, Impaired Gas Exchange, or Ineffective Breathing Patterns. For a patient with a left pulmonary contusion observed to demonstrate O_2 saturation changes when turned on the left side, a nursing diagnosis of impaired gas exchange related to left side positioning may be made. Once this nursing diagnosis is made, then nursing interventions can be planned to treat the problem, such as position changes from supine to right side only and continued correlation of changes in SvO_2 and patient activity; however, were the patient's SvO_2 dropped significantly, and this change was *not* associated with a change in position and could not be improved with nursing intervention, then this clinical change would require immediate referral to the physician for medical evaluation and treatment.

Systems Strategies. The systems in the critical care unit comprise the next group of implementation strategies. Unit systems should be designed, modified, or revised to support diagnosis-based nursing practice. Of particular importance are the systems for shift report, the model of nursing practice, the documentation system, and orientation of new personnel. One unifying issue for all of these systems in the critical care area is the sheer volume of data and information: the amount of patient data that must be communicated through these various systems and the complexity of the information create a need for well-designed systems.

A way of dealing with this volume of data in a manner that supports diagnosis-based nursing practice is the nurse-to-nurse shift report. The nurse who has cared for the patient provides a bedside report and demonstrates pertinent findings to the nurse on the next shift. This type of report system prevents the filtering of information that can occur when patient data are reported to the charge nurse for presentation to the next shift; moreover, the opportunity for the arriving nurse to verify patient findings or observations also decreases the possibility of misinterpretation or distortion of information. Finally, nurse-to-nurse report, at the bedside, provides a mechanism for the off-going nurse to establish a sense of accomplishment and completion of a job well done.

The use of a nurse-to-nurse report system is one part of a model of nursing practice that supports diagnosis-based nursing practice. In the critical care area, the smaller ratio of nurses to patients offers some assistance in designing a model for professional nursing practice.

Indeed, primary nursing or total patient care are easily implemented in the critical care area. The newly emerging model of case management may also have a role in the critical care area; however, this remains to be seen. In any event, the nurse-patient ratio and the unique nurse-patient interaction provide some assistance in designing a model for diagnosis-based nursing practice in the critical care area. (See Chapter 6 for further discussion of models of nursing practice.)

Documentation of nursing care activities plays an important role in the unit systems of the critical care area. An important issue is the volume of data and information that must be recorded and easily accessible. The use of flow sheets and special forms to document repetitive numerical data can greatly facilitate the more routine documentation aspects (See Chapter 7 for further discussion of documentation issues in general and flow sheets in particular.) Certainly, automation can provide assistance in the data-handling requirements for the volumes of data from physiologic monitoring equipment and repeated, standardized patient observations. Indeed, when computerized monitoring systems can provide printouts of heart rate, respiratory rate, blood pressure, and other physiologic parameters, it seems pointless for nurses to record these data manually. Furthermore, the time saved through the use of automated documentation can be used for professional nursing care activities. (See Chapter 9 for a discussion of information systems in diagnosis-based nursing practice.)

The existence of well-defined unit systems is very helpful in the orientation of new personnel. Clearly identified expectations for nursing practice, including shift report and documentation, are the foundation of an orientation program. When the unit systems are based on nursing diagnosis, then inclusion of nursing diagnosis in orientation is logical and relatively easy. In the critical care area, new nurses must be guided through the complexities of the patient's condition as well as the unit's systems. When both are phrased in nursing diagnostic language, conflict or confusion about which is more important—the patient or the paperwork—are minimized.

An orientation program for the critical care area should include clinical content about commonly occurring nursing diagnoses, the determination of nursing vs. medical conditions and interventions, and the technical aspects of care, such as monitors, lines, and tubes. Opportunities for the new nurse to practice patient assessment, formulation of nursing diagnoses, and selection of nursing interventions should be provided and supervised. Initially, this guided diagnostic and treatment activity should focus on stable, predictable problems, moving on to more complex patient situations as the new nurse's skill and ability increase. These supervised practice activities should also include participation in nurse-to-nurse report and documentation.

All of the educational and clinical strategies can be greatly enhanced through the availability of knowledgable clinical resources. Resource persons should be available to answer questions as they arise and to identify potential problems before they become unmanageable. It is helpful to have resources available at key times such as when charting is occurring, during nurse-to-nurse report, during patient care conferences, and in educational events to assist staff with problem solving. An advantage to having clinical resources who are immediately available is that they can assist staff with problem solving around such issues as which nursing diagnosis to use, differential diagnosis between similar nursing diagnoses, and when a nursing diagnosis is appropriate. They should also provide consistent feedback on an frequent basis.

Administrative Strategies. The last group is the administrative strategies. A complete discussion of this group is presented in Chapter 5, and the issues for critical care units are very much the same. Two particular aspects bear repeating, however, and these are the need for feedback and reward for nurses as they begin to work with nursing diagnosis and the importance of evaluating the change to diagnosis-based nursing practice.

Refreezing

Refreezing can best be facilitated by building nursing diagnosis into existing practice systems such as changing shift report. Critical care units which utilize bedside report for patients have an ideal opportunity to incorporate nursing diagnosis into the everyday care of the patient by sharing critical patient information based on nursing diagnosis. This same process can be expanded to include unit-to-unit reports on patients being transferred.

Charting is another excellent way to incorporate nursing diagnosis into day-to-day practice. This can occur in a progress note, nurse's note or in a computerized care planning system. Regardless of the place the charting occurs, it allows the nurse and other health team members to see the work of the nurse and the progress of the patient. It should be used in all conferences, interdisciplinary rounds, orientation, and continuing education. Creativity can be expanded to the limit in this phase of implementing nursing diagnosis.

In addition to building nursing diagnosis into practice systems, it should become part of the professional nurse job description and performance criteria. Feedback to staff from managers should occur as well at yearly intervals in regard to these criteria.

IMPLEMENTING NURSING DIAGNOSIS IN NEURO ICU: AN EXAMPLE OF THE CHANGE PROCESS

Especially for implementing nursing diagnoses in the critical care area is the clinical strategy of determining when a nursing diagnosis is required for a patient condition and when the situation should be described in medical terms. This strategy was used in the Neuroscience Intensive Care Unit (NSICU) of the Medical College of Virginia as a part of a larger change project that included the introduction of new documentation forms as well as the implementation of nursing diagnosis. The targeting of a particular nursing diagnostic label and criteria for its use was a major factor in the success of the change project for this intensive care unit.

Applying nursing diagnoses to the patient in the NSICU presents a number of complex dilemmas that involve identifying human responses that nurses can address, naming them, and determining which nursing interventions are most effective. An issue of particular concern to the nurses in this unit was the physiologic phenomenon of increased intracranial pressure (ICP). High-level technology and research protocols including ICP monitoring and measurement of cerebral blood flow were routinely employed, so that increased ICP was a problem that the nurses could easily identify, and there were a number of standing medical orders available for its treatment.

There is also a body of nursing research that identifies a relationship between nursing care modalities, patient activities, and ICP increases. These activities include turning and positioning, suctioning, straining, painful procedures, and conversation at the bedside.[23-28] The effect of these activities on an *individual* patient's ICP, however, are highly variable. The presence of an ICP monitor and the avoidance of these stimuli are important for patients where small changes in ICP may be significant. Indeed, much nursing time and energy in this NSICU was concerned with managing patients activity and stimuli to avoid or minimize ICP increases.

Determining which nursing diagnosis to use for the patient with increased ICP was preceded by a discussion of whether a nursing diagnosis was required for this group of patients, and, if so, under what circumstances. A series of group discussions, covering the better part of six months, focused on exactly what it was that nurses did for these patients. In these discussions, the types of nursing interventions used were explored and analyzed. In many of the discussions, all of the nursing interventions for a particular patient were listed and classified as to whether they were independent, interdependent, or dependent, and the goals of individual or groups of nursing interventions were identified.

A surprising result of the discussions was that very few nursing interventions were dependent, falling into the category of delegated medical activities. In fact many interventions these nurses used were independent, based on the unique responses of the patient to activity or stimuli and the nurse's expertise in identifying, avoiding, or minimizing these responses; furthermore, the majority of medical orders for the patients under discussion were PRN orders that required a great deal of nursing judgment and discretion for their execution. Examples of these interdependent nursing interventions were the specific timing of the administration of narcotic or paralyzing agents to control pain or motor activity, specific timing of ventricular drainage, and manual hyperventilation before or during certain activities. All of these nursing intervention strategies involved the execution of medical orders, but the timing, sequencing, or execution was directed by nursing judgment to provide highly specific and individualized nursing care.

The recognition that the majority of nursing interventions were *not* physician directed but rather concerned control of the patient's environment and activity to avoid ICP elevations led us to the conclusion that nursing care activities for the patient with increased ICP requires two distinct approaches. On one hand, there is the situation where a major clinical change in the patient's condition is detected—the patient stops following commands, begins to demonstrate motor posturing, or develops a dilated and fixed pupil. Here, nursing care responsibilities focus on careful monitoring of the patient so that changes can be detected early and known causes of increased ICP or reduced adaptive capacity such as coughing or jugular venous compression can be avoided.

In this situation, definitive treatment *must* come from the physician. Furthermore, these symptoms may result from another cause such as an expanding mass lesion. Here, nursing care falls within its standardized or protocol-directed activities. These include those nursing care activities that all patients would require, including neurologic assessment and proper positioning, and the implementation of dependent interventions ordered by the physician, such as medications or assisting with diagnostic tests.

The second nursing management situation for the patient with increased ICP is seen when an ICP monitor is available to provide data about the patient's ICP dynamics and responses to stimuli. Objective data permit the nurse to observe any specific stimuli or activity associated with ICP elevations in addition to detecting any critical elevations. The ability to control the patient's environment and activity, as indicated by ICP responses, considerably expands the patient's nursing care options.

Based on this analysis of two different situations for ICP management, it was decided that a nursing diagnosis would be appropriate for the second situation. This decision reflected the clinical knowledge and expertise of a group of nurses who were very familiar with the pathophysiology of increased ICP, as well as the conviction that nursing care played a significant role in avoiding and minimizing those critical ICP elevations that required medical management. This discussion and analysis provided the clinical framework for deciding which clinical situations require a nursing diagnosis and which should be referred to the physician. Major clinical changes and critical elevations of ICP that do not respond promptly to nursing interventions would be referred to the physician and named with medical terminology. Transient ICP elevations that are associated with activity or stimuli and can be managed with independent or interdependent nursing interventions would be named with a nursing diagnosis. The next question was which nursing diagnosis to use.

A number of nursing diagnostic labels for the patient who is at risk for or actually experiencing increased ICP have been suggested. These range from Altered Level of Responsiveness: Decreased Response,[29] Alteration in Cerebral Perfusion,[30] Potential for Increased ICP,[31] Potential for Organ Failure: Brain,[32] Potential for Secondary Brain Injury,[33] to Decreased Adaptive Capacity: Intracranial.[34] While these proposed nursing diagnoses offer some insight into the human response of the patient experiencing increased ICP, they are actually broad concept labels.

Another difficulty is that these nursing diagnoses are either unaccompanied by defining characteristics[35] or the ones listed are broad and non-specific. When defining characteristics are identified, they include parameters such as decreased responsiveness, confusion, generalized motor response to stimuli,[36] decrease in motor and sensory function not related to sleep/wake cycles, loss of brain autoregulatory mechanisms, and cerebral hypertension/cerebral edema.[37] The absence of a specific, consistent, and reliable cue cluster offers little guidance in deciding which nursing diagnosis fits the patient with increased ICP.

Further group discussion and analysis resulted in the selection of the nursing diagnosis Alteration in Cerebral Perfusion as most descriptive of the pathophysiology and clinical state of the patient population with increased ICP in the NSICU. An etiology statement was developed to accompany this diagnostic label based on an approach to nursing intervention that focuses on identifying and addressing those activities or stimuli associated with ICP increases to avoid any alteration in cerebral perfusion.

Three defining characteristics for the nursing diagnosis Alteration in Cerebral Perfusion related to activity or stimuli were also identified:

1. An ICP monitor was present to provide objective data about the patient's ICP and responses to activity or stimuli.
2. ICP elevations, above the treatment level determined by the physician, were observed.
3. ICP elevations were associated with activity or stimuli and could be successfully treated with independent or interdependent nursing interventions.

These defining characteristics maintained the focus of this nursing diagnosis as a patient response that could be treated by nursing intervention. When the patient's ICP elevation was accompanied by a significant clinical change or when it could not be promptly treated with nursing intervention, then the ICP management situation moved from a nursing diagnosis/nursing intervention situation to one where referral to the physician for medical diagnosis/medical intervention was required.

This nursing diagnosis and defining characteristics were displayed on a poster in the nurses' area of the NSICU, and nurses were encouraged to use this diagnostic label for appropriate patients. Both a neuroscience clinical nurse specialist and a unit-based nurse clinician were available to the NSICU nurses for consultation about the use of this nursing diagnosis. Sometimes the consultative process was initiated by the CNS and clinician in order to stimulate interest in and use of this nursing diagnosis. Regular patient care conferences and staff meetings also provided forums for continued discussion of application of this nursing diagnostic label to the patient population. The new documentation framework supported its use by incorporating nursing diagnosis into the unit's orientation program and the development of a number of clinical protocols.

Approximately one year after implementation of nursing diagnosis and the decision to use the Alteration in Cerebral Perfusion label, a descriptive study was conducted by the CNS and the clinician to identify those defining characteristics that NSICU nurses were using to make this nursing diagnosis and to examine nursing interventions used in treating this nursing diagnosis. The utility of a nursing diagnosis in clinical nursing practice is contingent upon a consistent, reliable cluster or pattern of defining characteristics that indicate when the nursing diagnosis should be made; furthermore, the necessary nursing interventions must be associated with the diagnostic label if it is to serve its purpose of directing nursing care. Research methods to examine the possible defining characteristics and interventions for this nursing diagnosis were a concurrent review of the patient record for demographic and clinical data and a nurse questionnaire.

As a result, two consistent findings were identified that could be used as defining characteristics for the nursing diagnosis Alteration in Cerebral Perfusion related to ICP increases with activity or stimuli. These findings both consisted of ICP responses, which were defined as any increase in ICP over 20 mmHg or the level ordered by the neurosurgeon for treatment. Two types of stimuli were consistently associated with ICP responses: an external stimulus, such as turning or suctioning, and a particular sign or symptom, such as pain, agitation, or restlessness. In addition, the observation of these ICP responses associated with specific stimuli was one of the most frequently cited reasons that NSICU nurses listed on the questionnaire for making this nursing diagnosis.[38]

Another predictive cue for this nursing diagnosis was the presence of a medical diagnosis with a high probability of increased ICP. The presence of an ICP monitor could also be considered a predictive cue. Based on these findings, a cluster of defining characteristics for this nursing diagnosis would be:

1. Presence of a medical diagnosis with a high probability of increased ICP
2. Presence of an ICP monitor to provide supporting data about ICP dynamics and responses
3. Observation of an actual ICP response (an ICP increase over 20 mmHg or the treatment level ordered by the physician) that is associated with an identifiable stimulus, sign, or symptom, and can be treated with independent or interdependent nursing interventions[39]

This cluster of defining characteristics consists of two predictive cues and one supporting cue and is very similar to the defining characteristics that were proposed when the use of this nursing diagnosis was begun.

The selection of the nursing diagnosis Alteration in Cerebral Perfusion related to ICP increases with activity or stimuli to describe a particular patient population in the NSICU was an important and effective strategy for implementing nursing diagnosis in that unit. By attacking the most challenging clinical problem head on, many issues that could have created problems and resistance to nursing diagnosis were addressed. Furthermore, the group analysis and decision-making strategies used contributed to increased knowledge about both nursing diagnosis and ICP dynamics, as well as providing opportunities to deal with many of the attitude and value issues that are often a pivotal part of the implementation process. Finally, this strategy was part of a comprehensive change project that included nursing documentation, nursing diagnosis, and a number of clinical systems in the unit. Each of these aspects of change supported and facilitated the other, and this was a very important factor in the success.

CONCLUSION

The successful implementation of nursing diagnosis in the critical care unit is not a simple endeavor. It is a process that requires thoughtful consideration and expert planning.

Three key ideas are paramount to the success of the implementation of nursing diagnosis in critical care. Involvement in the implementation process by the nurses working in the unit is one. Change is threatening to most individuals especially when the outcome of the proposed change is unknown. It is important to involve staff in decision making and planning to give them some control over their current practice and to promote the control of their future practice.

A second key strategy is commitment. Commitment must be made to a philosophy of how nursing practice will occur on the unit. The commitment to a philosophy guides the entire implementation process toward the expected outcome.

Finally, timing is a third key to success in implementing a nursing diagnosis-based practice in critical care. Nursing diagnosis-based practice is a way of thinking. Helping critical care nurses examine and define what they do takes time due to the complexity of the practice environment. Failure to provide sufficient time to examine practice will result in nursing diagnosis becoming just another task for the nurse to perform, instead of the foundation of diagnosis-based nursing practice.

REFERENCES

1. Hickey, M. Nursing diagnosis in the critical care unit. *Dimensions in Critical Care Nursing*, 1984, *84*, 2, 91
2. Hudack, C., Lolu, T., & Gallo, B. *Critical care nursing* (3d ed.). Philadelphia: J. B. Lippincott, 1982
3. *Ibid*
4. *Ibid*
5. Willis, S. & Tremblay, S. *Critical care review for nurses*. Boston: Jones and Barlett Publishers, 1988
6. Gordan, M. *Nursing diagnosis process and application*. New York: McGraw Hill, 1982
7. Kim, M.J. Without collaboration what's left? *American Journal of Nursing*, 1985, *85*, 281, 284
8. Hulbalik, K. & Kim, M.J. Nursing diagnosis associated with heart failure in critical care nursing. In M.J. Kim, G.K. McFarland, & A.M. McLane (Eds.), *Classification of nursing diagnosis: Proceedings of the fifth national conference*. St. Louis: C. V. Mosby, 1984
9. Kim, M.J. Physiologic nursing diagnosis: Its role and place in nursing taxonomy. In M.J. Kim, G.K. McFarland, & A.M. McLane (Eds.), *Classification of nursing diagnosis: Proceedings of the fifth national conference*. St. Louis: C. V. Mosby, 1984
10. Carpenito, L. Nursing diagnosis in critical care: Impact on practice and outcomes. *Heart and Lung*, 1987, *87*, 596
11. *Ibid*
12. Suhayda, R. & Kim, M.J. Documentation of nursing process in critical care. In M.J. Kim, G.K. McFarland, & A.M. McLane (Eds.), *Classification of nursing diagnosis: Proceedings of the fifth national conference*. St. Louis: C. V. Mosby, 1984
13. Carpenito, p. 595
14. Seybolt, J. Dealing with premature turnover. *Journal of Nursing Administration*, 1986, *86*, 27
15. *Ibid*
16. *Ibid*
17. Young, M.S. & Lucas, C. Nursing diagnosis: Common problems in implementation. *Topics in Clinical Nursing*, 1984, *84*, 72
18. Kim, M.J., Amoroso-Seritella, R., Gulanic, M., et al. Clinical validation of cardiovascular nursing diagnoses. In M.J. Kim, G.K. McFarland, & A.M. McLane (Eds.), *Classification of nursing diagnosis: Proceedings of the fifth national conference*. St. Louis: C. V. Mosby, 1984
19. Willis & Tremblay, p. 3
20. Lewin, K. Frontiers in group dynamics: Concept, method, and reality in social sciences; Social equilibrium and social change. *Human Relations*, 1947, *1*, 1, 5
21. Guzzetta, C. & Sherer, A.P. A unitary person assessment tool. Poster presented at the Eighth Conference on Nursing Diagnoses, St. Louis, March, 1988.
22. *Ibid*
23. Davenport-Fortune, P. & Dunnam, L.R. Professional nursing care for the patient with increased intracranial pressure: Planned or "hit and miss"? *Journal of Neuroscience Nursing*, 1985, *17*, 6, 367
24. Lipe, H.L. & Mitchell, P.H. Positioning the patient with intracranial hypertension: How turning and

head rotation affect the internal jugular vein. *Heart & Lung,* 1980, *9,* 6, 1031

25. Mauss, N.K. & Mitchell, P.H. Increased intracranial pressure: An update. *Heart & Lung,* 1976, *5,* 6, 919

26. Mitchell, P.H. Intracranial hypertension: Implications of research for nursing care. *Journal of Neuroscience Nursing,* 1980, *12,* 3, 145

27. Mitchell, P.H. & Mauss, N.K. Relationship of patient-nurse activity to intracranial pressure variations: A pilot study. *Nursing Research,* 1978, *27,* 1, 4

28. Mitchell, P.H., Ozuna, J., & Lipe, H.P. Moving the patient in bed: Effects on intracranial pressure. *Nursing Research,* 1981, *30,* 212

29. Alcorn, M.H. Altered levels of responsiveness: Decreased response. In M. Snyder (Ed.), *A guide to neurological and neurosurgical nursing.* New York: John Wiley & Sons, 1983

30. Kim, M.J., McFarland, G.K., & McLane, A.M. *Pocket guide to nursing diagnosis.* St. Louis: C.V. Mosby, 1984

31. Gettrust, K.V., Ryan, S.C., & Engelmann, D.S. *Applied nursing diagnosis.* New York: John Wiley & Sons, 1985

32. Steele D. & Whalen, J. A proposal for two new nursing diagnoses: Potential for organ failure and potential for tissue destruction. *Heart & Lung,* 1985, *14,* 5, 426

33. American Association of Neuroscience Nurses and American Nurses' Association. *Neuroscience nursing practice: Process and outcome criteria for selected diagnoses.* Kansas City: American Nurses' Association, pub. no. MS-13, 1985

34. Mitchell, P.H. Decreased adaptive capacity, intracranial: A proposal for a nursing diagnosis. *Journal of Neuroscience Nursing,* 1986, *18,* 4, 170

35. Kim, McFarland, & McLane

36. American Association of Neuroscience Nurses & American Nurses' Association

37. Steele & Whalen

38. Miller, E.R. & Williams, S. Alteration in cerebral perfusion: Clinical concept or nusing diagnosis? *Journal of Neuroscience Nursing,* 1987, *19,* 4, 183

39. *Ibid*

CHAPTER 14

Clinical Application of the Nursing Diagnosis: Powerlessness

Catherine S. Kedy

Nurses frequently direct their interventions toward preventing patient powerlessness but without identifying the goal of increasing patient power and control. Interventions that include teaching about a specific illness or a procedure, learning about the patient's unique response to illness as influenced by biopsychosocial factors, and helping patients to identify personal and social resources to promote coping with health-related issues, are all aimed at increasing individual adaptation, control, and power.

Individual autonomy is challenged as soon as the patient enters the health care system. The individual must assume the role of patient, which involves loss of personal belongings, clothes, usual daily routines, and privacy. The patient must accept institutional rules and is rewarded for deferring to the wishes and expertise of the health care team. Patients can respond in a variety of ways, including submission, fear, helplessness, or anger. These responses are not conducive to health promotion and wellness. While assumption of the sick role helps the patient to obtain needed assistance, the nurse must help the patient balance this with an amount of control, or the patient becomes helpless and powerlessness develops.

If power is "possession of control, authority, of influence over others,"[1] then powerlessness is being without influence. Powerlessness is defined as "the perception of the individual that one's own actions will not significantly affect an outcome. Powerlessness is a perceived lack of control over a current situation or immediate happening."[2] Certainly, in the health care system, there are many situations that can trigger a sense of powerlessness, and, if it continues, a cycle begins that leads to decreased self-esteem, depression, and helplessness.[3]

Powerlessness is a failure of adaptation. Roy's Adaptation Model[4] provides a conceptual framework for understanding the development of powerlessness and directs nursing interventions that increase patient power. The patient is viewed as a part of an interactive system that responds to the environment. When adaptation is threatened, the goal of nursing intervention is to manipulate parts of the system to promote and improve adaptation. The nurse interacts with the patient within four subsystems that facilitate adaptation: physiologic needs, self-concept, role function, and interdependence.

Adaptation in the subsystem of physiologic needs involves changes the body makes to respond to its environment, such as increasing heart rate as physical activity increases. The subsystem of self concept is defined by perceptions of oneself as the result of interactions with others. Confidence is one result of a positive self concept. The mode of role function involves how one responds to societal roles including the role of spouse, parent, worker, and hobbies. The last mode, interdependence, is the subsystem that deals with interpersonal interactions. How the individual obtains and asks for help and support from the environment is examined within this mode.

CONCEPTS RELEVANT TO POWERLESSNESS

Several concepts are closely related to the concept of powerlessness and will be discussed in further detail. These include control, helplessness, and hopelessness.

Positive Effects of Control

The positive effects of control have been shown to far outweigh the negative effects. Control tempers the effect of physiological and emotional stress even if the stressor is unchanged. Even the belief that an individual has control strengthens the ability to cope and decreases the stress of the event.

The availability of resources, both physical and social, is an important mitigating factor in coping with powerlessness. Predictability decreases the psychological stress of loss of control.[5] Since powerlessness is defined as a perceived lack of control, the effects, both positive and negative, of control are important factors.

Powerlessness has also been shown to effect learning. In a group of hospitalized tuberculosis patients, those who were high in powerlessness knew less about their disease and health maintenance than did those low in powerlessness. Nursing staff perceived the patients low in powerlessness as better informed. This same group was also less satisfied with information that had been given to them.[6]

Control has been shown to decrease anxiety.[7] Nurses are well aware that high levels of anxiety interfere with learning, therefore, allowing an appropriate level of control is imperative to controlling anxiety. The nurse must consider the level of powerlessness the patient is experiencing both in terms of situational responses and long-term personality traits. Planning structured programs in small increments is a helpful strategy for individuals with a high sense of powerlessness. In contrast, those with a low sense of powerlessness respond to having alternatives presented and being allowed to make choices about the most useful approach for them.[8]

Negative Effects of Control

On the other hand, some studies have concluded that control can have negative effects. This can occur if the individual does not have enough information to make a decision, [9,10] or if the individual has excessive feelings of responsibility.[11] An individual may also respond negatively to control if the long-term personality style is one of powerlessness. This person would probably find having control as highly stressful as it would be outside the repertoire of responses.

Helplessness

Helplessness is defined as the condition of lacking strength or effectiveness and is considered synonymous with powerlessness.[12,13] Seligman studied responses to helplessness and developed his theory of learned helplessness.[14] The theory describes helplessness (powerlessness) as resulting from repeated, uncontrollable events. It is learned that relief cannot be obtained no matter what actions are taken. In fact, helplessness is often difficult to unlearn. The individual may experience decreased initiation of voluntary responses and motivation, negative beliefs about resolution of problems, decreased aggression, and physiologic changes. Feelings of anxiety and depression may occur. Nurses have observed how this spiraling process affects their patients.

Hopelessness

Hopelessness is "a subjective state in which an individual sees limited or no alternatives or personal choices available and is unable to mobilize energy on own behalf."[15] It is a sense of giving up.[16] If powerlessness continues, hopelessness can develop.[17] The depression and apathy that accompany powerlessness promote the sense that the patient has no hope for the future.

Hopelessness has been identified as a factor in unexpected death. Lefcourt documents such a case where powerlessness and hopelessness precipitated the death of a psychiatric patient who had been mute for ten years.[18] She was a resident of the "hopeless" floor and was moved to a different unit while renovations were made. Prior to the move, she underwent a physical examination that revealed excellent health. The new unit housed patients that were close to discharge and had many unit privileges. While on the new unit, the woman became more socially involved and began talking within two weeks. When renovations were completed, she was returned to the "hopeless" unit. Within a week, she collapsed and died. An autopsy found no pathology. Lefcourt concluded that having a sense of control and the belief that one can exert choice has a positive effect in maintaining life.

LOCUS OF CONTROL

Locus of control refers to the way an individual perceives the cause of events and is closely tied to the concept of powerlessness. Someone with an internal locus of control believes in self-determination and personal initiative as causes for events. An individual with an external locus of control sees events as the result of chance or fate.[19] For example, the internally-controlled person who receives a job promotion would see this as a result of personal work, while the person with external control would view the promotion as a result of luck, friendship, or some external factor outside the individual's control.

Locus of control is considered a stable personality trait, while powerlessness may be stable over time (trait powerlessness) or situationally dependent.[20] Trait powerlessness refers to a long-term pattern or a lifestyle of helplessness, while situational powerlessness refers to feelings of helplessness that occur in a normally empowered person. The person whose style is to be dependent and submissive would be an example of trait powerlessness and most likely have an external locus of control. The situationally powerless individual might be someone who functions adaptively but feels out of control when hospitalized. This person might have either an external or internal locus of control.

Locus of control affects patient responses that nurses encounter (see Table 14–1). Externally-controlled individuals consistantly have higher anxiety levels and report it more readily. Internals perceive unpleasant events as less stressful when they are able to predict when and how these events will occur.[21] Nurses need to consider that internally- and externally-controlled individuals may experience changes in health quite differently. Information seeking is also effected by locus of control.[22] Individuals who valued health and were internally controlled were more likely to seek out health information than were those who valued health and were externally controlled. (See Table 14–2.)

TABLE 14–1. COMPARISON OF RESPONSES BY LOCUS OF CONTROL

	Internal Locus	External Locus
Fear of Disability	*Fear emotional disability*	*Fear physical disability*
Health Information	*More likely to request*	*Less likely to request*
Approach for Nursing Intervention	*Self-directed programs*	*Group programs*
Coping with a Crisis	*Effective problem solving*	*Less task-oriented, higher stress level*
Response to Pain	*Higher tolerance*	*Lower tolerance*

Coping with a crisis was also influenced by locus of control. After a hurricane, owner-managers of small businesses were studied.[23] Externals experienced higher stress and displayed less task-oriented behavior, while the coping behavior of internals resulted in more successful solutions of problems. Nurses need to consider that patients may respond to hospitalization as a crisis. Externally-controlled individuals may require nursing assistance to help initiate and sustain coping strategies.

The effects of locus of control on tolerance to painful stimuli were found to differ between internally- and externally-controlled subjects. Internals had greater tolerance to increasing intensities of electric shocks given by the researcher than did externals.[24] Externally-controlled individuals may not be receptive to our exhortations to make changes to improve health.[25] A post-myocardial infarction patient may see no need to decrease stress if it is believed that one cannot alter destiny. This patient might respond to recommendations if the health care provider's expert power can be used to an advantage. The patient may view the changes, recommended by the nurse as another external control, and accept and utilize suggestions "because the nurse said to do it."

POWERLESSNESS: CONTRIBUTING FACTORS AND PATIENT RECEPTIONS

Many factors can contribute to powerlessness in hospitalized patients. Environmental factors such as enforced confinement and separation from family, hospital routines and schedules, and loss of personal belongings and clothes all help to create a sense of loss of control. The patient must also cope with the illness that caused the hospitalization. It may be an acute illness, a traumatic injury, or an exacerbation of a chronic condition. With an acute illness, the patient must deal with anxiety about what the diagnosis might be and the implications it will have for future recovery and health.

A traumatic injury may cause feelings of powerlessness over one's life. An individual, in control of all other aspects of life, may experience self-doubt about the ability to remain in

TABLE 14–2. NURSING ASSESSMENT OF PATIENT LOCUS OF CONTROL

1. *Does the patient ask questions about health, prognosis, and changes in lifestyle?*
2. *Does the patient ask or demonstrate a desire to participate in self-care activities?*
3. *Does the patient begin anticipating needs or changes in lifestyle?*
4. *Does the patient believe individual actions and health behaviors can make a difference in wellness?*
5. *Does the patient develop ideas about how to solve problems?*

control of the situation and cope with the injury. Furthermore, trauma alters the family and social system as well and effects these usual supports.

The chronically ill must cope with the unpredictability of symptoms, multiple treatments, and strain on family and personal coping.[26] These patients constantly struggle to maintain control over their illness and long to be "normal."

In an attempt to cope with her own surgery and to explore the subjective experience of patients, Kritek[27] documented her own feelings of powerlessness while hospitalized. During her hospitalization she kept notes of her perceptions and used French and Raven's[28] bases of power (coercive, legitimate, referent, expert, and reward) to analyze her data.

The largest number of her experiences fell into the coercive power category. She describes her perceptions of the health care system as having unfair control and having the ability to punish her in some way. She felt angry, and later became preoccupied with thoughts of leaving against medical advice when her anticipated surgery went unscheduled for four days. She also felt she was denied medical information about her status, and little information was given in response to her questions. She noticed irritation on the part of her care givers when she pressed. To avoid further alienating her care takers, she asked fewer and then no questions by the end of her hospitalization.

When a nurse employed coercive power instead of enlisting her cooperation, Kritek became oppositional and indifferent. Another response that she noted was that of over-conformity. Her ability to reciprocally communicate was diminished, and her only way to express disagreement was by being the perfect patient.

The exercise of legitimate power was also a frequent occurrence. This power base refers to the authority that one individual grants to another. Kritek admits, reluctantly and gradually, accepting the role of "patient." As she did this, she conceded the health care system's authority over her. Kritek described her cooperation with and praise for those individuals who took a personal interest in her and who shared her own value of providing patients with information. This response is in direct contrast with her response of noncompliance to coercive power.

Kritek was also able to exert legitimate power as a patient. She knew it was expected that patients complain about the prescribed postoperative diet, and, after gradually escalating her complaints, her diet was changed. At other times she compromised her own wishes so she could fit the norm and utilize legitimate patient power. Rather than admitting her ambivalence about discharge, she eagerly requested written discharge information.

Referent power is based on an individual's identification with another. Kritek's experience is atypical because she too was a nurse and identified strongly with nursing staff. She found herself excusing behaviors and care that didn't suit her needs. She wasn't given information because it was assumed she already knew it, even when she stated that she did not know. She found herself being given too much independence and again was unable to express her anger. This time she remained quiet, not because of fears of retribution, but because she identified with the nurses and criticizing them would be equivalent to criticizing herself.

Expert power is based on the belief that an individual has superior knowledge and expertise. Kritek notes that there were few incidents classified in this category that may also be attributed to her own nursing and medical knowledge. She did refer to the health care system's expert power when she consented to evaluation, treatment, and surgery. Some nurses commanded expert power, but, on the whole, she felt she did not benefit from the nurses' expertise as staff didn't obtain enough data about her to make an accurate diagnosis and provide nursing treatment.

She observed that even though she was reluctant to initiate discussion about her fears, she wished that her nurses would have recognized her unspoken needs. She regretted that she never was able to utilize the knowledge and expertise of her care givers. So, inspite of her outward appearance of being self-sufficient, she wanted her nurses to recognize her need for reassurance and information intuitively. Kritek provides an excellent example of the internally-controlled person who is reluctant to admit anxiety.

The last type of power identified by French and Raven, reward power, is based on the ability to disperse rewards. This category had the fewest number of incidents. Kritek notes that this is due to her perception that the only possible reward that could be conveyed was discharge. The promised reward (discharge) was what propelled her to work towards a fast recovery.

An important implication from Kritek's analysis is that awareness and practice are the different patient responses to the use of legitimate, expert, and coercive power. The response to coercive power was noncompliance or overcompliance and anger while legitimate and expert power engendered cooperation and patient comfort. All patients respond in some way to the loss of control that results from hospitalization. Nurses need to assume an active role in minimizing loss of control.

Three types of control that have implications for minimizing this loss: behavioral, cognitive, and decisional.[29] Behavioral control is the ability and knowledge to act to gain control of a situation. Cognitive control is the ability to modify perceptions and the way an event might be interpreted. Decisional control is having the opportunity to make choices. Miller[30] gives patient examples of factors that decrease behavioral, cognitive, and decisional control. (See Table 14–3.) Corrective nursing interventions are also suggested (See Table 14–4.)

TABLE 14–3. EXAMPLES OF FACTORS DECREASING BEHAVIORAL, COGNITIVE, AND DECISIONAL CONTROL IN HOSPITALIZED PATIENTS

Behavioral Control	Cognitive Control	Decisional Control
Blind patient was left in a wheelchair in the center of the waiting room and was not told where she was or how long she must wait.	*Patient was reprimanded for leaving waiting room to go to restroom after waiting 2 hours. "If you aren't here when we call you, you will miss your turn."*	*Appointment scheduled in ambulatory care department without asking patient if date and time is convenient.*
Patient was left alone in X-ray room on hard table in cold room, only partially covered.	*Patient was not informed of his daily lab values although she had requested that this be done.*	*Patient in X-ray department told to "try to hold it" when he asked location of bathroom.*
	Health-care personnel more knowledgeable about patient's illness and treatment than he is.	*Diagnostic and treatment procedures scheduled without asking patient or explaining why they were being done.*
	Health-care personnel walked into patient's room without knocking.	*Patient has little or no choice about who will share room.*
	Health-care personnel talk "over" patient about their personal activities.	*Little choice over scheduling activities: eating, sleeping, bathing, and treatment.*
	Health-care personnel are not wearing name tags.	

(Reprinted by permission of Miller, J.F., Coping with Chronic Illness: Overcoming Powerlessness. *Philadelphia: F.A. Davis, Co., © 1983 by J. F. Miller and Publisher, p. 52*)

TABLE 14—4. EXAMPLES OF FACTORS INCREASING BEHAVIORAL, COGNITIVE, AND DECISIONAL CONTROL IN HOSPITALIZED PATIENTS

Behavioral Control	Cognitive Control	Decisional Control
Nursing care plan: "Allow patient to sleep until breakfast trays arrive; do not awaken for TPR."	Patient informed of weight, blood pressure, lab values.	Patient given access to refrigerator to get own soft drinks.
	Patient taught about medications.	
Patient moved to another room at request because roommate smoked.	Nursing care plan: Detailed description of how to do patient's dressing change had been worked out with the patient.	Patient given list of all U.S. dialysis centers and given full responsibility for making own arrangements.
Patient in X-ray was told, "We can see you through the window. Hold up your hand if you need something."	Patient given feedback about lab values, taught how to record results on a flow sheet.	Medications left at bedside for patient to take when ready.
After patients were taught specific procedures, expectation given for them to take full responsibility for catheter care, urine testing, dressing change, shunt care.		

(Reprinted by permission of Miller, J.F., Coping with Chronic Illness: Overcoming Powerlessness. *Philadelphia: F.A. Davis, Co.*, © 1983 by J.F. Miller and Publisher, p. 53)

Another factor that may contribute to patient powerlessness is nurse powerlessness. Nurses have a history of being physicians' handmaidens and being dependent on physicians for direction. Nurses were recognized for their ability to provide comfort for the patient, but they still relied on physicians to give instruction. While nursing practice continues to have dependent functions, such as administering scheduled medications and treatments, nurses also have independent and interdependent functions.

Nursing has grown from these roots and is assuming more responsibility in caring for patients. One way nurses are claiming power is by utilizing nursing diagnosis as a way to identify the nurse's unique contribution to patient care. As nurses treat the patient's nursing problems, they increase their power, both individually and collectively. When this is done, nursing's contribution to patient care can be identified and valued. It is essential that not only colleagues and patients but also nursing peers recognize the knowledge and power that nurses possess.

While these changes are developing, nurses may be recognized as employees rather than colleagues. It is not coincidence that this dependent role has occurred in nursing, which is a predominantly female profession. Women have not been recognized as having power until recently. The traditional, hierarchical system of the hospital contributed to the powerlessness of the nurse. The only individual with less power than the nurse was the patient. No wonder nursing has been reluctant to "share" it's limited power with the one person over whom they could exert power.

In order to be able to share power, nurses must feel confident in their own role. Certainly sharing knowledge and expertise is the best way to empower patients, thereby improving their health. Power should not be feared but recognized and utilized to the nurse's and the patient's advantage.

THE DIAGNOSTIC PROCESS

The nursing process consists of five steps: assessment, diagnosis, planning, implementation of nursing interventions, and evaluation. The diagnostic process consists of the data collecting and critical thinking process that are used to formulate a nursing diagnosis from assessment data and clinical knowledge. (See Chapter 4.) If a diagnosis of Powerlessness is suspected, the nurse begins the diagnostic process by assessing the patient's past and present coping strategies, including loss of control, recent stressors, and life changes. The nurse also assesses the meaning hospitalization and illness have for the patient and family. One patient may find the hospital a reassuring place to recover while another may be threatened by the experience.

Assessing Power Resources of the Patient

An effective way to assess coping style is to gather information about the patient's power resources. These sources of strength enhance individual coping and include physical strength, psychologic stamina, self concept, energy, knowledge, motivation, and personal belief system.[31] By utilizing this approach, the nurse obtains data about coping strengths and weaknesses. The nurse then helps the patient and family to support existing strengths and works with them to reinforce areas of weakness. Each power resource will be discussed with examples.

Physical strength includes current functioning and potential strength for recovery and rehabilitation.[32] The individual's preexisting physical strength must be considered along with current physical condition, be it a degenerative or time-limited illness. The patient with an acute illness who was previously physically active will have more physical strength and reserve than a patient with a long history of congestive heart failure with a limited tolerance for activity.

Psychologic stamina refers to the ability to maintain emotional equilibrium inspite of illness.[33] Social support as well as personal attributes are widely acknowledged as mitigating factors in adjusting to illness. The patient with a concerned and interested family and a conviction that whatever is encountered can be handled is psychologically better prepared than the individual with no family and overwhelming fears of illness.

Psychologic stamina is also influenced by recent stressors. If the patient has experienced loss or significant changes within recent years, coping ability may be compromised. If past crises were not constructively resolved, they may reappear at times of stress and inhibit current psychologic coping. For example, if a middle-aged woman denied her emotional loss at the time of her mother's death, her grief might be rekindled five years later when she is admitted to the hospital where her mother died. Another factor to consider is the temporal proximity of life events to one another. One major loss may not be as stressful as several less stressful changes or events that occur in a short period of time.

The power resource of self concept consists of the individual's total thoughts and feelings about oneself.[34] Self concept consists of body image, role function, idealized self, and self-esteem.[35] When hospitalized an individual's self concept is challenged in many ways. Body image may be threatened by a traumatic injury or impending surgery, with resultant fears about the return of normal function and appearance.

Idealized self includes conscience, morals, and expectations for self.[36] Under stress personal beliefs and usual coping strategies are challenged. If the individual responds in a manner that is inconsistent with personal ideals and standards of behavior, self concept is altered. For example, a woman who has always seen herself as emotionally strong is hospitalized and becomes tearful and anxious; because she doesn't respond as she believes she should, her idealized self concept is altered.

Self-esteem, the last component of self concept, is the value or worth the individual holds for oneself.[37] Self-esteem includes self-approval and self-confidence. Confidence about personal ability to cope with illness and hospitalization is empowering for the patient and is generally the result of past successful experiences with coping.

To assess the power resource self concept, the nurse listens for the patient's fears about change in appearance and usual roles. The nurse also asks for the patient's subjective opinion about personal coping. Is this an overwhelming situation or is the patient confident in the ability to cope? Does the patient feel that coping is inadequate and that others would handle the same situation in a better manner?

Energy is also a power resource and refers to the ability to do physical or mental work. When ill, the balance between energy expended for healing and recovery may exceed energy stored. If this is the case, the patient may have little energy for learning or coping with the stress of illness.[38]

Knowledge and insight are powerful coping resources. When the patient is informed and able to make decisions about the plan of care, anxiety is decreased and powerlessness is avoided.[39] Individuals differ in the amount of information required to feel empowered; therefore, the nurse must take note of the patient's desire for information as well as the response to information that is given and the patient's ease with that information. Patients that are internally controlled will most likely request more information and should be included in decision making about their treatment. Externally controlled patients may not ask as many questions and may defer to the judgment of their care givers.

Motivation, a patient power resource, is a need or desire that causes a person to act.[40] Motivation prompts the patient toward improved well-being. During assessment, the nurse looks for signs of high motivation such as appropriate questions and active participation in personal care. Signs of low motivation include disinterest or hopelessness.

The power source of personal belief system consists of spiritual beliefs, confidence in care givers, therapeutic regimes, and self.[41] The patient who derives strength from a personal belief system demonstrates high levels of trust in staff and obtains strength from faith that is based on personal beliefs. A patient deficient in belief system strength might be distrustful of care givers and experience a decrease in spirituality or self confidence.

By gathering information about power resources (see Table 14–5), the nurse learns a great deal about how the patient and family are prepared to cope with hospitalization and illness. If areas of weakness are discovered, the patient is at risk for developing powerlessness. During assessment, the nurse listens for the indicators or defining characteristics that indicate feelings of loss of control. The criteria for making the diagnosis of Powerlessness are included in Table 14–6.

Miller suggests that a diagnosis of Powerlessness can be made when one of the severe indicators is identified.[42] The signs and symptoms classified as moderate and low are indicators of powerlessness but alone might not be sufficient to make the diagnosis. Two or more of the moderate and/or defining characteristics, however, provide enough support to make the diagnosis. Other defining characteristics have also been identified (See Table 14–7.) The second step in the diagnostic process is determining the nursing diagnosis. During this step, the nurse examines the defining characteristics and chooses a nursing diagnosis.

TABLE 14–5. ASSESSMENT OF POWER RESOURCES

Physical Strength
What is the patient's prognosis for recovery?
What was the patient's physical condition prior to hospitalization?
Is the condition time-limited or degenerative?

Psychologic Stamina
What are the patient's social supports?
Are there recent stressors?
What is the patient's response to cumulative stressors?
What are the patient's past coping strategies?

Self Concept
Has the patient's body image been altered or threatened?
What are the patient's concerns about body image?
What are the patient's social roles?
How have the patient's roles been altered by hospitalization?
How does the patient perceive personal coping ability?
What are the patient's personal expectations for coping?
Is the patient confident about the ability to cope?

Energy
Does the patient have the physical and emotional energy for recovery?
Does the patient have energy for learning?

Knowledge/Insight
Does the patient ask appropriate questions?
Does the patient have an external or internal locus of control?
Is the patient able to retain information?

Motivation
Does the patient participate in personal care?
Does the patient show interest by asking questions?

TABLE 14–6. POWERLESSNESS: DEFINING CHARACTERISTICS

Severe:
1. Verbal expressions of having no control or influence over situation
2. Verbal expressions of having no control or influence over outcome
3. Verbal expressions of having no control or influence over self care
4. Depression over physical deterioration that occurs despite patient compliance with regimes
5. Apathy

Moderate:
1. Nonparticipation in care or decision making when opportunities are provided
2. Expressions of dissatisfaction and frustration over inability to perform previous tasks and/or activities
3. Does not monitor progress
4. Expression of doubt regarding role performance
5. Reluctance to express true feelings, fearing alienation from care givers
6. Passivity
7. Inability to seek information about care
8. Dependence on others that may result in irritability, resentment, anger, and guilt
9. Does not defend self-care practices when challenged

Low:
1. Expression of uncertainty about fluctuating energy levels.

Kim, M.J., McFarland, G., & McLane, A. Pocket Guide to Nursing Diagnosis (2d ed.). St. Louis: C. V. Mosby, 1987

TABLE 14—7. SUGGESTED DEFINING CHARACTERISTICS OF POWERLESSNESS

1. *Low orientation to learning control—relevant information*
2. *Lack of knowledge about own illness*
3. *Low planned use of health services*
4. *Acknowledges failure readily*
5. *Rationalizes failure*
6. *Displays aggression when goal achievement frustrated*
7. *Devalues desired goal when achievement frustrated*
8. *Withdrawal*
9. *Resignation*
10. *Fatalism*
11. *Aimlessness*
12. *Anxiety*
13. *Restlessness and uneasiness*
14. *Sleeplessness*
15. *Malleability*
16. *Sadness or crying*
17. *Inappropriate aggression*
18. *Low self-esteem*
19. *Mistrust of others*
20. *Low self-reliance*
21. *Asks many questions*
22. *Loss of control over personal behavior*
23. *Inappropriate or immature coping abilities for developmental stage*
24. *Projects blame on others and environment*
25. *Seeks immediate rewards in favor of long-term goals*

Bowers, A., Hirsch, J., McFarland, G., et al. Clinical Nursing. St. Louis: C. V. Mosby, 1986, p. 1829

DETERMINING THE ETIOLOGY

Once the choice of a nursing diagnosis has been made, the next part of the diagnostic process is the selection of the etiology statement. (Etiology is discussed in Chapter 3.) When choosing a diagnostic label, the etiology statement is an important component. The etiology statement allows the nurse to identify the most likely cause or contributing factor for the patient's condition and to direct nursing interventions toward alleviating or ameliorating powerlessness.

Four etiology factors have been suggested for the diagnosis of Powerlessness[43]: health care environment, interpersonal interaction, illness-related regimen, and lifestyle of helplessness. Two of these etiologies, health care environment and illness-related regimen are clinically useful. The first suggested etiology, health care environment, is appropriate when the patient is responding to a loss of control related to hospitalization. This situation describes the patient as a normally powerful individual who is temporarily out of control due to the event and routines of hospitalization. For instance, an executive who is admitted for evaluation of chest pain and who resists following instructions for bedrest and persists in managing his office by telephone from his hospital bed.

The second etiology suggested for diagnosis of Powerlessness, illness-related regimen, would include individuals with complex medical treatments, progressive loss of physical strength, loss of independence, and loss of control of daily living. The patient is particularly at risk for powerlessness if these events occur in conjunction with adherence to the prescribed treatment plan. This diagnosis would apply to the hemodialysis patient who follows diet recommendations, keeps dialysis appointments, and feels that his life is controlled by fate rather than his personal choice. Powerlessness would be increased if he developed persistent leg cramping during and after dialysis.

The etiology of illness-related regimen can be used in acute or chronic situations. It is intended for use when the health care routine precipitates the response of powerlessness. In fact, this etiology may be used while the individual is hospitalized but is responding to the prescribed regimen and not the experience of hospitalization. In contrast, the etiology of health care environment is generally used in acute situations when the individual is responding to the hospital environment.

The etiologies interpersonal interaction and lifestyle of helplessness are incomplete diagnostic labels. The nursing diagnosis names the human response and the etiology makes a statement about the possible cause and is intended to direct nursing interventions. (See Chapter 3.) The diagnostic label Powerlessness related to interpersonal interaction does not provide any direction for nursing interventions. The nurse is left unable to make any inferences about the cause of the patient's powerlessness or begin planning nursing care. The etiology, lifestyle of helplessness, describes the patient's experience and, therefore, is a defining characteristic of powerlessness and not an etiology. Both statements, lifestyle of helplessness and interpersonal interaction, are attempting to describe the patient with a long-term experience of powerlessness and who, as a result, responds in a maladaptive manner.

Additional Suggested Etiologies

A more descriptive and directive etiology is recommended: low self-esteem. This etiology provides the nurse with both a causative factor and guide to appropriate interventions. The patient with long-term powerlessness most likely views the self as weak and interpersonally inadequate. The etiology of low self-esteem is indicated for the patient who feels a lack of control, is nonassertive, or expects failure.

Another suggested etiology is chronic illness, indicated for use with the individual who experiences a sense of powerlessness over health or lifestyle as a result of long-term illness. Chronic illness may be confused with the etiology illness-related regimen. The former is used with individuals who respond to the loss of control that may result from the uncertain nature of exacerbations of chronic illness. The patient with multiple sclerosis who has to alter plans for a vacation after a flare-up of this illness would be appropriate use of this etiology. Illness-related regimen would be used when the individual feels powerless due to the required nursing and medical procedures necessary to promote maximum wellness.

The last suggested etiology, situational crisis, is an important factor in the diagnosis of Powerlessness. Many normally-empowered individuals may feel a sense of powerlessness when confronted with a situational crisis. For example, a woman who practices preventive health behaviors such as self breast exam, exercises regularly, modifies her diet to decrease salt and cholesterol, and obtains regular physical examinations, may feel very powerless when, in spite of her efforts, she is told she has hypertension.

Although the etiology health care environment addresses some aspects of hospitalization as a situational crisis, hospitalization is often a crisis experience itself. There are very specific nursing interventions for the patient who responds to hospitalization as a crisis that warrant a separate etiology. The nurse must determine the meaning and consequences of the hospitalization that will help the patient to gain control by modifying health care environment.

The etiology of situational crisis would also be used when the loss of control is not caused by the health care environment but by some other event in the patient's life. Although it may be a contributing factor, hospitalization may be the last in a series of stressors that creates the feeling of powerlessness, or hospitalization may be the first step toward regaining power and control. A patient may have experienced situational crisis such as a marital separation and loss

TABLE 14–8. ETIOLOGIES FOR NURSING DIAGNOSIS: POWERLESSNESS

Health Care Environment
Illness-Related Regimen
*Low Self-Esteem
*Chronic Illness
*Situational Crisis

*Etiologies suggested by author

of employment that precipitated an episode of depression. The goal of hospitalization would be to restore personal coping ability and for the patient to learn new coping strategies. In this case, the nurse would not focus on the crisis of hospitalization but rather the crisis experienced outside the hospital and use the etiology of situational crisis. The diagnosis could also be used to plan nursing care in the community after hospital discharge. (See Table 14–8 for the list of etiologies for the nursing diagnosis of Powerlessness.)

Planning and Implementation

The next step in the nursing process is planning. The overall goals for the nursing diagnosis of Powerlessness are to increase the patient's sense of control and to identify the feeling of powerlessness. These expected outcomes can be made more specific depending on the patient's response. (See Tables 14–9 to 14–13 for selected outcomes and interventions.)

After expected outcomes are identified, it is necessary to select and implement those nursing interventions that will be most effective in accomplishing the desired outcomes. Making a diagnosis of Powerlessness directs nursing care toward increasing the patient's

TABLE 14–9. NURSING DIAGNOSIS: POWERLESSNESS RELATED TO HEALTH CARE ENVIRONMENT

For use with patient responding to loss of control as a result of being hospitalized.

Expected Outcomes:
• Patient will state feeling more in control of situation
• Patient will participate in self-care activities
• Patient will identify feelings of powerlessness

Nursing Interventions:
1. Obtain patient's input into planning daily routine
2. Offer patient education materials as appropriate
3. Provide for patient's privacy (knock on door before entering room)
4. Assess patient's understanding of procedures and rationale and explain as necessary
5. Offer patient choices
6. Avoid power struggles with patient
7. Encourage independent activities as appropriate
8. Avoid coercing patient or being overly directive
9. Place necessary items within patient's reach (call bell, telephone, urinal)
10. Allow patient to talk feelings of powerlessness
11. Help patient identify controllable and uncontrollable events
12. Help patient set realistic goals
13. Help patient to problem solve and try alternate coping strategies
14. Identify improvements to condition
15. Ask for patient's views and opinions before giving information
16. Encourage patient to ask questions
17. Maintain a predictable routine
18. Have staff wear name tags and introduce themselves when interacting with patient
19. Avoid technical language

TABLE 14–10. NURSING DIAGNOSIS: POWERLESSNESS RELATED TO ILLNESS-RELATED REGIMEN

For use with individuals who have complex treatments that interfere with daily routine, progressive loss of physical or mental ability, or lack of progress in spite of adherence to regimen.

Expected Outcome:
• Patient will state feeling increased control over health care regimen
• Patient will discuss feelings of powerlessness over routine
• Patient will identify changes in routine that will increase control

Nursing Interventions:
1. Help patient to plan daily routine to include pleasurable activities
2. Obtain patient's input in planning daily routine
3. Identify procedures that patient can manage independently and those that require assistance
4. Help patient to problem solve about ways to increase independence
5. Help patient to problem solve about more efficient ways to manage regimen
6. Avoid being coercive or overly directive
7. Allow patient to talk about feelings of powerlessness
8. Help patient set realistic goals
9. Identify successful attempts to resolve problem
10. Ask for patient's views and opinions before giving information
11. Encourage patient to ask questions
12. Have needed items accessible to patient
13. Maintain a predictable routine

feeling of control and improving the patient's adaptation. The etiology statement guides the nurse in selecting appropriate interventions based on the individual's unique response. The nurse needs to adapt interventions to the patient's locus of control. Care plans that allow a high degree of choice and autonomy are indicated for internally-controlled individuals while externally-controlled patients need structure and slower paced instructional plans.

The nurse does not employ every possible intervention but chooses the ones that will be most effective and can be implemented within the constraints of time, environment, nurse's

TABLE 14–11. NURSING DIAGNOSIS: POWERLESSNESS RELATED TO LOW SELF-ESTEEM

For use with the patient who feels a lack of control, is nonassertive, or expects failure.

Expected Outcomes:
• Patient will state feeling an increased sense of control
• Patient will participate in decision making
• Patient will identify personal strengths

Nursing Interventions
1. Encourage patient to make choices
2. Encourage independent behavior
3. Involve patient in decision making about plan of care
4. Help patient identify and discuss feelings of powerlessness
5. Help patient identify realistic goals
6. Plan tasks and activities to insure patient success
7. Teach patient problem-solving strategies
8. Identify past coping strategies and discuss effectiveness
9. Identify and teach alternate coping strategies
10. Help patient identify personal preferences, wants, feelings, values, attitudes
11. Help patient identify and use strengths
12. Teach assertive communication skills
13. Provide positive reinforcement for adaptive behaviors
14. Discuss with patient possible family/significant other reactions to new behaviors

TABLE 14–12. NURSING DIAGNOSIS: POWERLESSNESS RELATED TO CHRONIC ILLNESS

For use with the patient who experiences a loss of control over his/her health or lifestyle as a result of long-term illness.

Expected Outcomes:
- *Patient will state feeling an increased sense of control over chronic illness*
- *Patient will discuss feelings of powerlessness over illness*
- *Patient will participate in self-care activities*

Nursing Interventions:
1. *Obtain patient's input in planning care and daily routine*
2. *Provide for patient privacy (knock on door before entering room)*
3. *Allow patient to wear own clothes*
4. *Offer patient choices*
5. *Avoid power struggles with patient*
6. *Avoid coercing patient or being overly directive*
7. *Encourage independent activities*
8. *Place necessary items within reach*
9. *Allow patient to talk about feelings of powerlessness*
10. *Help patient identify controllable and uncontrollable events*
11. *Help patient set realistic goals*
12. *Help patient identify activities that can still be enjoyed*
13. *Allow patient to express grief over loss of normalcy*
14. *Help patient to problem solve and try alternate coping strategies*
15. *Ask patient for views prior to giving information*
16. *Encourage patient to ask questions*
17. *Maintain a predictable routine*
18. *Help patient plan daily routine to include pleasurable activities*

skill and ability, and the patient's coping style. When developing a therapeutic nursing care plan, more is not necessarily better.

Evaluation

The final step in the nursing process is evaluation. The nurse examines the effectiveness and appropriateness of nursing interventions based on the identified expected outcomes. For the diagnosis of Powerlessness, the nurse looks for signs and listens for statements that indicate

TABLE 14–13. NURSING DIAGNOSIS: POWERLESSNESS RELATED TO SITUATIONAL CRISIS

For use with the patient who feels out of control as the result of an identified stressor.

Expected Outcomes:
- *Patient will state feeling an increased sense of control over crisis*
- *Patient will discuss feelings of powerlessness*
- *Patient will identify coping strategies*

Nursing Interventions:
1. *Help patient to identify and utilize past coping strategies*
2. *Identify available resources (community and hospital)*
3. *Allow patient to make choices*
4. *Include patient in decision making*
5. *Identify feelings of powerlessness*
6. *Allow patient to discuss feelings of loss of control*
7. *Help to identify controllable and uncontrollable events*
8. *Help patient to problem solve and identify new coping strategies*
9. *Ask for patient's input in plan of care*
10. *Identify patient's strengths*

the patient feels more in control. Data that would demonstrate the accomplishment of increased patient control and adaptation might include verbalization of feeling more control, assumption of self activities, improvement in mood and confidence, ability to make well thought out decisions, and participation in the health regime.

If the nurse does not find that there is a response to intervention, several possible explanations exist. First, enough time may not have elapsed for the patient to respond. Interventions may not have been consistently utilized, which would interfere with patient response and improvement. Lastly, the nurse must examine if the correct diagnosis was made. Loss of control is an element of many patient responses. The nurse must recognize when powerlessness is the diagnosis or a contributing factor. For example, the nurse might have to decide if loss of control over one's body or pain is the patient's main problem. The issue of differential diagnosis will be described in the next section.

DIFFERENTIAL NURSING DIAGNOSIS

One of the greatest challenges for nurses is determining if a correct diagnosis has been made. The nurse must decide if loss of control is the critical factor or merely contributory. Several diagnoses may be considered in addition to Powerlessness; frequently included are the diagnoses of Grief, Alteration in Self Concept, Ineffective Coping, and Hopelessness. Each of these diagnoses will be discussed with a patient example.

Powerlessness

Powerlessness can present itself quite differently. This makes accurate and careful assessment essential. For example, Mr. Adams is admitted to the hospital after a car accident in which he was not at fault. He sustained multiple, severe injuries that required hospitalization for six months. During this time he spent two months in an intensive care unit. He underwent life-saving surgery, venipunctures, painful wound care every eight hours, and constant monitoring of his hemodynamic status.

His locus of control was external. He consistently looked to his family for decision making and obtained his emotional support from them. These traits were present prior to his injury and continued during his hospitalization. A young man of few words, he became progressively more withdrawn as time wore on. He expressed his feelings only when coaxed. He admitted that he felt he had lost control of his body and his daily routine. He was lonely as his family lived an hour's distance away and could visit only three days a week. After many episodes of infection, he began to doubt if he would ever recover and became less aware of reasons for specific treatments and his clinical condition.

The diagnosis of Powerlessness related to health care environment was made. Nurses structured interventions to gradually allow him to feel in control because of his external locus of control. Nursing actions include working with Mr. Adams to plan activities for each shift and posting of a schedule of the agreed upon plan. Nurses informed him of impending procedures and what to expect in advance. He was given simple choices, such as when he would receive his injections.

He also had constant, abdominal pain that was exacerbated by caring for his wound. This contributed to his feelings of powerlessness, and interventions were planned to increase his control over the pain. By administering a long-acting narcotic on a schedule, providing additional medication prior to wound care, planning activities during the peak effect of the medication, and using relaxation techniques, nurses were able to significantly improve pain control.

This, in turn, helped him regain feelings of control over his body as he was more comfortable and able to participate in his recovery.

At times, both nurses and Mr. Adams became frustrated due to the slow progress he was making, but, with persistence and time, results were apparent. Toward the end of his hospitalization, when he physically felt better and had more energy, he was optimistic about his ability to cope with his situation and began planning a new business.

Mr. Barnes had a very different manifestation of his sense of powerlessness although both patients had some commonalities. Mr. Barnes was also involved in a traumatic injury that required hospitalization for two months. While Mr. Adams had no culpability in his accident, Mr. Barnes did. He was the owner of a small electrical firm, which was doing very well due to his hard work. While hurriedly showing an employee how to perform a wiring job, he sustained an electrical injury to his right hand and arm. His treatment involved immobilization of his dominant right hand and arm.

Mr. Barnes was well educated and highly respected in his community. He was internally controlled and very much the self-made man. He was no longer in control of himself or his situation after his accident. He attempted to regain control in several ways. He refused to take pain medicine in order to prove that he could handle the pain. He was overly preoccupied with dressing changes and punitively challenged the slightest deviation from usual procedure. He was sexually suggestive with female nurses at times and once patted a nurse on her buttocks with his free hand. His mood quickly changed from pleasant to sarcastic and angry when he was questioned.

Mr. Barnes quickly became a problem for nurses who were uncomfortable with his behavior and dreaded being assigned to him. When staff examined and discussed his behavior, they were able to recognize that these were Mr. Barnes' attempts to reestablish equilibrium in his world. The diagnosis of Powerlessness related to situational crisis was made because he was responding to hospitalization as a crisis along with the crisis of his inability to control his body (loss of function of his right arm) and his loss of social status as a patient in the hospital.

Interventions included asking Mr. Barnes for his input about the best way to change his dressings, avoiding power struggles, asking him to discuss his job, focusing on his expert knowledge, and recognizing his behaviors as an attempt to gain control and not as a personal attack. The staff didn't expect to change his underlying personality, but, with their interventions, they were able to make hospitalization tolerable for Mr. Barnes as well as the staff.

Grief

Grief and powerlessness both involve loss. When deciding between the two diagnoses, the nurse must decide if the patient is responding to a loss or potential loss, or if the individual's lack of control over the event is primary. The selection of the correct diagnosis is influenced by the patient's response, personal characteristics, and history.

Grief and Powerlessness also have a number of common defining characteristics. These include withdrawal, inability to carry out activities of daily living, feelings of despair, inability to make decisions, dependency, anger, guilt, and anxiety. The critical defining characteristic in the differential for the diagnosis of Grief is an actual or potential loss. The loss can be a person, possession, social status, job, a body part, or function.[44] The loss itself may not appear to be significant but it may rekindle past unresolved experiences with grief.

Ms. Carter, an elderly widow with peripheral vascular disease, presented such a diagnostic dilemma. She was admitted with a sore on her calf which wouldn't heal. She eventually required a below-the-knee amputation and when it did not heal, an above-the-knee amputation was necessary. Throughout her hospitalization she was sad and, at times, tearful. She never actively participated in her care and became progressively more dependent on staff to meet her needs, both physical and emotional. It was learned that prior to her admission, she rarely left her home. She had been active in her church's Sunday school, but she had lost interest in this and no longer even went to services. Her husband died four years earlier and, since that time, her daughter who was chemically dependent lived with her. Ms. Carter was not able to rely on her daughter to perform household tasks or to help her with physical care. As her hospitalization dragged on, it became apparent that she no longer would be able to return to her home and care for herself. Reluctantly Ms. Carter agreed to nursing home placement after all family members stated they would be unable to care for her.

Ms. Carter's ability to cope with her family's rejection, the loss of her leg, and her home, was complicated by her preexisting, unresolved sense of grief for the loss of her husband. She was overwhelmed by her losses and was grieving. Her sadness and grief were what her nurses diagnosed and treated. Nurses allowed her to talk about her losses and permitted crying. They reminisced with her about more pleasant times and encouraged her to reestablish contact with her closest church friends. Nurses talked with Ms. Carter about her impending move to a nursing home and how she felt about leaving her home. They also discussed how Ms. Carter envisioned life at the nursing home and were able to correct misconceptions.

Alteration in Self Concept

Self concept and powerlessness are interrelated in complex ways. Self concept is defined as the individual's total thoughts and feelings about oneself.[45] The self concept includes body image, role function, idealized self, and self-esteem. When an individual experiences powerlessness, this feeling alters self concept by challenging the person's perception of body image, role function, idealized self and/or self-esteem. Miller[46] identifies a positive self concept as a patient power resource that helps mitigate the effects of powerlessness.

Distinguishing between Alteration in Self Concept and Powerlessness can be a challenge. Defining characteristics for Alteration in Self Concept: Body Image include negative feelings about body, preoccupation with change or loss, feelings of unreality, and not looking at or touching the affected body part. While these characteristics appear straight forward, diagnostic decisions can be complicated by the fact that denial and feelings of hopelessness and powerlessness are also defining characteristics in the diagnosis of Self Concept. So, while powerlessness and grief may be associated with an alteration in self concept, the nurse must make a decision about which diagnosis best describes that patient's response.

Mr. Davis was a 25-year-old single man who was injured while a passenger in a car accident when returning home from college. As a result, his spinal cord was completely severed at the level of the eighth thoracic vertebra. During his hospitalization, he underwent surgery for stabilization of his spine and was instructed in self-care activities such as intermittent urinary catheterization and dressing techniques. He participated in physical therapy after his recovery from surgery.

The main nursing challenge was his emotional response to his accident. Initially, he maintained that he would walk again and asked everyone he encountered if his spinal cord was completely severed. He preferred to sleep rather than cope with daily routine and kept his window shades drawn.

After two weeks, he began talking about not being able to walk but remained hopeful that he would experience a miraculous return of motor function. He also asked questions about his ability to have sexual intercourse and have children. He was able to talk about these changes with his fiancee and received her support and encouragement. He expressed anger about why this had to happen to him and if he could have done anything to avoid the accident.

His nurses identified grief, denial, sadness, withdrawal, and feelings of powerlessness, but a diagnosis of Alteration in Self Concept: Body Image related to spinal cord injury was chosen because all these responses were a result of the traumatic bodily injury and his adjustment to the changes it brought about. Nurses treated his response to his illness by allowing him to express his feelings about his altered body and provided him with information about his condition. They brought up the subject of sexuality and gave him permission to ask questions about alternative sexual practices. Nurses encouraged him to talk about his goals that would be changed as well as those that he could still achieve.

Past coping strategies were reviewed with Mr. Davis, and it was identified that he used physical activity to release tension, and, because of this, physical therapy became not only a way to restore his strength but also a way to cope. Mr. Davis found that after an hour of upper body exercises in physical therapy he was less anxious. He used his excess energy as a way to promote recovery.

These interventions were aimed at helping Mr. Davis deal with his changed self-image. Nursing actions were not primarily focused on his grief or powerlessness but the treatment of these responses was subsumed in the care plan for Alteration in Self Concept: body image.

Ineffective Coping

The diagnosis of Ineffective Coping may be confused with the diagnosis of Powerlessness. A patient responding to feelings of powerlessness may be viewed by health care professionals as coping ineffectively. This diagnosis has the potential for being used as a negative label rather than a descriptive one. When the patient copes with a situation in an unusual manner, or if nurses judge patients by their own values and perceive patient behavior as inappropriate, the diagnosis of Ineffective Coping would be in error.

Ineffective individual coping is defined as the impairment of adaptive behaviors and problem-solving abilities of a person in meeting life's demands and roles.[47] Ms. Evans demonstrates usage of the diagnosis in a way that is descriptive rather than judgmental. She was a 39-year-old divorced mother of two daughters ages 12 and 14. Since her separation from her husband, she worked sporadically as an office temporary. Her former husband paid no child support and showed little interest in the children. Ms. Evans had started business college six months earlier, but she dropped out prior to the first semester exams. Her income consisted of aid to dependent children. Since her divorce she had been drinking and smoking heavily. By the time she was hospitalized with nausea, vomiting, and elevated liver enzymes, she was drinking six cans of beer a day and smoking more than a pack a day of cigarettes. Her diet consisted mainly of coffee and junk food. She had isolated herself from her friends and had no plans for the future.

After examining the data, Ms. Evans' nurses identified her use of maladaptive behaviors and impaired problem-solving abilities and made the diagnosis of Ineffective Individual Coping related to multiple life changes. The goals for Ms. Evans were helping her to develop effective coping strategies and to utilize available resources. Nurses talked with her about her feelings about her situation and worked with her on other, more appropriate coping skills such as physical activity and relaxation techniques. She was encouraged to use available resources such as Alcoholics Anonymous and her community mental health center. Her nurses helped her to make food selections to improve her nutritional status and teach her about the foods she needed. They also confronted her, when necessary, with her responsibility as a parent and her daughters' need for a physically and emotionally healthy parent.

Ms. Evans was responding to her situation with powerlessness, but, in addition to this, she employed self-destructive coping strategies. Before her nurses helped her deal with her feelings of loss and powerlessness, they treated her maladaptive behaviors.

Hopelessness

The nursing diagnosis Hopelessness was accepted by the North American Nursing Diagnosis Association in 1986.[48] It is a subjective state in which an individual sees limited or no alternatives or personal choices available and is unable to mobilize energy on his or her own behalf. Hopelessness and powerlessness are closely related and present a diagnostic challenge for nurses.

When powerlessness continues it may develop into hopelessness. The depression that results from powerlessness contributes to low self-esteem and then hopelessness.[49] Nursing interventions that help the patient to reestablish hope also help the patient to regain power and control. When the nurse works to prevent or treat powerlessness, hopelessness is also prevented. Hope in itself is a powerful resource.[50]

Mr. Foster demonstrated the delicate balance between powerlessness and hopelessness. He was a 38-year-old manual laborer hospitalized with cholestatic pancreatitis. He had a hospital stay of over six months. During this time, he underwent multiple surgeries to drain pseudocysts and stayed in intensive care for a total of two months. Just when he improved enough to leave the ICU for a few days, he developed an infection that required returning to the ICU. This scenario took place three times. Initially, the diagnosis of Powerlessness related to health care environment was made, based on his verbalization of frustration with multiple and unpredictable procedures, sadness over his condition, passivity, and nonparticipation in self care. No matter what he did, his condition failed to improve. His psychological condition also deteriorated.

After three months of hospitalization, he began to say that he wanted to die. He avoided eye contact and was apathetic, unable to problem-solve, or make decisions. At this point, his nursing diagnosis was changed to Hopelessness related to prolonged illness. The critical defining characteristic in making this change was his desire to give up and die. While nurses still directed their interventions toward giving him a feeling of control, he was less able to participate because of his hopelessness. His nurses worked to convey that they had hope for him and weren't going to give up. They helped him initiate activities that he couldn't because of his sadness. They identified and qualified the progress he had made and set realistic, attainable goals so he could experience success.

CLINICAL APPLICATION

Often, nurses desire to make a diagnosis of Depression. This label is more useful as a medical diagnosis than a nursing diagnosis. While depression and sadness may be responses to an event, it is difficult to infer causation. When identifying the etiologic statement, is a situational crisis identified such as a divorce, or is an imbalance of neurotransmittors identified? Do nurses really treat a divorce or the chemical imbalance? No, physicians treat a decrease of dopamine by prescribing antidepressants, and no one can "treat" a divorce but rather the emotions it precipitates. Therefore, nurses should identify and treat the human responses of the patient. Using this approach, the depressed mood is a symptom or defining characteristic but not the diagnosis itself. Feelings of sadness and depression are typically present in the nursing diagnoses of Powerlessness, Hopelessness, Alteration in Self Concept, and Ineffective Coping. The nurse must examine all the defining characteristics and make a diagnostic decision based on clinical judgment.

In clinical practice, a differential diagnosis may be difficult to make. Human responses are complex and not necessarily discrete. Nurses must carefully consider defining characteristics, cluster the data according to various diagnoses, and make decisions about the clinically relevant data and the diagnoses that result from this process. It is critical that only the most relevant diagnoses are selected and implemented. It dilutes the impact of professional practice to identify too many diagnoses and try to implement them all. With limited time and resources, it is better to select the critical one, two, or three diagnoses and concentrate nursing efforts to treat these problems.

Acquisition of Skills

This reinforces the importance of thoughtful consideration of nursing diagnoses and ongoing evaluation. Obviously, acquiring skill with differential diagnosis is a developmental process. Blooms' Cognitive Taxonomy[51] illustrates how the acquisition of skills proceeds. The first level is knowledge. The nurse knows about the nursing process and individual diagnoses, including Powerlessness. The nurse is aware of the definition of powerlessness and can cluster relevant clinical data such as verbalizations of no control, prolonged hospitalization, and lack of initiative. The second level is comprehension. The nurse also has a conceptual framework that includes knowledge of the causative factors and theories that support the diagnosis. The nurse knows what powerlessness means.

The third level is application. The nurse can apply and utilize a particular nursing diagnosis, Powerlessness. Comprehension of the information promotes accurate application, but application may occur without comprehension. The nurse may recognize the defining characteristics and select the diagnosis of Powerlessness related to health care environment but still not comprehend why it, or another, diagnosis was appropriate. If the nurse chooses the wrong diagnosis, when evaluation occurs the correct one may be chosen. So even without comprehension, the nurse may stumble on the correct diagnosis through trial and error if the nurse is able to apply the knowledge.

The fourth level, analysis, occurs when the nurse can use the clinical data, appropriate theories, and conceptual framework to make decisions about patient care. The fifth level of synthesis allows the nurse to integrate knowledge, comprehension of several similar diagnoses such as Powerlessness, Hopelessness, and Grief, and analyze the relevant information to make a differential diagnosis. The analysis and synthesis levels of the taxonomy allow nurses to utilize nursing diagnosis at a very sophisticated level.

Skill Development

Obviously, not all nurses will be able to participate in the diagnostic process at the same level. The nurse's experience and skill is an important factor. Benner[52] applied the Dreyfus model of skill development to nursing. Five levels of proficiency are described: novice, advanced beginner, competent, proficient, and expert. The novice practitioner uses context-free rules because there are no past experiences to draw upon. The practice of the novice is rigid and limited. In fact, the novice is often limited by the rules on which she relies. The novice does not have the skill to adapt to any deviation from the rule.

The advanced beginner has some experience that allows the identification of aspects or the common characteristics of a situation. The nurse now formulates guidelines for practice rather than rules. The novice and the advanced beginner need assistance in formulating nursing diagnoses. They may have knowledge of the diagnosis of Powerlessness and the defining characteristics, but they are not able to prioritize the significance of various aspects of the patient's response.

The novice and the advanced beginner also have difficulty differentiating between similar diagnoses such as Powerlessness and Hopelessness. They lack the experience to know the difference between a patient who is frustrated by loss of control and the patient who is sad and has given up due to feeling hopeless. The competent nurse has two to three years experience in one area of practice and is able to visualize individual nursing actions as a part of an organized plan. This nurse is organized, deliberate, and can handle the exigencies of nursing practice. The competent nurse best learns from decision-making exercises and simulations of patient care.

The proficient nurse views the clinical situation as a whole rather than individual aspects. Experience allows the nurse to recognize abnormalities and adjust the plan of care. The nurse is able to prioritize and make judgments by examining only pertinent data. To help the proficient nurse develop diagnostic skills, case studies and care conferences can be utilized. These nurses need complicated cases that tax their ability to analyze patient responses as well as help them begin to synthesize data, and, because of the proficient nurse's ability to assess the whole situation, having an opportunity to "take apart" case studies helps them to understand the decision-making process that they use. These nurses are also excellent teachers for novices, advanced beginners, and the competent nurse. They can be identified as informal unit teachers as well as facilitators of case conferences.

The expert nurse is truly able to synthesize patient information to make a nursing diagnosis. The expert has extensive experience and no longer relies on rules or analysis to make clinical decisions. The situation is assessed intuitively and without contemplating extraneous information. When asked to describe the process used, the expert may have difficulty putting it into words. It is essential that the expert nurse be prompted to do just this. By making the expertise visible, other nurses with differing skill levels can emulate the expert's performance. This is the nurse to select to role model the utilization of nursing diagnosis for all practitioners. The expert is able to challenge other nurses to develop assessment and diagnostic skills. The expert has the skill to help others identify pertinent data and exclude extraneous information. For example, in making the diagnosis of Powerlessness, verbalization of loss of control would be pertinent while the patient's place of residence might be extraneous.

The expert nurse might make the diagnosis of Powerlessness when the less experienced, rule-oriented practitioner would not consider it. Powerlessness is a concept as well as a human response and encompasses other more concrete diagnoses such as Alteration in Self Concept, Alteration in Comfort, Grief, Ineffective Coping, and Hopelessness. The novice or advanced beginner may choose the more concrete and easily identifiable diagnosis of Alteration in Self Concept related to change in role performance rather than selecting Powerlessness related to illness-related regime.

For example, Mr. Gray was started on renal dialysis after three months of declining renal function. He is married and the father of two school-age children. He is an upper-level manager of a local business firm and has always prided himself on being able to handle whatever situation arose. He is respected by his peers for his ability to lead and take charge when the unexpected occurs. During his visit to dialysis, he is frustrated and angry. He expresses concern about his ability to support his family financially and psychologically. He states that dialysis is too big a challenge for him. He is fearful because he has never experienced those feelings before.

The diagnosis Alteration in Self Concept related to change in role performance could be made and would not be in error. Mr. Gray would benefit from being able to discuss his feelings about the changes in his health and family roles as well as helping with his own care. The expert nurse, however, selects the diagnosis of Powerlessness related to situational crisis instead. This nurse weighs the importance of patient data based on the context of the situation[53] and makes a more precise diagnosis.

Powerlessness is chosen because it directs nursing actions toward the cause of Mr. Gray's alteration in self concept, his feelings of loss of control. He has always been an empowered man and is now temporarily powerless. In addition to the interventions of allowing him to express his feelings, his nurses plan ways for him to regain control. Mr. Gray agrees to participate in the self-care dialysis program and is gradually taught about his own care. Before long, he is able to utilize his own personal strengths to help him cope with his change in health. Plans are begun for home dialysis, which would give Mr. Gray and his family more control and flexibility.

The expert nurse was the one who identified the patient's whole response to his situation and planned the most appropriate interventions. While the diagnosis of Alteration in Self Concept related to change in role performance was not wrong, the diagnosis of Powerlessness related to situational crisis allowed the nurse to treat the problem in the most effective and efficient manner. If the Alteration in Self Concept diagnosis had been made, the evaluation process would help the nurse identify if another diagnosis was needed. This is dependent on whether the nurse has the knowledge or comprehension of the concept of powerlessness to apply the diagnosis to a clinical situation. Again, the role of the expert nurse as role model and teacher is essential for the development of less experienced nurses.

CONCLUSION

The nursing diagnosis of Powerlessness is extremely useful in the practice of nursing. In order to use it effectively, nurses must recognize its defining characteristics and realize the importance of increasing patient control and power. In addition, nurses must explore their own feelings and responses to power before they can share power with patients.

Sachs describes his feelings of powerlessness while a patient especially when his care takers minimize his concerns.

> . . . yet I couldn't shake off the nightmare feeling which had lain on me, doubtless to some extent since admission, but which became acute and specific when communications broke down—when the surgeon said, with authority, that there was "nothing," and so contradicted and questioned and doubted my (most elemental) perceptions—perceptions on which my most elemental sense of "I," self-integrity, was based. When I felt physically helpless, paralyzed, contracted, confined—and not just contracted, but contorted as well, into roles and postures of adjection.[54]

Nurses have a responsibility not only to recognize powerlessness but to prevent it. By doing so, nurses can directly improve their patients' adaptation and improve health and even prolong life.

REFERENCES

1. *Webster's new collegiate dictionary.* Springfield, MA: G. & C. Merriam, Co., 1973
2. North American Nursing Diagnosis Association. *Taxonomy I.* St. Louis: North American Nursing Diagnosis Association, 1986
3. Miller, J. F., Ed. *Coping with chronic illness.* Philadelphia: F. A. Davis, Co., 1983, p.51
4. Riehl, J. P., & Callista, R. *Conceptual models for nursing Practice* (2nd ed.). New York: Appleton-Century-Crofts, 1980

5. Rodin, J. Aging and health: Effects of the sense of control. *Science,* 1986, *233,* 1271
6. Seeman, M. Alienation and learning in a hospital setting. *American Sociological Review,* 1962, *27,* 772
7. Perlmuter, L. C., & Monty, R. A. Effect of choice of stimulus on paired associated learning. *Journal of Experimental Psychology,* 1973, *99,* 120
8. Miller
9. Rodin, J., Rennest, K., & Tolomon, S. K. Applica-

tions of personal control. In A. Baun & J. E. Singu (Eds.), *Advances in environmental psychology,* vol. 2. Hillsdale, NJ: Erlbaum, 1980, p. 131

10. Rodin
11. Averill, J. Personal control over aversive stimuli and its relationship to stress. *Psychological Bulletin,* 1973, 80, 286
12. *Webster's New Collegiate Dictionary*
13. Miller
14. Seligman, M. *Helplessness: On depression, development, and death.* San Francisco: Freeman & Co., 1975, p. 82
15. Hurley, M. E., Ed. *Classification of nursing diagnosis: Proceedings of the sixth conference.* St. Louis: C. V. Mosby, 1986
16. Engel, G. A life setting conducive to illness: The giving up–given up complex. *Annals of Internal Medicine,* 1968, *69,* 293
17. Miller
18. Lefcourt, H. The function of the illusion of control and freedom. *American Psychologist,* 1973, *28,* 417
19. Rotter, J. B. Generalized expectancies for internal vs. external control of reinforcement. *Psychological Monographs,* 1966, *1,* 80
20. Stephenson, C. Powerlessness and chronic illness: Simplifications for nursing. *Baylor Nursing Education,* 1979, *1,* 1, 17
21. Miller
22. Wallston, B.F., Wallston, K.A., Kaplan, G.D., & Maides, F.A. Development and validation of the health locus of control scale. *Journal of Consulting and Clinical Psychology,* 1986, *44,* 580
23. Anderson, C. Locus of control, coping behavior and performance in a stress setting: A longitudinal study. *Journal of Applied Psychology,* 1977, *62,* 450
24. Craig, K. & Best, A. Perceived control over pain: Individual differences and situational determinants. *Pain,* 1977, *3,* 133
25. Zahn, J. Some adult attitudes affecting learning: Powerlessness, conflicting needs and role transition. *Adult Education Journal,* 1969, *19,* 91
26. Miller
27. Kritek, P.B. Patient power and powerlessness. *Supervisor Nurse,* 1981, 26

28. French, J. & Raven, B. The bases of power. In E. Hollander & R. Hunt (Eds.), *Current perspectives in social psychology.* (3rd ed.). New York: Oxford University Press, 1971, p. 525
29. Averill
30. Miller
31. *Ibid.,* p.5
32. *Ibid*
33. *Ibid.,* p.6
34. Driever, M. Theory of self-concept. In R. Callista (Ed.), *Introduction to nursing: an adaptation model.* Englewood Cliffs, NJ: Prentice Hall, 1976, p. 169
35. Miller
36. *Ibid*
37. *Ibid.,* p.8
38. *Ibid*
39. *Ibid*
40. *Ibid.,* p.9
41. *Ibid.,* p.10
42. *Ibid.,* p.55
43. Kim, M.J., McFarland, G., & McLane, A. *Pocket guide to nursing diagnosis* (2nd ed.). St. Louis: C. V. Mosby, 1987
44. *Ibid*
45. Driever
46. Miller
47. Kim, McFarland, & McLane.
48. McLane, A., Ed. *Classification of nursing diagnosis: Proceedings of the seventh conference.* St. Louis: C. V. Mosby, 1987
49. Miller
50. *Ibid.,* p.388
51. Bloom, B.S., Ed. *Taxonomy of educational objective: The classification of educational goals by a committee of college and university examiners,* vol. I. New York: D. McKay, Co., 1956
52. Benner, P. *From novice to expert—excellence and power in clinical nursing practice.* Menlo Park, CA: Addison-Wesley, 1984
53. *Ibid*
54. Sachs, O. *A leg to stand on.* New York: Summit Books, 1984, p. 158

North American Nursing Diagnosis Association (NANDA) Approved Nursing Diagnostic Categories

This list represents the NANDA-approved nursing diagnostic categories for clinical use and testing (1988). Changes have been made in 15 labels for consistency.

PATTERN 1: EXCHANGING

1.1.2.1	Altered Nutrition: More than body requirements
1.1.2.2	Altered Nutrition: Less than body requirements
1.1.2.3	Altered Nutrition: Potential for more than body requirements
1.2.1.1	Potential for Infection
1.2.2.1	Potential Altered Body Temperature
**1.2.2.2	Hypothermia
1.2.2.3	Hyperthermia
1.2.2.4	Ineffective Thermoregulation
*1.2.3.1	Dysreflexia
#1.3.1.1	Constipation
*1.3.1.1.1	Perceived Constipation
*1.3.1.1.2	Colonic Constipation
#1.3.1.2	Diarrhea
#1.3.1.3	Bowel Incontinence
1.3.2	Altered Patterns of Urinary Elimination
1.3.2.1.1	Stress Incontinence
1.3.2.1.2	Reflex Incontinence
1.3.2.1.3	Urge Incontinence
1.3.2.1.4	Functional Incontinence
1.3.2.1.5	Total Incontinence
1.3.2.2	Urinary Retention

#1.4.1.1	Altered (Specify Type) Tissue Perfusion (Renal, cerebral, cardiopulmonary, gastrointestinal, peripheral)
1.4.1.2.1	Fluid Volume Excess
1.4.1.2.2.1	Fluid Volume Deficit (1)
1.4.1.2.2.1	Fluid Volume Deficit (2)
1.4.1.2.2.2	Potential Fluid Volume Deficit
#1.4.2.1	Decreased Cardiac Output
1.5.1.1	Impaired Gas Exchange
1.5.1.2	Ineffective Airway Clearance
1.5.1.3	Ineffective Breathing Pattern
1.6.1	Potential for Injury
1.6.1.1	Potential for Suffocation
1.6.1.2	Potential for Poisoning
1.6.1.3	Potential for Trauma
*1.6.1.4	Potential for Aspiration
*1.6.1.5	Potential for Disuse Syndrome
1.6.2.1	Impaired Tissue Integrity
#1.6.2.1.1	Altered Oral Mucous Membrane
1.6.2.1.2.1	Impaired Skin Integrity
1.6.2.1.2.2	Potential Impaired Skin Integrity

PATTERN 2: COMMUNICATING

2.1.1.1	Impaired Verbal Communication

PATTERN 3: RELATING

3.1.1	Impaired Social Interaction
3.1.2	Social Isolation
#3.2.1	Altered Role Performance
3.2.1.1.1	Altered Parenting
3.2.1.1.2	Potential Altered Parenting
3.2.1.2.1	Sexual Dysfunction
3.2.2	Altered Family Processes
*3.2.3.1	Parental Role Conflict
3.3	Altered Sexuality Patterns

PATTERN 4: VALUING

4.1.1	Spiritual Distress (distress of the human spirit)

PATTERN 5: CHOOSING

5.1.1.1	Ineffective Individual Coping
5.1.1.1.1	Impaired Adjustment

*5.1.1.1.2	Defensive Coping
*5.1.1.1.3	Ineffective Denial
5.1.2.1.1	Ineffective Family Coping: Disabling
5.1.2.1.2	Ineffective Family Coping: Compromised
5.1.2.2	Family Coping: Potential for Growth
5.2.1.1	Noncompliance (Specify)
*5.3.1.1	Decisional Conflict (Specify)
*5.4	Health Seeking Behaviors (Specify)

PATTERN 6: MOVING

6.1.1.1	Impaired Physical Mobility
6.1.1.2	Activity Intolerance
*6.1.1.2.1	Fatigue
6.1.1.3	Potential Activity Intolerance
6.2.1	Sleep Pattern Disturbance
6.3.1.1	Diversional Activity Deficit
6.4.1.1	Impaired Home Maintenance Management
6.4.2	Altered Health Maintenance
#6.5.1	Feeding Self Care Deficit
6.5.1.1	Impaired Swallowing
*6.5.1.2	Ineffective Breastfeeding
#6.5.2	Bathing/Hygiene Self Care Deficit
#6.5.3	Dressing/Grooming Self Care Deficit
#6.5.4	Toileting Self Care Deficit
6.6	Altered Growth and Development

PATTERN 7: PERCEIVING

#7.1.1	Body Image Disturbance
#**7.1.2	Self Esteem Disturbance
*7.1.2.1	Chronic Low Self Esteem
*7.1.2.2	Situational Low Self Esteem
#7.1.3	Personal Identify Disturbance
7.2	Sensory/Perceptual Alterations (Specify) (Visual, auditory, kinesthetic, gustatory, tactile, olfactory)
7.2.1.1	Unilateral Neglect
7.3.1	Hopelessness
7.3.2	Powerlessness

PATTERN 8: KNOWING

8.1.1	Knowledge Deficit (Specify)
8.3	Altered Thought Processes

PATTERN 9: FEELING

#9.1.1	Pain
9.1.1.1	Chronic Pain
9.2.1.1	Dysfunctional Grieving
9.2.1.2	Anticipatory Grieving
9.2.2	Potential for Violence: Self-directed or directed at others
9.2.3	Post-Trauma Response
9.2.3.1	Rape-Trauma Syndrome
9.2.3.1.1	Rape-Trauma Syndrome: Compound Reaction
9.2.3.1.2	Rape-Trauma Syndrome: Silent Reaction
9.3.1	Anxiety
9.3.2	Fear

* New diagnostic categories approved 1988
** Revised diagnostic categories approved 1988
# Categories with modifed label terminology
North American Nursing Diagnosis Association, *Nursing Diagnosis Newsletter,* 1988, 15, *1*

Index